THE PUBLIC HEALTH
QUALITY IMPROVEMENT
HANDBOOK

Also available from ASQ Quality Press:

Solutions to the Healthcare Quality Crisis: Cases and Examples of Lean Six Sigma in Healthcare
Soren Bisgaard, editor

On Becoming Exceptional: SSM Health Care's Journey to Baldrige and Beyond
Sister Mary Jean Ryan, FSM

Journey to Excellence: Baldrige Health Care Leaders Speak Out
Kathleen Goonan, editor

A Lean Guide to Transforming Healthcare: How to Implement Lean Principles in Hospitals, Medical Offices, Clinics, and Other Healthcare Organizations
Thomas G. Zidel

Benchmarking for Hospitals: Achieving Best-in-Class Performance without Having to Reinvent the Wheel
Victor Sower, Jo Ann Duffy, and Gerald Kohers

Lean-Six Sigma for Healthcare: A Senior Leader Guide to Improving Cost and Throughput, Second Edition
Greg Butler, Chip Caldwell, and Nancy Poston

Lean Six Sigma for the Healthcare Practice: A Pocket Guide
Roderick A. Munro

Improving Healthcare Using Toyota Lean Production Methods: 46 Steps for Improvement, Second Edition
Robert Chalice

Root Cause Analysis: Simplified Tools and Techniques, Second Edition
Bjørn Andersen and Tom Fagerhaug

5S for Service Organizations and Offices: A Lean Look at Improvements
Debashis Sarkar

To request a complimentary catalog of ASQ Quality Press publications, call 800-248-1946, or visit our Web site at http://qualitypress.asq.org.

THE PUBLIC HEALTH QUALITY IMPROVEMENT HANDBOOK

*Ron Bialek, Grace L. Duffy,
and John W. Moran*

ASQ Quality Press
Milwaukee, Wisconsin

American Society for Quality, Quality Press, Milwaukee 53203

© 2009 by ASQ

All rights reserved. Published 2009

Printed in the United States of America

15 14 13 12 11 10 09   5 4 3 2 1

Library of Congress Cataloging-in-Publication Data

The public health quality improvement handbook / [compiled by] Ron Bialek,
  Grace L. Duffy, and John W. Moran.
      p. cm.
  Includes bibliographical references and index.
  ISBN 978-0-87389-758-7 (hard cover : alk. paper)
  1. Health services administration—United States—Quality control—Handbooks,
manuals, etc. 2. Medical care—United States—Quality control—Handbooks, manuals,
etc. 3. Public health—United States—Quality control—Handbooks, manuals, etc.
  I. Bialek, Ronald G. II. Duffy, Grace L. III. Moran, John W., 1944–

  RA399.A3P825 2009
  362.1068—dc22   2009011244

ISBN: 978-0-87389-758-7

Publisher: William A. Tony
Acquisitions Editor: Matt T. Meinholz
Project Editor: Paul O'Mara
Production Administrator: Randall Benson

ASQ Mission: The American Society for Quality advances individual, organizational, and
community excellence worldwide through learning, quality improvement, and knowledge
exchange.

Attention Bookstores, Wholesalers, Schools, and Corporations: ASQ Quality Press books,
videotapes, audiotapes, and software are available at quantity discounts with bulk purchases
for business, educational, or instructional use. For information, please contact ASQ Quality
Press at 800-248-1946, or write to ASQ Quality Press, P.O. Box 3005, Milwaukee, WI 53201-3005.

To place orders or to request a free copy of the ASQ Quality Press Publications Catalog,
including ASQ membership information, call 800-248-1946. Visit our Web site at www.asq.org
or http://www.asq.org/quality-press.

Printed in the United States of America

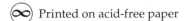 Printed on acid-free paper

Quality Press
600 N. Plankinton Avenue
Milwaukee, Wisconsin 53203
Call toll free 800-248-1946
Fax 414-272-1734
www.asq.org
http://www.asq.org/quality-press
http://standardsgroup.asq.org
E-mail: authors@asq.org

Table of Contents

List of Figures and Tables

Foreword

Dennis Lenaway, PhD, MPH, and Liza C. Corso, MPA
Office of Chief of Public Health Practice,
Centers for Disease Control and Prevention

The past several decades have brought new public health challenges that redefined the role and expanded the visibility of public health. Past achievements such as vaccinations, fluoridation of drinking water, and reduced maternal mortality have given way to threats from terrorism, emerging diseases, and escalating chronic conditions and obesity. While we may not be able to foresee future challenges to the public's health, it does raise the question of how we can most rapidly transform a complex partnership of federal agencies working in collaboration with state and local health departments, with significant contributions from nongovernmental organizations, into a 21st-century public health system. As public health leaders and practitioners, we are being challenged to provide a level of performance commensurate with our new role and new expectations.

The concept of performance in public health is well understood. Reawakened in the late 1980s, public health has gone on to define its essential services, craft systemwide model standards and assessment tools, develop performance management tools and frameworks, and voluntarily engage the broader public health community to create and implement a national accreditation program for health departments. In similar fashion, workforce competencies have been explored, defined, and promoted. Each of these important endeavors has sought to focus attention on a means for improving public health. The foundation laid by such efforts has been coupled with the opportunity offered by adoption and adaptation of the quality improvement techniques and tools successfully used in healthcare, industry, and other sectors. The principles of quality improvement in public health—so well defined in this handbook—hold great promise for more effective public health systems and services, which ideally will lead to achieving more sustainable results and, ultimately, better health outcomes.

How then do we expand the use of quality improvement tools and techniques in public health? We believe that the federal governmental public health system has an opportunity, and a responsibility, to embrace quality improvement and promote its use among its many programs, services, and funding mechanisms. Properly constructed incentives that flow from federal to state and local agencies can induce the public health system toward greater interest in, and use of, quality improvement methods. It bears mentioning that the Centers for Disease Control and Prevention (CDC) has been actively exploring several approaches to embedding quality improvement into programs and funding streams. The National Public Health Performance Standards Program, as well as model standards and improvement programs in areas such as laboratory systems and environmental health, are built upon the precepts of quality improvement. CDC supports the newly-emerging national program for accreditation of state and local health departments, which has great potential for marrying the needs of accountability and quality improvement in an effective and efficient manner. Newly drafted State Strategic Management Agreements, in which CDC and state leaders agree upon targeted goals and objectives, have ample opportunity to create incentives for quality improvement. Indeed, the list is nearly inexhaustible given the range of possibilities across CDC programs, offices, and centers.

By acknowledging the importance of quality improvement, then, we must tackle several important issues. We need to clearly define what quality improvement is, identify what methods are most appropriate and effective for public health, provide access to expert technical assistance, create incentives and rewards, and research the impacts on performance and health outcomes. Most importantly, we need to create a culture of quality improvement wherein it becomes both a deliberate and instinctive way of doing business at all levels—in programs and services, in our organizations, and in our public health systems. In the same way that quality improvement should be understood and embraced at all levels of an organization, it should also be understood and embraced at all levels of governmental public health—local, tribal, state, and federal in order to successfully contribute to the transformation of our public health system

The concepts, techniques, and experiences presented in this handbook provide an invaluable resource for accelerating our journey down this path. If we are to truly achieve a healthier America, then we need to collectively recognize the value of quality improvement and begin in earnest to improve our workforce, our programs and services, our organizations, and our public health systems. By doing this, we will create a new and improved "21st-century public health system" that will improve the health of the individuals and communities that we serve.

Preface

Ron Bialek
President, Public Health Foundation

Public health has some of the most dedicated and hardest workers you will find in any field. We work tirelessly to get the job done, no matter what it takes. Why do we do this? The answer is simple. We care about the public's health and are committed to seeing it improved.

Because of this hard work and dedication, we go home each day knowing that we have made a difference—we have indeed improved the public's health. Is this reality, or just a wish that we have for the work we do? How do we measure our success? Do we really understand the root causes and address them in a way that will indeed make a measurable difference?

For too long we have focused our efforts on working hard, not necessarily on achieving a defined and measurable set of results. Just looking at the health of the United States compared to the world, and the health of most every community, we know that we can, and must, do better. We are not seeing the types of health outcomes we desire and that the public and policymakers are demanding.

What can we do to truly make a difference in the public's health? With the effective use of quality improvement (QI) tools and techniques we can, and will, see our hard work and dedication produce better results. We are seeing tremendous excitement throughout the country around the use of QI tools and techniques. Public health agencies and systems are learning these techniques, exploring and experimenting with them, and developing new and even better approaches to public health QI. And yes, we are seeing results—improved processes, efficiencies, and community health status.

Applying QI tools and techniques to improve the public's health will help us realize the promise of initiatives such as public health voluntary accreditation and the National Public Health Performance Standards Program. These programs are helping us to better understand and assess agency and system capacity and performance. It is the effective use of QI tools and techniques, however, that is helping us to make systematic and long-term improvements that will achieve the types of results we desire and the public deserves.

Central to the mission of the Public Health Foundation is to help public health agencies and systems achieve measurable improvement and better results. This *Public Health Quality Improvement Handbook*, full of examples, tools, and techniques, will make an important contribution to our community and the public's health as we continue on our quality voyage.

There has never been a better time or a more important one for us to harness the energy, enthusiasm, hard work, and dedication of our public health workforce to make a lasting difference. By effectively using QI tools and techniques, we can, and will, improve our nation's health and the health of the many communities we serve.

Acknowledgments

The editors thank each of the authors who have contributed to making this *Public Health Quality Improvement Handbook* a reality. The authors worked under a very tight deadline and were gracious enough to share their knowledge, skills, experience, opinions, and lessons learned about how to make quality improvement (QI) work in the public health field.

Each author contributed a segment to this handbook. Approaches covered include:

- The strategic view

- The operational view

- Developing the conditions to make QI thrive

- Involving community stakeholders

- Using tools and techniques to make improvements

- Sponsoring and using improvement teams effectively

- Measuring results

- Incorporating QI into daily work

- Tying QI to accreditation and national and state quality awards

These gifted authors give the reader a comprehensive reference on all aspects of quality improvement in their public health organization. The case studies and storyboards developed by practitioners provide examples of the quality improvement process in actual use in a variety of public health settings.

We will update this handbook over time, and encourage any reader who would like to contribute to a future edition to contact the editors to discuss the contribution. The more we share our successes and lessons learned, the more we advance quality improvement in public health.

The editors were privileged to work with such a dedicated, knowledgeable group of public health quality improvement professionals. Their contributions made this handbook a reality. Again, to each chapter author, a heartfelt thank-you for working so cooperatively with us over the past few months.

Ron Bialek, President, Public Health Foundation
John Moran, Senior Quality Advisor, Public Health Foundation
Grace Duffy, President, Management and Performance Systems,
Public Health Foundation Quality Improvement Consultant

Prologue

Pamela Russo, MD, MPH
Senior Program Officer, Robert Wood Johnson Foundation

T he publication of the *Public Health Quality Improvement Handbook* is a significant milestone for the public health field. Performance management is not a new concept in public health, as evidenced by the history of programs like Turning Point and the National Public Health Performance Standards. What is new in this handbook is the demonstration that quality improvement techniques from other sectors are rapidly and successfully being adapted to the public health context. Particularly notable are the case studies in the handbook that begin to connect the dots between process improvement and improved community health outcomes.

When the Robert Wood Johnson Foundation committed to improving quality in public health, our strategy was informed by 20 years of experience in building the field of healthcare quality improvement. At first, the knee-jerk reaction of many experts was that the healthcare experience with quality improvement (QI) could be directly applied in public health. This did work for some of the ambulatory prevention, control, and screening functions that many health departments offer, but the healthcare experience did not translate for the majority of public health functions and services. The evidence base for applying QI techniques to public health needed major expansion. In addition, there was a crucial need to have examples of application to issues that are familiar and relevant for public health practitioners in order for training to be successful. This handbook helps fill that gap for public health.

The Robert Wood Johnson Foundation is committed to improving the performance and impact of public health and building the evidence for what works to improve the quality and effectiveness of public health practice and policy. A cornerstone of our strategy is national voluntary public health accreditation, and working with our public health partners we have supported the establishment of the Public Health Accreditation Board. We believe that national voluntary accreditation of health departments will establish standards and benchmarks for essential public health services and engage health departments in ongoing quality improvement. This concept is well described in Chapter 10 of the handbook, "Accreditation As a Means for Quality Improvement."

To help health departments prepare for accreditation and to improve the overall quality and impact of governmental public health, the Foundation is working to ensure that local, state, and tribal health departments receive training and technical assistance on quality and performance improvement. In 2008, the Foundation invested in a third round of "A Multistate Learning Collaborative: Lead States in Public Health Quality Improvement." This initiative brings state and local health departments together with other stakeholders to improve public health services and the health of their communities by implementing quality improvement practices and preparing for national accreditation. The progress of the Multistate Learning Collaborative made to date is concisely summarized in Chapter 19, "Creating the Conditions for Quality Improvement." This is just one of a number of programs the Foundation is supporting to offer training, technical assistance, and the exchange of knowledge about the use of quality improvement in public health. A new initiative is under way to evaluate the effects of applying QI on not only process and health outcomes but also on staff and organizations. Many of the chapters in this handbook describe approaches to overcoming barriers and successfully engaging public health staff in meaningful quality improvement efforts. Several chapters also describe how QI can help public health departments work effectively and efficiently to meet the heightened need in these uncertain fiscal times.

The Robert Wood Johnson Foundation views this handbook as an important step in establishing a culture of continuous quality improvement in public health. The publication of the handbook by the American Society for Quality, an international leader in quality recognition and training, will also increase awareness in other sectors of the dedication to quality of public health practitioners working at the local, state, and national levels. It heralds a coming of age of quality improvement in public health.

Introduction

Paul Borawski

Executive Director and Chief Strategic Officer,
American Society for Quality

There is a current surge in quality improvement efforts among city, county, and state public health departments in the United States. This increased activity has been prompted by a number of factors, including reduced budgets, increased community needs and an aging government workforce. These factors are all too familiar to the members of ASQ, the professional society for which I serve as executive director and chief strategic officer.

According to a press release dated July 17, 2008, by the Trust for America's Health (TFAH), a small strategic investment in disease prevention could result in significant savings in U.S. healthcare costs. In its report entitled *Prevention for a Healthier America: Investments in Disease Prevention Yield Significant Savings, Stronger Communities*, TFAH finds that an investment of $10 per person per year in proven community based programs to increase physical activity, improve nutrition, and prevent smoking and other tobacco use could save the country more than $16 billion annually within five years. This is a return of $5.60 for every $1.00 spent.

"Healthcare costs are crippling the U.S. economy. Keeping Americans healthier is one of the most important, but overlooked ways we could reduce these costs," said Jeff Levi, PhD, executive director of TFAH. "This study shows that with a strategic investment in effective, evidence-based disease prevention programs, we could see tremendous returns in less than five years—sparing millions of people from serious diseases and saving billions of dollars."

Public health leaders are searching for effective and efficient tools to help their departments address issues such as disease prevention, substance abuse, infant health, and environmental safety. Scarce resources and growing needs dictate a culture of "Doing the best with what you have." Leveraging the resources and talents at hand is the mission of quality techniques such as the plan–do–check–act improvement cycle, lean enterprise, data-based management, teams, statistical process control, and balanced scorecard.

WHY ASQ AND THE PUBLIC HEALTH FOUNDATION ARE WORKING TOGETHER

ASQ and Public Health Foundation have a lot in common. As an executive, I would love to have a cookbook that I could open and select just the right recipe for leadership, strategic planning, process improvement, resource balancing, and client support or employee motivation. As a realist, I know that is not going to happen. *The Public Health Quality Improvement Handbook* comes pretty close, however. It is not a "how to" book. It is an anthology of chapters written by subject matter experts in public health who are successfully meeting client needs, working together to maximize outcomes, and expanding their collaboration with community partners to encourage better health within neighborhoods, counties, and states.

ASQ has long promoted a strategy dedicated to supporting quality within both the local and the global community. Current social responsibility discussions suggest that the tools and culture of quality are critical to every segment of the community. Public health departments around the United States are actively involved in integrating the concepts of quality improvement into every function of their organizations. Corporations, not-for-profit organizations, hospital systems, medical clinics, governments, faith-based groups, and community associations are joining forces to address the societal needs of today.

The main focus of the Public Health Foundation (PHF) is to improve public health infrastructure and performance through innovative solutions and measurable results. This focus drives PHF to collaborate with a complex and interrelated set of community partners to assess the strengths and needs of individuals and organizations and provide a balanced, effective set of programs to support assessed opportunities. ASQ and PHF have agreed to pursue a stronger relationship around quality improvement, community health, and social responsibility goals to help public health agencies be more successful in their community support efforts.

IMPROVING PERFORMANCE WITHIN PUBLIC HEALTH SERVICES

Two of the major topics of business literature now are "improvement" and "performance." How do we anticipate improvement? How do we plan for it? How do we implement it and get employee participation? How do we keep riding the leading wave of performance assessment and improvement? These questions are the grist of many news channel talk shows. The need for innovation is clear as competition intensifies for new technologies, scarce resources, and broader client support.

These challenges are not new to management. The pace at which we are bombarded by these challenges is. Managers do not have the time to sit in a quiet office and consider multiple alternatives. We must elicit ideas from those around us, generate options, and drive the best opportunity forward to success. We need quality improvement models and tools to assist us in making decisions. We need a fast and reliable source of techniques for success.

Topics in this anthology address the challenges public health leadership faces in our current environment. Chapter 1, "Daily Management," provides tools and approaches for increasing performance in our office and work places. Then Chapter 2, "Managing Performance to Improve Health," Chapter 3, "Strategic and Operational Planning," and Chapter 4, "Public Health Program Design and Deployment," take an increasingly broad view of performance improvement through measurements, strategic planning, and program design.

Chapter 5, "The Baldrige Criteria for Performance and Excellence As a Framework to Improve Public Health," Chapter 8, "Reporting: Telling Your Story," Chapter 12, "Already Doing It and Not Knowing It," Chapter 23, "Using Influence to Get Things Done," Chapter 24, "Orange County Health Department STD Quality Improvement Case Study," and Chapter 25, "The Minnesota Public Health

Collaborative for Quality Improvement," are all written by public health leaders who lived the scenario they write about. Chapter 26, "Translating Clinical Quality Improvement Success to Public Health," is a strong message for expanding quality applications from core functions to administrative and support activities. These chapters are the real thing. They are success stories and lessons learned. They are the crowning achievement and also the scar tissue that reflect the day-to-day responsibilities all of us accept when we enter the world of public health.

Other chapters provide more strategic wisdom related to management of the public health organization. Chapter 6, "Measures for Public Health," and Chapter 13, "Data Management and Basic Statistics," are significant guides for using fact- and data-based decision making to improve organizational performance in a reliable, repeatable, and documented way. Chapter 7, "Leading and Lagging Indicators," Chapter 17, "Community-Focused Performance Management," Chapter 18, "Community Balanced Scorecards for Strategic Public Health Improvement," Chapter 20, "Performance Management in Action," and Chapter 27, "Risk Management," give specific techniques and examples for using data to identify operational priorities and allocating resources effectively.

EXPANDING PUBLIC HEALTH STATURE IN THE COMMUNITY

A newly rising public health improvement effort is the realization of the impact of our efforts within the community. Like many service organizations, when the public health department is doing its job, we are not noticed. It is only when a crisis occurs that we are visible in the news or within city, county, or state conversations. There is a much stronger story available concerning the role public health plays in the long-term viability of our communities.

Chapter 9, "Creating Lasting Change," Chapter 10, "Accreditation As a Means for Quality Improvement," and Chapter 11, "Improving and Enhancing Community and Client Relationships," each highlight the strength a public health department (PHD) adds to the overall structure supporting the citizens of a geographic community. The current accreditation initiative championed by the National Association for City and County Health Organizations (NACCHO), PHF, and their partners, is a seminal project to create a baseline of service performance across all PHDs within the United States. Once this baseline is established and validated, it will serve as an operational definition for dialog among public health leadership, much as the Malcolm Baldrige Performance Excellence Model and the National Customer Satisfaction Index serve for the quality community in the United States.

QUALITY IMPROVEMENT TOOLS FOR PUBLIC HEALTH

The middle chapters of the *Public Health Quality Improvement Handbook* focus on how to use the tools of quality to improve specific processes within our function. Chapter 14, "Basic Tools of Quality Improvement," introduces the seven basic quality tools, including real-life examples of how these tools have been used in recent PHD quality improvement projects. Chapter 15, "Advanced Tools of Quality Improvement," takes the reader to a higher level of data-gathering, analysis, and decision making with more qualitative and intuitive decision-making approaches. Again, examples based on actual public health data and situations are included.

Chapter 16, "Applying Lean Six Sigma in Public Health," describes an excellent application of a performance improvement model frequently implemented within successful corporate and financial businesses around the world. This model is effective for any organization, whether complex or simple. Quality improvement is not a new way of doing things. It is a culture that becomes interwoven into what we do every day. Quality is not an "add on"; it is a different way of doing the things we do every day. When done effectively, it returns time to our schedules rather than increasing our responsibilities.

The final three chapters in the center of this handbook return to the behavioral aspect of performance. Chapter 19, "Creating the Conditions for Quality Improvement," Chapter 21, "Roles and Responsibilities for Teams," and Chapter 22, "The Reality of Teams in Resource-Constrained Public Health," share ideas for creating a motivating environment in which a workforce is energized toward the goals of public health in the community. Quality improvement is about increasing our ability to meet client needs and leveraging the resources necessary to meet our operating requirements. The tools of quality are not just flowcharts and measurement reports. Attitude is a tool. Positive thinking and effective communication are critical to reducing tension and disruption in our work environment. The better we work together within the PHD and with our community partners, the more effective we are in attaining the goals we set for ourselves.

EXPANDING OUR VISION

The final messages in the *Public Health Quality Improvement Handbook* look to the future of our function. Social responsibility and ethics are frequent topics on television, in major journals, newspapers, and books. Little is accomplished within an organization without trust. Quality improvement is not just about using tools, gathering data, or building effective processes. Unless the human beings who use processes trust each other and the organization in which they work, little will be achieved. Chapter 28, "The Ethics of Quality Improvement," addresses the critical topics of trust, responsibility, and accountability. How we work with each other is more important than what tools we use. Getting the job done is important. Getting it done in a way that others will accept is even more important. Public health has a strong history of success and service. The professionals within public health have a special sense for the impact of their efforts. Ethics is a core value within this community. This value must be incorporated into any performance or improvement effort we undertake.

SUMMARY

Little in the current world is simple. The higher we go in the organization, the more complex our challenges become. Nothing comes in a box for us to add water and stir. There are those, however, who have been successful and who are willing to share their success. The messages in the *Public Health Quality Improvement Handbook* are from leaders, physicians, practitioners, academics, consultants, and researchers who are successfully applying what they share with us in the pages of this book.

Quality improvement is the foundation for sustainable results. Improvement is something we can lead. The chapters of this book are written to support the leaders and workforce of our public health community.

This book is written to be read as you need the information. If you wish to start at Chapter 1 and move sequentially through the book, you will most certainly enjoy the journey. You might also find there is value in starting with a chapter that especially fits your current challenge. Where a chapter overlaps another, the author makes reference so the reader can branch out for additional reading, if desired.

Whatever approach you take in using the tools offered in the *Public Health Quality Improvement Handbook*, you will benefit from the information. This is a foundation work for the public health community. The Public Health Foundation and the American Society for Quality are honored to make it available to you.

Chapter 1

Daily Management

John W. Moran and Grace L. Duffy

WHAT IS DAILY MANAGEMENT?

Aristotle, Greek philosopher and scientist, once said that "Quality is not an act. It is a habit." *Daily management* is the overarching philosophy of incremental change in the day-to-day work we all do to meet the needs of our clients and the marketplace. It is a cornerstone of a total quality management system. Daily management has to be a habit for it to be effective. People doing the work have to make daily incremental improvements in their work processes to constantly keep up with shifting client demands.

Daily management is a process to help you manage your job and not let your job manage you. Daily management puts control and change in the hands of those doing the work. Daily management is the system that focuses process improvement at the lowest level possible—those who do the work. It is the utilization of the tools and techniques of quality improvement in day-to-day work activities by those doing the work.

Daily management is composed of two subparts:

1. *Daily improvement,* which is the continuous, never ending quest of uncovering work process improvement opportunities to improve our effectiveness, efficiency, productivity, and our ability to deliver timely services to our clients.

2. *Daily control,* which is the establishment of a measurement system composed of metrics we utilize to monitor our work processes to ensure they are in control and delivering the services our clients want and need in a timely and seamless manner.

Daily management must be supported by the organization's reward and recognition structure to encourage employees to constantly be looking for areas to improve in their process. To help employees to be able to identify new improvement opportunities on a regular basis, it is important to have an active and timely:

1. Measuring and monitoring system in place in the key areas of the process.

2. Client surveying system in place where we actively monitor our client to ensure we are providing them with the services they need. Since a majority of public health processes interact directly with a client it is easy to set up a survey process to capture data at each interaction. A simple survey either verbal or written can capture real-time data that can be used to gauge our client's satisfaction with services being received.

Daily management is a continuous, never ending process of improvement because the clients we serve and the marketplace we deliver our services in are forever maturing and changing. There is an old saying that you must "constantly innovate or die in the marketplace." To keep our work processes up to date and in tune with our clients and the marketplace we must:

- Understand our process and its elements

- Know the boundaries of our process

- Understand the lines of process responsibility and make them clear

- Monitor the process with metrics to understand its normal variation

- Constantly look for wasteful steps, delays, and waits to improve our response time to our clients

- Understand our clients and their wants and needs

- Communicate our wants and needs to the suppliers of our process's inputs

- Continually keep up on current and future changes in the marketplace that could impact the way we deliver our services

CULTURE REQUIRED TO SUPPORT A DAILY MANAGEMENT SYSTEM

Organizations have a culture just like civilizations do. Culture is generally defined as: patterns of human activity and the symbolic structures that give such activities significance and importance.[1]

Senior leadership in an organization establishes and maintains a culture based on the behaviors visible to employees, customers, suppliers, and stakeholders. Cultures evolve over time. What is done by senior management is stronger than what is said or published by the marketing department. The old adage of "I can not hear what you are saying because what you are doing speaks so much louder" is completely appropriate in studying organizational culture. Culture is what establishes the mind-set of people working in a company. Culture sets expectations of behavior over time.

Attention to daily management is a mind-set. As mentioned at the beginning of the chapter, daily management is a process to help you manage your job. Daily management puts control and change in the hands of those doing the work. Senior management either trusts those assigned to accomplish a critical task or they don't.

Trust within an organization is a major cultural condition. Empowering workers at the lowest possible level of responsibility to accomplish significant operational goals maximizes the resources of the organization. Doing more with less means using every skill, talent, idea, and ounce of energy available to meet customer needs. Resources are wasted when work is performed by a higher paid or more skilled employee than necessary.

Generating a culture of trust is a long-term accomplishment. Trust must be integrated into every level and every function within the organization. Trust, empowerment, accountability, and recognition are all combined as a cultural characteristic of management. Management has the responsibility for providing an environment in which the workforce feels supported to assess daily situations, analyze opportunities, and take appropriate risks to meet changing requirements of customers and stakeholders. The workforce has the responsibility to take advantage of training, empowerment, and flexibility within the scope of their position to maximize the use of company resources to meet organizational goals.

The ongoing interaction between management and workforce creates the culture of trust and empowerment within the organization. Effective daily management is a significant indicator of a successful organizational culture.

DEFINING YOUR CRITICAL PROCESSES

Whenever we flowchart a process we are always looking for those few key elements that define the success of the output of the process. Every process is composed of many tasks that are integrated together in a pattern of activity that has one building upon another. When we analyze a flowchart we need to look for those few very important tasks that can spell success or failure if they are not executed properly. These few important processes are called *critical processes*. Every process contains a set of critical processes that are the key determinants of whether or not our client is satisfied with the output of our process.

Critical processes are the very important sets of tasks that determine if we successfully meet our client's wants and needs. Critical processes have the following characteristics:[2]

1. They are few in number, usually five to 10

2. They are linked horizontally and vertically

3. The critical processes of an individual's job should capture 75 to 80 percent of the factors that determine the success of that position

4. They can be mapped or diagrammed

5. They can be measured

6. They can be improved

When a process is done on a repeated, daily basis it is easy to map it, define the discrete activities that compose it, determine the critical processes, and determine the process variation and problem areas. At the managerial and supervisory level it is sometimes difficult to understand what your critical processes are since they are not done in a repeatable, daily manner. Some managerial and supervisory critical processes may be done weekly (payroll), monthly (budgets), or quarterly (performance reviews) but they are critical to how your organization performs. Some managerial and supervisory critical processes may be quite broad and comprehensive, and if that is the case it may be helpful to think in terms of "critical systems," which are a collection of critical processes that must occur simultaneously across the organization. One such critical system is the human resource system, which may consist of a number of critical processes such as hiring, training, development, recognition, and compensation.

One approach to get a handle on what your managerial or supervisory critical processes is to keep an activity log as shown in Figure 1.1.

Over time you will begin to see a pattern of activities that consumes the largest percentage of your work time. These can be your initial critical processes since they have the highest percentages of time spent. Then the process of analysis begins where you take the top two or three processes and begin to analyze them by mapping out the tasks it takes to complete them. Once you have mapped out the tasks involved in a critical process it is time to determine if there are any problem areas that need to be resolved, what the causes of those bottlenecks are, what can be done to improve them, and finally what can be measured to show that the gains from a change have been accomplished and sustained.

As you improve your managerial and supervisory critical processes, a key question you should be asking of each task identified is "Should I be doing this or should a subordinate be doing it?" Too often as managers and supervisors we take over tasks from subordinates because they are not capable to do them. Rather than invest the time and effort to train them or replace them we wind up doing the task. This is a time to make sure that the tasks you are doing are appropriate and need to be done at your level. These extra tasks we pick up add stress to our jobs and work life that can be rectified by putting the task back at the appropriate level in the organization and investing the time to make sure it gets completed in the manner you need it.

Critical processes will change over time so it is a good idea to keep tracking your time spent on a weekly basis to see how things evolve over time as changes are made, technology improves, client needs change, and organizational strategy evolves. Nothing is constant in the world of work.

Activity	How often	Time spent	Percent of total time
Budget review	Once per week	12 hours	15 percent
Performance reviews	Quarterly	40 hours	20 percent
Payroll	Weekly	10 hours	10 percent
Review meeting preparation	Monthly	20 hours	25 percent

Figure 1.1   Managerial activity log tracker.

A useful tool to use is the table shown in Figure 1.2 in which you analyze the tasks of a critical process and decide which ones you should continue doing (delivering value to the client), should start doing (missing steps found during the process analysis and improvement phase, which is described later in this chapter, or requested by your clients), or stop doing (the non-value-added elements).

The "Assign to" column is used to indicate what happens to tasks we decide to stop or start doing. We may decide to start doing new tasks to improve the output of our process and need to indicate who will be doing it in the future. If we transfer a task from ourselves to a subordinate, we need to indicate the transfer. If a task is no longer being done we need to indicate that it has been terminated in the "Why" column. This tracker will give you a record of what changes you have made, when, and why.

UNDERSTANDING YOUR PROCESS

The SIPOC diagram is used during the initial definition of a process. It depicts the high-level logic of how requirements flow into the process and how items flow out of the process to the customer. Figure 1.3 gives a visual representation of a SIPOC diagram. SIPOC is an acronym consisting of the first letter of each of the components of the diagram: supplier, inputs, process, outputs, and customers. Occasionally you will see the term reversed to "COPIS" to reflect the desire to put the "customer" first. Suppliers and customers are people or organizations. Inputs and outputs are tangible items such as products, services, information, and data.

Date	Task	Continue doing	Start doing	Stop doing	Assign to:	Why

Figure 1.2 Task analyzer.

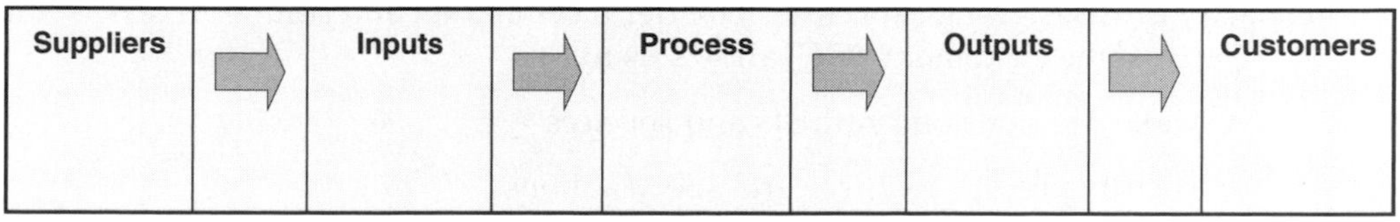

Suppliers	Inputs	Process	Outputs	Customers

Figure 1.3 SIPOC diagram.

Some benefits of using a SIPOC are that it:

- Allows a multifunctional team to review the organizational process "at 30,000 feet"

- Provides an opportunity to recognize where bottlenecks occur

- Encourages participants to identify corrective actions or opportunities for improvement

- Offers a visual platform from which to analyze process parameters

It is helpful to involve a team of people who know the process under study to identify the different components of the SIPOC. The SIPOC tool is an excellent base for exploratory dialog around different perceptions of the process from those involved in process activities. Steps in creating a SIPOC are:

- Involve representative stakeholders.

- Address the premier customer base; do not attempt to include every detail.

- List the main suppliers of products or services.

- Identify the major inputs to the process.

- List key process steps that transform inputs to added-value outputs.

- Include any external resources or outsourcing required under inputs or suppliers.

- List the target markets for outputs under the customer category.

- Maintain a database of information gathered during this activity for analysis and trending.

- Research best practices from other organizations, either internal or external, for long-term process capability.

The *voice of the customer* is a tool used to describe a detailed plan to gather and collect customer needs and customer perceptions. Customer requirements are identified and documented through a series of surveys, focus groups, individual interviews, data gathering, and analysis. The requirements are then mapped to the organization's ability to meet these requirements. The resulting matrix of needs and internal processes provides a working checklist for enhancing internal capacity or redesigning processes to better meet market and competitive needs.

Voice of the customer (VOC) allows us to:

- Make decisions on products and services

- Identify product features and specifications

- Develop baseline metrics on customer satisfaction

- Focus on improvement plans

- Identify customer satisfaction drivers

The quality improvement community has identified six generic *critical-to-business outcomes* through voice of the customer activities. These six outcomes are:

1. Importance
2. Perceptions
3. Characteristics
4. Relationships
5. Trade-offs
6. Targets

These outcome categories provide us with suggested next steps for improving internal processes. VOC input suggests priorities for targeting processes for improvement. *Importance* and *perceptions* identify areas of greater priority. *Characteristics, relationships,* and *trade-offs* offer areas for further discussion with the customer. These discussions serve two purposes. One is to establish specific functionality of products and services. The other is to improve customer relationship management through better communication and engagement with customer personnel and leadership. *Targets* suggest priorities for balancing internal resources appropriate to customer-stated requirements.[3] Knowing which requirements are most critical from a customer perspective is essential if you have to make trade-offs or sacrifice one requirement to meet another.

A process for collecting VOC data is:

- Identify customers and their needs.
- Collect and analyze reactive data.
- Consider proactive approaches for anticipating customer needs.
- Convert collected data into customer needs.
- Sort out the most important attributes.
- Obtain specifications for the critical-to-quality characteristics.

Some examples of critical-to-quality characteristics are:

- Performance
- Price
- Design
- Ease of use
- Access
- Color
- Defect free
- Friendly service

How do you know what your customer wants? One of the best ways is to ask. There are a number of other approaches that are appropriate depending on the situation and whether you are meeting the customer face to face or seeking input from a large population.

Some suggestions for gathering VOC data are:

- Ask customers to list their requirements.

- Identify what measurements the customer uses.

- Find out your customer's highest priority.

- Find out your customer's biggest complaint.

- Determine what process of yours would cause the most problems for your customers.

- Determine what improvement would give your customer a competitive edge.

- Determine whether your customer's requirements are possible.

- Discuss and try to agree on targets, and so on.

There is another related tool called the *voice of the supplier* (VOS). The process for identifying and gathering the information is the same as for the VOC. The only change is that we are the "customer" in this scenario. The benefits are basically the same. We have the opportunity to improve our relationship with the supplier through increased communication and partnering in order to meet the final end user requirements in the supply chain we both support.

The final voice addressed in this section is the *voice of the process* (VOP). There are many tools developed over the last 60 years to identify, analyze, improve, and monitor processes within the organization and those that include interactions with suppliers, customers, and related stakeholders. Statistical process control techniques calculate the control limits and capability of an existing process. Advanced tools highlight areas for redesign and breakthrough improvement. Once the current process is mapped and measured, the next step is to identify priority areas for improvement.

DAILY MANAGEMENT IMPROVEMENT

Daily management is the system that focuses process improvement at the lowest level possible: those who do the work. It is the utilization of quality improvement in day-to-day work activities by those doing the work.

Involving multiple levels of workforce and management in the analysis of current process performance is helpful in gaining different perspectives and expectations for the output of a particular process. Tools such as the SIPOC, flowcharts, run charts, checklists, and audits provide quantitative and tangible evidence of process stability and reliability. Once the current state of the process is known, the next action is to plan for improving the process to better meet customer needs.

Steps to improve processes and services are:

1. Identify internal customer interfaces

2. Establish internal customer's needs and requirements

3. Ensure that the internal and external customer requirements support each other

4. Document service-level agreements

5. Establish improvement goals and measures

6. Implement systems for tracking and reporting

There is also a cycle for sustaining and standardizing a process when it is performing adequately to meet the voice of the customer. Figure 1.4 shows a combined SDCA/PDCA cycle of *standardize–do–check–act* and *plan–do–check–act*.

The plan–do–check–act cycle was made popular by Dr. W. Edwards Deming, who is considered by many to be the father of modern quality control; however, it was always referred to by him as the "Shewhart cycle," after Walter Shewhart, from whom Dr. Deming learned the process.

PDCA should be repeatedly implemented in spirals of increasing knowledge of the system that converge on the ultimate goal of process excellence, each cycle closer to excellence than the previous one. The power of Deming's cycle lies in its apparent simplicity.

The SDCA and PDCA cycles are separate but integrated. Once we have made a successful change we standardize and hold the gain. When the process is not performing correctly we go from SDCA to PDCA, and once we have the process performing correctly we standardize again. This switching back and forth

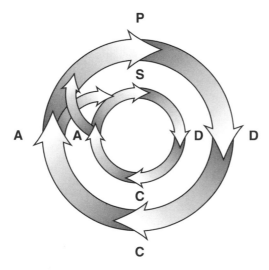

Figure 1.4   The SDCA/PDCA cycle.

between SDCA and PDCA provides us with the opportunity to keep our process customer-focused.

The *continuous improvement* phase of this process is where you make a change in direction. The change usually is necessary because the process output is deteriorating or customer needs have changed. The *plan* or *standardize* phase of the two cycles is the only real difference. The individual plan–do–check–act steps are:

Plan

- Identify what opportunities and priorities are to be realized through the improvement cycle.

- Establish measures and objectives for the improvement action.

- Involve a team of participants from different areas of the organization impacted by the change.

Do

- Implement the process improvement initiative, taking small steps in controlled circumstances.

- Get sponsors' approval and their support if implementing means going outside your personal area of responsibility.

- Document the changes so the process can be duplicated/standardized.

Check

- Continually check the results as the process is initiated and after it is in place to determine if the changes are meeting requirements.

- Determine if the measurements used to determine success are adequate.

- If not, define the required measurements and how these data can be developed.

- Remember to automate data gathering if at all possible.

Act

- Take action to standardize or improve the process.

- If the process changes are meeting requirements, continue to monitor occasionally.

Standardize the changes through implementation of the SDCA cycle. If the process still isn't meeting requirements, investigate additional process improvement opportunities. The *maintenance and standardization* phase of a process is where we hold the gains. If our process is producing the desired results, we standardize what we are doing.

How do we know whether a process is worth improving or even maintaining? Are the resources dedicated to the process being used for maximum benefit of the organization?

There are two key questions to ask:

1. Does the process under study support the organization's strategic mission?

2. Is the process under study necessary to meet the demands of our customers?

If the answer to both of these questions is no, strongly question whether it is worth continuing to perform the process.

ALIGNING DAILY MANAGEMENT IMPROVEMENT GOALS TO ORGANIZATIONAL GOALS

The flow of daily management is based on the concept of alignment as discussed in the balanced scorecard model.[4] Organizational measurements must be guided by the voice of the customer as discussed earlier in this chapter. The external customer and other key stakeholders provide strong input to the major goals of the organization. These goals are then cascaded down through senior leadership to middle management where they are translated into operational objectives, tasks, and measures of performance and results. This cascading identifies the lines of responsibility through which authority is granted for daily management activity.

First-line management, teams, and individuals establish performance plans based on the cascaded measurements. These performance plans are tracked on a daily, weekly, monthly, and quarterly basis, with reports provided upward to management, which ties the reported results to the respective key drivers at the corporate level.

Figure 1.5 gives a visual concept of alignment of the corporate vision and goals from the executives, management, and team leaders to the workforce. The workforce assesses overall goals, establishes tasks, actions, and dates for achievement, and provides feedback up through management to validate the ability of the organization to provide the desired results. The concept of daily management uses the alignment model to drive activities to the lowest level of the organization where the skill and capacity exists to accomplish the task.

Daily management uses the measures and indicators established by the front-line worker, teams, and supervisors to drive short-term achievements consistent with the long-term planning of senior management. Another term used with *balanced scorecard* is *direct line of sight* management. The idea is that all activity at the daily level can be tied up through the chain of management to the strategic goals and objectives of the organization.

The concepts of lean enterprise and value stream mapping use this alignment approach in comparing any activity with the value placed upon it by the customer of the process it supports. Lean enterprise concerns itself with reduction of waste

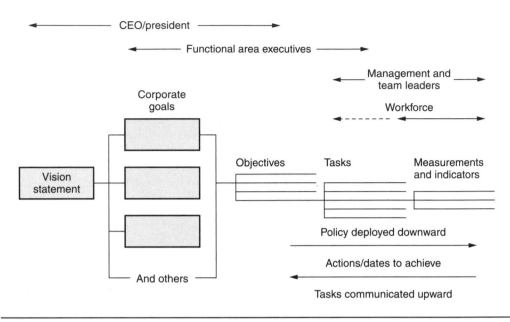

Figure 1.5   Aligning daily activities to organizational goals.

and redundancy. All activity within the organization should either directly support the requirements of an external or internal customer or be a requirement of doing business within our chosen markets. Mapping a process to the goals of the organization or the value expected by our customers is a significant tool for eliminating or reducing the use of any resource for other than essential activities.

Use the concept of daily management to organize department activities around the contributions made by an individual employee or team member to the core mission and requirements of the company—the specific requirements for which the department supervisor or team is responsible. Tie objectives described in any job description to the required outcomes of the department to which it is assigned. Daily management tracking will then serve as an effective audit function to ensure that resources are allocated in the best possible way to meet customer needs.

SUMMARY

Henry Ford is quoted as saying that "Quality means doing it right when no one is looking." This is the motto of daily management. Daily management when done well is done all the time in the organization, day in and day out. Daily management is a system that becomes acculturated into an organization and is not seen visibly except perhaps for some measurement and monitoring charts on a wall that are up-to-date, some employees meeting to solve a common problem using quality improvement tools, employees making a presentation where some of the tools and techniques of quality improvement can be seen, or a conference room with a fishbone diagram or flip chart on display. The visible signs of daily management in action are subtle.

As managers there are signs to look for that will indicate that daily management is not yet a reality in your organization:

- The quality of the output or client service of a process is different from shift to shift, location to location, person to person. This indicates a lack of standardized methods, poor training, or a lack of accurate metrics.

- The same problems keep reoccurring, and you keep fixing them over and over again.

- Work processes were never planned out but sort of evolved over time by the different people doing the job.

- Different areas doing the same work have different forms, collect different data, and may have different technology systems.

- Interacting processes have different goals and objectives so there is not smooth handoff and things get lost or delayed often.

- You are always in a crisis mode of operation.

- You blame the people for the problems that occur.

- Clients complain about a lack of service or long waits.

- You have poor documentation of changes made to the process, and most of the time those changes are not communicated clearly to those involved.

- When veteran employees take a vacation or leave, many problems arise since you do not know how they accomplished various tasks.

- Employees complain about how demanding their clients are. "They are never satisfied" is a common expression.

For daily management to be effective everyone must have an understanding of how their process works and interacts with the other processes in the organization, and how it contributes to the strategic direction of the organization. Everyone must feel an ownership of their process and its output. Measurement must be a way of life and used to improve and not punish. Everyone must have a customer/supplier orientation through which they communicate and understand their wants and needs. Equally important is that everyone must develop an attitude and willingness to change often since we are now in a fast-changing and evolving society in which the status quo is constantly being challenged.

Chapter 2

Managing Performance to Improve Health

Grace L. Duffy and John W. Moran

THE IMPORTANCE OF MANAGING PERFORMANCE

Performance management processes have measurably improved quality, outputs, and outcomes of public health services. The coordinated efforts of performance management strategies can impact an agency in a number of ways. Some of the ways performance management can positively influence a public health agency include:

- Better return on dollars invested in health

- Greater accountability for funding, and increase in the public's trust

- Reduced duplication of efforts

- Better understanding of public health accomplishments and priorities among employees, partners, and the public

- Increased sense of cooperation and teamwork

- Increased emphasis on quality rather than quantity

- Improved problem solving

RESULTS IN PUBLIC HEALTH

According to the February 2002 Performance Management National Excellence Collaborative (PMC) Survey, *Performance Management Practices in States: Results of a Baseline Assessment of State Health Agencies,*[1] 76 percent of responding state health agencies reported that their performance management efforts resulted in improved performance. Most reported performance improvement pertained to:

- Improved delivery of services (program, clinical preventive, and the 10 essential public health services)

- Improved administration/management, contracting, tracking/ reporting, and coordination

- Improved policies or legislation

Specific examples from the PMC survey of states that used performance management practices and saw results include:

Tennessee. Improved outcomes in rates of immunization.

North Dakota. Improved performance in several maternal and child health indicators.

New Jersey. Improved managed care organization performance, including customer satisfaction and outcome measures, improved survival rates for coronary bypass surgery, including risk-adjusted mortality for hospitals and individual surgeons, and improved nursing home performance, including inspection results and complaint data.

Massachusetts. Increased funding for substance abuse, tobacco, breast cancer, pregnancy prevention, school health, and other programs.

Texas. Increased awareness of and accountability for the provision of public health services among program managers and staff.

Over the last decade, the Florida Department of Health improved outcomes in several areas of health. Between the years of 1991 and 1998, rates of congenital syphilis decreased by approximately 87 percent.[2] In the same period of time, rates of tuberculosis cases decreased by 33 percent.[3] Florida's Department of Health also cut infant mortality rates in minority populations more than any other state.[4] The state attributes these changes to a movement away from a focus solely on quality assurance to a more comprehensive quality improvement process. The quality improvement process implements the components of performance management, including an emphasis on customers, examining processes, involving employees, benchmarking, and making decisions based on data.

On the local level in Florida, one of the authors has been involved with the Orange County Health Department (OCHD) since 2006 in a series of process improvement team efforts focusing on improving testing processes for sexually transmitted diseases (STDs) and immunology, reducing cycle time of septic system permitting, and implementing an integrated quality system across the total health department. A case study of the OCHD STD 2006 project is available in Chapter 26 of this text.

OCHD began their efforts on a project-by-project basis supported by grants through the Public Health Foundation and local supporting organizations. Because of the success of the initial project improvements, senior management has now moved to an integrated systems approach for using quality improvement to manage performance across the whole county Department of Health.

In order for these results to be achieved, performance management practices must be integrated or institutionalized into routine public health processes, and all players within an agency or program need to understand and be invested in his or her role within a larger system. Many later chapters in this text identify successful approaches and tools to support this systems view of quality and performance management.

RESULTS IN OTHER FIELDS

Examining the results of performance management practices in other fields, such as the business sector, can help public health professionals gain a better understanding of the importance of the processes of performance management. It is not enough to look at the end results or outputs of a system. Strong evidence from profitable U.S. companies suggests that getting results also requires careful attention to performance in areas such as human resources, information systems, and internal processes.

Performance excellence models such as the Baldrige National Performance Excellence program supported by the U.S. Department of Commerce (www.NIST. gov) and many state assessment and recognition programs are actively soliciting applications from not-for-profit and health organizations. Chapter 5 in this text has a summary of the national and several state programs as they relate to issues important to public health.

HOW MANAGERS CAN USE PERFORMANCE MEASURES

Quality improvement efforts are critical at all levels of the organization. Certainly the commitment of senior management in setting and maintaining a culture of performance and quality is imperative to long-term success. Likewise is the effectiveness of involving the direct workforce in the identification and resolution of performance problems on a daily basis. Line and staff management are in a good position to see both the strategic direction coming from senior officers as well as the individual contribution of the line worker. Some of the important contributions of middle managers in performance management are:

- Identify aspects of the work that have and have not resulted in satisfactory results.

- Identify trends.

- Further investigate the nature of particular problems.

- Set targets for future periods.

- Motivate managers and staff to improve performance and increase their interest in better serving clients.

- Hold managers and staff accountable.

- Develop and improve programs and policies.

- Help design policies and budgets and explain these to stakeholders.[5]

For example, the seven performance Criteria for the Malcolm Baldrige National Quality Award Program (see Chapter 5) for business, education, and healthcare are used by thousands of organizations for self-assessment and training and as a tool to develop performance and business processes. Using the criteria can result in better employee relations, higher productivity, greater customer satisfaction, increased market share, and improved profitability for many organizations.

Baldrige award winners who excel in the seven areas have over the last decade created tremendous shareholder value. The "Baldrige Index," a hypothetical stock fund made up of publicly traded U.S. companies that received the Baldrige Award, has consistently outperformed the Standard & Poor's 500 by approximately three to one.[6]

According to a report by the Conference Board, a business membership organization, "A majority of large U.S. firms have used the criteria of the Malcolm Baldrige National Quality Award for self-improvement, and the evidence suggests a long-term link between use of the Baldrige criteria and improved business performance."[7]

IMPROVING PERFORMANCE IS ABOUT USING DATA

Performance management is the practice of actively using performance data to improve the public's health. This practice involves strategic use of performance measures and standards to establish performance targets and goals. Performance management practices can also be used to prioritize and allocate resources, to inform managers about needed adjustments or changes in policy or program directions to meet goals, to frame reports on the success in meeting performance goals, and to improve the quality of public health practice.

Performance management as described in the Performance Management Model developed by the Turning Point Performance Management National Excellence Collaborative includes the following components (see Figure 2.1):

1. *Performance standards.* Establishment of organizational or system performance standards, targets, and goals to improve public health practices.

2. *Performance measurement.* Development, application, and use of performance measures to assess achievement of such standards.

3. *Reporting of progress.* Documentation and reporting of progress in meeting standards and targets and sharing this information through feedback.

4. *Quality improvement process.* Establishment of a program or process to manage change and achieve quality improvement in public health policies, programs, or infrastructure, based on performance standards, measurements, and reports.

The four components of performance management can be applied to:

- Human resource development
- Data and information systems
- Customer focus and satisfaction
- Financial systems
- Management practices
- Public health capacity
- Health status

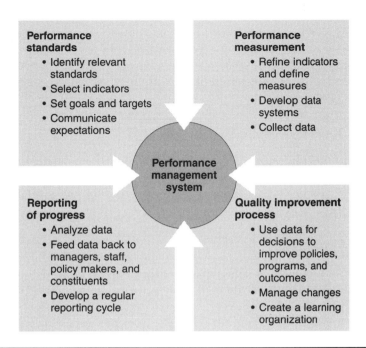

Figure 2.1   Performance management framework and components.
Source: Public Health Foundation, "Turning Point: From Silos to Systems."
http://www.phf.org/pmqi/silossystems.pdf

A performance management system includes the continuous use of all of the above practices so that they are integrated into an agency's core operations. Performance management can be carried out at multiple levels, including the program, organization, community, and state levels.

DOES YOUR AGENCY HAVE A PERFORMANCE MANAGEMENT SYSTEM?

There are a series of questions the Public Health Foundation has identified to assist public health leadership in assessing the effectiveness of their performance management system. The following questions are strongly related to a quality and performance excellence culture at the organizational level:

- Do you set specific performance standards, targets, or goals for your organization? How do you determine these standards? Do you benchmark against similar state organizations or use national, state, or scientific guidelines?

- Do you have a way to measure the capacity, process, or outcomes of established performance standards and targets? What tools do you use to assist in these efforts?

- Do you document or report your organization's progress? Do you make this information regularly available to managers, staff, and others?

- Do you have a quality improvement process? What do you do with the information gathered in your progress report or document? Do you have a process to manage changes in policies, programs, or infrastructure that is based on performance standards, measurements, and reports?

EXAMPLES OF THE FOUR COMPONENTS

A successful performance management system is driven by state and local needs and designed to closely align with a public health agency's mission and strategic plans. Public health agencies have applied the four components in a variety of ways.

Performance Standards

Public health agencies and their partners can benefit from using national standards, state-specific standards, benchmarks from other jurisdictions, or agency-specific targets to define performance expectations. The National Public Health Performance Standards Program (NPHPSP) defines performance in each of the 10 essential public health services for state and local public health systems and governing bodies. The NPHPSP supports users of the national standards with a variety of technical assistance products including online data submission and an analytic report back to the user jurisdiction. Some states such as Ohio, West Virginia, and Washington have developed their own performance standards for health departments. These state standards serve a variety of purposes, such as to provide a benchmark for continuous quality improvement, to determine eligibility for state subsidies, or for self-assessments in meeting established standards.

It is important to set challenging but achievable targets. Achieving performance targets should require concerted efforts, resources, and managerial action. If targets can be achieved easily despite budget cuts and limited efforts, there is little motivation to improve performance or to invest in additional agency efforts.

Performance Measures

To select specific performance measures, public health agencies may consult national tools containing tested measures (such as Tracking Healthy People 2010) as well as develop their own procedures to help them assess performance. Washington performs field tests with state and local health departments to determine how well its measures work for evaluation. Texas created an intranet reporting system for its agency users, which helped to increase efficiency and accuracy of reporting on its performance measures. The Texas Performance Measure Management Group meets quarterly to discuss measures and reporting. Because quantitative data sometimes are not available to measure performance indicators, New Hampshire includes a provision in its performance-based contracting system requiring contractors to describe activities for which they can not provide data to assess their performance. Contractors are advised to develop systems to capture the data needed for the performance measures.

Terms to know:

Performance standards are objective standards or guidelines that are used to assess an organization's performance (for example, one epidemiologist on staff per 100,000 population served, 80 percent of all clients who rate health department services as "good" or "excellent"). Standards may be set based on national, state, or scientific guidelines, by benchmarking against similar organizations, based on the public's or leaders' expectations (for example, 100 percent access, zero disparities), or other methods.

Performance measures are quantitative measures of capacities, processes, or outcomes relevant to the assessment of a performance indicator (for example, the number of trained epidemiologists available to investigate, or percentage of clients who rate health department services as "good" or "excellent").

Performance indicators summarize the focus (for example, workforce capacity, customer service) of performance goals and measures often used for communication purposes and preceding the development of specific measures.

Performance targets set specific and measurable goals related to agency or system performance. Where a relevant performance standard is available, the target may be the same as, exceed, or be an intermediate step toward that standard.

Reporting of Progress

How a public health agency tracks and reports progress depends on the purposes of its performance management system and the intended users of performance data. In Ohio, the Department of Health publishes periodic reports on key measures (identified by Department staff) that are used by the agency for making improvements. Relevant state and national performance indicators are reviewed by representatives of all interested parties. Casting a wider net for reporting and accountability, Virginia established a Web site to make performance reports and planning information accessible to policy makers, public health partners, agency employees, and citizens.

Saginaw County Michigan uses the results of their MAPP-based community-wide assessments to enhance the measures consistently gathered through their partnership with the University of Michigan and national public health data sources. See Chapter 10 for a case study of Saginaw County's 2008 MAPP assessment staff leadership and community partner training project.

Quality Improvement Process

An established quality improvement process brings consistency to the agency's approach to managing performance, motivates improvement, and helps capture lessons learned. An established quality improvement process may focus on one aspect of performance, such as customer satisfaction, or cut across the entire health agency. Rather than leave the use of performance data to chance, some states have instituted processes to ensure they continually take actions to improve performance and accountability. In its highly dynamic process for systemwide improvement, the Florida Department of Health charges its Performance Improvement Office with coordinating resources and efforts to perform regular performance management reviews and provide feedback to managers and local county administrators. As part of the state's quality improvement process, state and local staff collaboratively develop agreements that specify what each party will do to help improve performance in identified areas. New Hampshire has a process to redirect program dollars to reward quality and contractors' performance in serving the target population.

THE PERFORMANCE MANAGEMENT CYCLE

The ideas of "continuous quality improvement" and a cycle of "performance-based management" are not new. In the 1950s, W. Edwards Deming, a professor and management consultant, transformed traditional industrial thinking about quality control with his emphasis on employee empowerment, performance feedback, and measurement-based management. Deming believed the following:

- Inspection measures at the end of a production line ignore the root causes of defects and result in inefficiencies. Discarding defective products creates more waste than "doing it right the first time."

- Defects can be avoided and quality improved indefinitely if these root causes are discovered and addressed through ongoing evaluation processes. Companies should adopt a cycle of continuous product and process improvement, often referred to as *plan–do–check–act*.

- All business processes should be part of an ongoing measurement process with feedback loops. Managers, working with employees, should examine data fed back to them to determine causes of variation or defects, pinpoint problems with processes, and focus attention on improving specific aspects of production.

Many subsequent models, such as total quality management in the 1980s, take root in Deming's philosophy.

In public health, the "production line" to create healthy communities has many aspects that must continually be managed with feedback loops:

- Although those working in public health are mission-driven with a focus on health outcomes, checking only health status and other outcomes will not help to identify root causes of health problems or inefficiencies. To create high-performing agencies, the efficiency and quality of related inputs and outputs leading to better outcomes must be managed. The Assessment Protocol for Excellence in Public Health (APEXPH) Health Problem Analysis model, used by Florida in its performance management system, is an example of an approach to examining root causes and contributing factors for health problems.

- Donabedian's[8] assessment framework of structures, processes, and outcomes can help public health agencies examine performance in distinct aspects of their system. An optimal performance management approach creates feedback loops around all three aspects. Public health performance should be managed for:

  1. Structures such as financial and information resources

  2. Processes such as health promotion and epidemiology services

  3. Outcomes such as health status and cost savings

For an illustration of a continuous performance feedback loop involving structural capacity, processes, and outcomes related to public health, refer to the performance measurement model in Figure 2.2.

In the model described in Figure 2.2, the macro, or community, context of public health translates into an integrated system of structural capacity and process guided by the public health system mission and purpose. This integrated system drives the effectiveness, efficiency, and equity of the outcomes of the local public health system.

Each local public health system is dependent on the community it serves. The Public Health Foundation performance management system describes four components used to define and analyze community needs, compare these needs to nationally tested standards, and identify appropriate measures and targets to guide local health department efforts in their goal of addressing communitywide public health needs.

The four components of performance management (see Figure 2.1)—performance standards, measures, reporting, and quality improvement processes—are

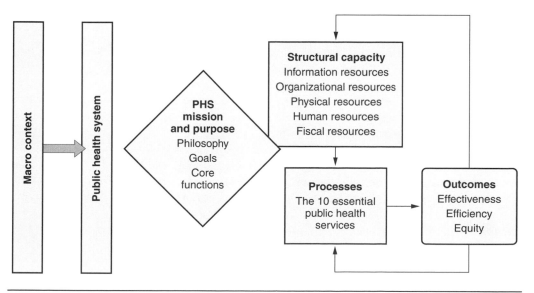

Figure 2.2   Conceptual framework of the public health system as a basis for measuring public health systems performance.[9]

practical tools to help public health agencies put performance feedback loops into operation.

Performance management can be used across a larger system (for example, to improve state and local public health agency collaboration or efficiency) or to improve the performance of one aspect within a smaller system, (for example, to improve outcomes of an anti-tobacco campaign, or to improve restaurant managers' compliance with an agency's food safety program). However it is applied, the performance management cycle is a tool to improve health, increase efficiency, and create other benefits and value for society.

IS THIS A SCIENCE OR AN ART?

Performance management should focus on a mix of structure, process, and outcome measures—but what is the right mix? What performance indicators and measures are most related to improved outcomes? On what processes should managers and employees focus their energies? It is vital to consult scientific literature and guidelines when choosing indicators and making management decisions. In clinical care and many health promotion areas, for example, there are well-established relationships between professional practices and certain outcomes, making management of shorter-term indicators a sound and cost-effective approach. Currently there is little science to help public health professionals optimally manage performance of a public health system overall, underscoring the need to conduct further research in this area and share experiences from the field. As researchers and practitioners gather more data, public health professionals can look forward to using more evidence-based approaches to performance management.

The *Public Health Quality Improvement Handbook* is a foundation work intended to begin the dialog in a systematic way to define a standardized approach to gathering and analyzing data related to the effectiveness of performance management in public health. The authors invited to contribute to this work are the industry leaders in public health and communitywide needs assessment.

Performance management is a well tested and proven approach for meeting the needs of our customers and clients. The Public Health Foundation model for performance management, Turning Point, is designed to provide a working structure through which local public health departments can realize improved outcomes in their communities and at the same time share best practices with their peers at the national level.

The four components of the Public Health Foundation Turning Point model are the scientific part of the equation. How each local public health agency interprets and applies the model is the art of the equation. The following chapters offer a series of tools, techniques, and concepts to support local leadership in weaving an effective blanket of both science and art into their community efforts.

Chapter 3

Strategic and Operational Planning

John W. Moran and Grace L. Duffy

The *strategic plan* of an organization is a document that sets forth the course for an organization to follow over a long-range horizon of usually up to five years. It is a statement of the potential an organization could reach in the future based on an environmental assessment conducted by the senior management of the organization.

Usually the strategic plan is a bold and inspiring statement that has been built by the senior management of the organization after careful assessment and consideration of the forces of change, currently in play and in the future, that will shape the arena where the organization will deliver its products and services.

In developing a strategic plan, an organization needs to understand how its current resources and capabilities position it in the environment in which it operates. It is best to start with an environmental assessment of how the organization is situated in its current marketplace. The focus should be on the strengths and weaknesses of the organization and the most pressing organizational needs at the time. We need to assess how these strengths, weaknesses, and needs are impacting the organization's:

- People
- Processes
- Performance
- Culture
- Morale
- Stakeholders

Once an organization understands its strengths and weaknesses it should then focus on the future opportunities and threats it will face and need to overcome if it is to reach its full potential. Figure 3.1 shows a SWOT (strengths, weaknesses, opportunities, threats) matrix that can be utilized to accomplish this type of analysis. The results of the SWOT analysis will enable an organization to conduct a gap analysis between its current resources and resources required to reach its

Strengths	Weaknesses	Opportunities	Threats
Reputation	Lack of access to key resources and limited funding	Unfulfilled customer needs	Other service providers

Figure 3.1 SWOT analysis.

Political	Environmental
Legislation	Local disaster potential
New administration	Pollution increase
Sociological	**Technological**
Less-qualified workers	Mismatched systems can not share data
Demographics	

Figure 3.2 PEST analysis.

future desired state. This gap analysis will then help develop a plan to acquire the needed resources.

Public health agencies should also conduct a PEST analysis, as shown in Figure 3.2, which helps to identify those *political, environmental, sociological,* and *technological* attributes that affect the organization's ability to achieve its strategic plan and to improve and protect its community position. A thorough PEST and SWOT analysis will provide a public health agency with a good overview of its current stable and potential future state to begin developing a strategic plan.

Developing the strategic plan is a facilitated process that may take many months of data analysis, customer interviews, and executive meetings to develop a consensual agreement of the future state and direction of the organization. It is beyond the scope of this chapter to define a detailed strategic planning process, but we will discuss the deployment of the strategic plan and the pitfalls associated with the process. Specific approaches for public health strategic planning are offered in Chapter 17, "Community Focused Performance Management."

When the strategic plan is developed it demonstrates what the strategic intent of the organization is to be in the future. The strategic intent[1] is developed to provide a common direction that those in the organization can align around to focus their organization work and efforts. The strategic intent, when it is deployed systematically organizationwide, provides the vehicle to align all the parts of the organization in a common direction. This alignment process is shown in Figure 3.3.

The deployment of the strategic intent to the rest of the organization is one of the most vital and critical components in aligning the organization. If the strategic intent is not deployed successfully, the organization tends to be confused, drifting, and wandering, which results in no action being taken that supports the strategic

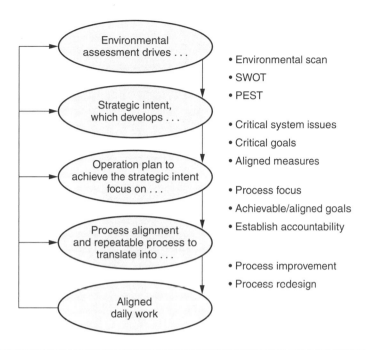

Figure 3.3   Deployment and alignment model.

intent. The management of the organization needs to translate the strategic intent yearly into one-year objectives to be achieved to reach the desired future state, which are deployed to the operating departments to develop their yearly plans.

The operating units then develop operational plans to reflect how they will support the yearly objectives. It should be noted that the operating units do not have to support each of the objectives, just the ones they can impact. Deployment of the strategic intent is a process that requires the operating units to have the opportunity to interpret the objectives as to how they apply to their unit. The operating units develop their yearly plans and through a dialogue process with their management come to agreement on exactly what they will be accountable to achieve. This dialogue process may take much iteration. It is a process of negotiation and fact finding on both sides to come to an agreement. It should be noted that the long-term and yearly plans can be modified if conditions underlying the original yearly plan change dramatically. This deployment process is shown in Figure 3.4. Chapter 18, "Community Balanced Scorecards for Strategic Public Health Improvement," provides a comprehensive example of an aligned plan—from strategic through tactical to operational—based on the needs of a community as identified by national and local data and trends.

When things are clear and focused, the organization creates alignment between the strategic intent and operational directions, which are then focused with the same purpose to the future desired state. Creating this alignment is not an easy process and requires the management group to constantly test and retest whether the organization is focused on the same future direction and making

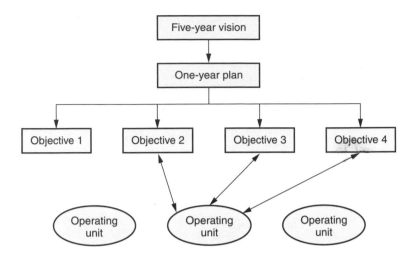

Figure 3.4   Strategic intent deployment process.

any corrections, clarifications, and amplifications to make sure that direction is always clear. Over time as an organization becomes comfortable with this process the plan will drive the budget and not the other way around. Today most organizations make their plans after the budget is set. Chapter 7, "Leading and Lagging Indicators," provides excellent discussion on measurement techniques available to the management group for continuous monitoring.

Reviewing the progress of the operational units is a bottom-up process, as shown in Figure 3.5. The review process should be one that rolls up from the bottom and is focused on how much progress each unit is making toward achieving their yearly objectives. The purpose of the review process is not to punish but to accomplish the following:

- *Assist* operating units in achieving their objectives

- *Validate* that operating units are on course

- *Assure* that objectives are and will be achieved

- *Applaud* effort that is being made

- *Identify* areas needing attention or improvement so that things stay on track.

The review process is one that should be done on a monthly basis to ensure that the operating units are on track and the future state that the organization wants to achieve will be a reality.

The preceding was an overview of the strategic planning process. The remainder of this chapter will discuss the problems that organizations encounter when doing strategic planning, with some suggestions on how to overcome those pitfalls.

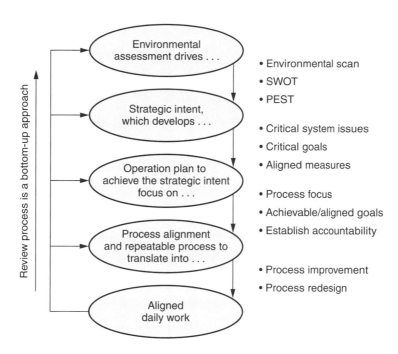

Figure 3.5   Reviewing progress of operational units.

THE PITFALLS ASSOCIATED WITH STRATEGIC AND OPERATIONAL PLANNING AND HOW TO OVERCOME THEM

We have all experienced strategic planning sessions that have been at best boring, poorly planned and executed, and had no follow-up to all the work that was done at the various sessions. Usually we leave strategic planning sessions frustrated and with less hope for the organization's survival than when we entered the session. Most of these strategic planning sessions are doomed from the outset because the planners have not adequately considered all the potential pitfalls that can happen.

Over the years the authors have been able to interview many participants in failed strategic planning sessions to identify what the participants felt was the reason for failure. The many reasons for failure have been grouped into like categories designated as pitfalls. Thirty pitfalls are presented in this chapter. At the end of the chapter is a self-assessment form for you to rate how your organization does today on strategic planning. This self-assessment can also be used as a checklist to plan for effective and productive strategic planning sessions in the future by avoiding the pitfalls presented here.

If your favorite pitfall is not included, please e-mail it to us at jmoran@phf.org and it will be included in a future edition.

Pitfall 1: Mix-Up

The mix-up occurs when an organization sets out to do planning. Long-range planning is often substituted for strategic planning. Strategic planning develops the intent of the organization—what it will be, where it is going—and long-range planning determines how it is going to get there. Developing the strategic intent takes courage since you must stake out the future marketplace and then drive the organization to it utilizing your core competencies. It means understanding key customer requirements and aligning organizational capabilities toward meeting those requirements. This is fundamentally different from long-range planning.

Frequently, management has trouble deciding if they want a breakthrough path for the organization or to tweak a set of operational measures for continuous improvement. Everyone wants and talks "breakthrough," but because of lack of focus or resources settles for small continuous incremental improvements. These small incremental continuous improvements never move or accelerate the organization to the point where it can capitalize on a few big breakthrough gains that would help it leapfrog its competition, realize substantial operating results, or develop new and innovative products for market leadership.

The strategic intent and long-range planning mix-up also causes us to collect the wrong data to make decisions. Developing the strategic intent requires an ongoing effort to collect information about our marketplace, competition, and economic trends, and changes that might shift our consumer's focus and needs. Long-range planning to some is to review last year's operating results and then set unrealistic goals that are 10 to 20 percent higher without making any changes in the existing infrastructure of the organization. Long-range planning tends to keep our planning sights at too low a level, and we get caught up in the day-to-day reasons why we can not make change.

Devoting the time and the resources to developing a strategic intent gives the organization a lever that can be used to accelerate their business and marketplace successes. Developing the strategic intent is intended to be a process that involves teamwork on the part of the top executives of the organization, and is not designed for individualism. The top of the organization must make fundamental decisions that will set the organization on a course for the future not bound by the past or current problems or successes.

Pitfall 2: No Linkage

The strategic goals become lost in the middle of the organization. The middle of the organization seems like the Bermuda Triangle to many top executives. They know they sent the goals to everyone in middle management but they seem to have never gotten there.

The strategy and goals sit on the shelf of the middle-level executive's credenza with little or no relation to day-to-day operations. It's almost as if middle management greeted the strategy process with a yawn and said, "We'll wait until this phase passes—it won't have anything to do with us."

The problem is that the middle of the organization has no process to translate the strategy and goals into operational responses. Plans are developed at the top of the organization, but there is no automatic mechanism to effectively deploy them and link them to the processes that will be needed to deliver the results. No real action takes place, it takes longer and longer to get results, and there is frustration at the lack of progress both at the top and the bottom of the organization.

The employees in the organization feel isolated from the decision-making process since they are not able to effectively participate. They hear pronouncements from management that their ideas are valuable and wanted but no one ever sets up a forum for them to deliver their ideas. At best, a brainstorming session is held to see how many ideas we can come up with to cut costs, and the department with the most ideas gets an award. These types of input sessions do not allow input to the direction of the organization. We tend to do episodic employee involvement on short-term issues and not the long-term strategic ones where we really need to cultivate their commitment and ownership.

Developing the ability to effectively deploy strategy and goals to the middle of the organization is a process that requires executives to invest time and energy in communication. Executives need to constantly clearly state and communicate what the goal is and what is expected in return and by when. They need to also have a structured deployment process with trained facilitators to assist middle managers in developing their aligned operational plans. Then they need to do regular reviews to ensure that the operational plans are aligned and delivering the expected results. Attention to the details of the deployment and review process is what makes the strategy happen and the goals a reality. Refer to Chapter 18, "Community Balanced Scorecards for Strategic Public Health Improvement," in this text for an excellent discussion of alignment and measures to ensure middle management involvement in strategic planning and execution.

Pitfall 3: Data Gathering

Data gathering is usually done at one of the following extremes:

- Too much irrelevant data
- Too little relevant data

In the data-gathering phase organizations usually gather so much data that no one uses it or so little data that everyone involved in the planning process does not feel comfortable making a decision based on such limited information, so they use their experience and opinion. When executives in a planning situation start using their opinion instead of data it often leads to pitfall 24: "O.K. Corral."

In our experience the data-gathering phase of strategic planning is a crucial one. One of the principles of breakthrough thinking is *limited information collection,*[2] which focuses on determining the purpose the information will serve in the planning process. If we collect reams of market data and then do operational planning, or we gather all the performance measures for a strategic planning session and do not find it useful, this is a clear indication that the data collection preceding strategic or operational planning needs to be focused on the purpose of the process or to inform the members of the planning team.

We frequently find that data is too old. The data is out of date before it is used. We find executives who have notebooks full of statistics and reports but do not know what to do with it. We have found that the best data is that which challenges executive's opinions. This is usually the data that is overlooked and not utilized because it is controversial; controversial data delivers the wrong message, not the politically correct one.

The presentation of the data is also a key variable in how useful it will be to a senior executive. Those who collect the information must have a data management strategy in place that effectively translates, consolidates, and communicates the information in a timely manner. The authors have found that the preparation of a briefing book that is well organized with appropriate executive summaries brings the data to life.

Pitfall 4: Meeting with no purpose

The *meeting with no purpose* (MWNP) happens quite often in organizations and is not exclusively a phenomenon of strategic planning. The MWNP is not always obvious when it begins, but after a short time someone in the meeting will ask, "Why are we here?" It is then that the MWNP has officially begun. The MWNP has no agenda, no designated output, and success can be declared at any time. Some organizations have a number of individuals who have made a career out of either leading or attending a constant stream of MWNPs. They constantly put out meeting notices to a large group of invitees that are politically correct. They know that most of the top-level invitees will either not attend but ask for a summary memo or have to leave after making an appearance. The professional leaders of MWNPs co-opt their attendees by giving them the appearance of being well connected and important. They do not want their attendees' participation but rather their quick appearance so they can say to the group, "Sue and Bill are really behind this and want results." In reality Sue and Bill do not have a clue as to why they were invited, it just appeared on their schedule. Sue felt, "If Bill is going, I should attend for a few minutes," and Bill felt likewise.

The MWNP and pitfall 7 (Wallpapering) are closely aligned. Since there is nothing to do at a MWNP, we might as well wallpaper the walls with easel paper and pretend that something productive is going on in the meeting. The professional leaders of MWNPs know that this type of meeting should not last too long. The meeting should last just long enough for the top executives to appear, show support, and leave. The leader knows that once they have the politics covered it is time to create a committee to study the ramifications that this meeting has brought forth. Everyone quickly agrees since they want to leave, and nominates a lower-level person in their area to participate. The leader now has reason for existence for the next few months and then it will be time to call another MWNP.

The MWNP is an exercise in futility that happens too often in the strategic planning process. Many false starts occur until someone sets the direction. These MWNPs are a waste of an organization's resources that should be put to more productive use. MWNPs can be eliminated in strategic planning by clearly setting the strategic direction, defining roles and responsibilities of those involved, establishing milestones, and assigning accountability.

Pitfall 5: Roles and Responsibilities

Who does what in the planning process is a problem that we often encounter. Do the planners prepare the plan or provide data? Do the executives prepare the plan with the input of the planners? Not having clear roles and responsibilities helps pitfall 3 (Data Gathering) flourish. If there is no data management strategy in place then we usually collect reams of irrelevant data that are difficult to consolidate and usually have little bearing on the needs of the strategic planners.

Determining who does what in the planning process is key to avoiding confusion and duplication of work. Turf fighting over who controls the planning process only causes further delays in making rapid and timely responses to market changes. Organizations that want to use the strategic planning process as a competitive lever need to establish a clear mandate for intelligence gathering. For the strategic intent–setting process we need intelligence about the marketplace. The intelligence is in the form of quantitative analysis of where the marketplace is heading and it involves testing scenarios and hypotheses, "what if" assumptions, and drawing out the experience and thoughts of senior executives about the future. Few organizations ever make the distinction between data and intelligence. Every organization is full of data but usually lacking in the depth of their intelligence-gathering ability.

An organization needs to invest the time and resources in establishing a small data- and intelligence-gathering department to support the strategic intent, operational planning, and executive education effort. The purpose of this department is to monitor the economy, social trends, marketplace shifts, competitive position, product development efforts, and the overall performance of the organization. This group should also do selective benchmarking studies to focus on areas needing improvement. This group should prepare and deliver monthly and quarterly executive summaries showing the progress toward the strategy, goal deployment, results achieved, and highlighting areas needing immediate attention.

Organizations today are under enormous time pressure to respond quickly to resolve critical issues. Deciding our future position in the marketplace quickly can help shape the future rather than react to it when it arrives. Being able to accomplish this requires a thorough clarifying of roles and responsibilities concerning data and intelligence gathering so we can pay attention to the ultimate issue—the customer and their continued loyalty to our organization's products and services!

Pitfall 6: Involvement

A number of organizations today want to create the illusion that they have a participative structure and involve everyone in the decisions of the organization. What they really want is everyone to be good soldiers and buy in to the top executives' ideas without comment. They do not really want to hear any dissenting opinions.

Both of the authors attended a meeting where a senior executive was to hold a Town Hall with one of the organization's manufacturing plants. The executive had been overheard in the hallway just before the meeting by a group of employees stating that he had been ordered to do this and just wanted to get it over with.

The executive made it seem sincere but the rumor of what he had said had been circulated to everyone. No one spoke or responded to pleas for questions or concerns. The meeting had been scheduled for two hours but was over in 45 minutes. Everyone was unhappy and mad. Most employees, looked upon it as a waste of time since nothing new was heard and the future was beginning to look just like the past. "Do as I say." The senior executive just confirmed his opinion that his people have nothing to contribute and not to waste his time in the future doing this type of participative meeting.

Under the guise of open communication and consensus decision making, a chief executive will frequently decide to expand the strategy formulation group beyond his or her own direct reports. Attendees at the strategy work session should be limited to the small group that the chief executive can trust and has given major organizational responsibility. At times there will be an additional individual or two that the chief executive uses as a sage advisor or expert who may be used to consult with the strategy group. These individuals also can be included in the session to provide advice but not to set strategy. The role of these individuals has to be clear since they can sometimes be a disruptive influence to the overall group. In addition, anyone being invited in such a role should be fully briefed so they can make a meaningful contribution.

The purpose of the strategy meeting is to create a shared vision of the future among the executive team and not necessarily the sage advisors or trusted friends. The executive group then becomes responsible for the deployment of that vision to the rest of the organization and must have complete buy-in to it in order to make for meaningful deployment and attainable results.

Pitfall 7: Wallpapering

Before beginning a wallpapering meeting you must have the following supplies: five new easel chart pads, 25 multicolored scented markers with smells that annoy the participants, four large rolls of masking tape, and three uneven easel stands needing repair. The wallpapering process uses an activity-based measurement system to determine if it is successful. The success measure is to get as many pieces of easel chart paper as possible posted on every available amount of wall space in the conference room where the meeting is held. From these multiple posted easel chart sheets, prioritized to-do lists are developed and success is declared. No follow-up ever happens. The next step is to get the easel charts typed and distributed.

You can always tell the leader of a wallpapering meeting in the hallway since they are the one carrying two and a half armloads of rolled-up easel paper with a half ton of masking tape sticking out in all directions and catching onto anything that they pass by. This leader then goes back to his department and asks a secretary to type the sheets up. It usually takes two days to unravel the easel charts and repair the damage done by all the masking tape. For days we see easel paper hung from the secretary's cubical and littering out to the hallway. For days the secretary tries to figure out if A-4 follows 3-A. Another secret of a wallpapering meeting is that there is no consistent coding process since we are never going to use the information anyway.

Finally, the leader and the secretary, after wasting 40 hours on this task, have all the easel charts collated, typed, copied, distributed, and filed. Then they roll up and store the easel sheets. They store this large bunch of easel sheets in a corner of the secretary's cubical where everyone who enters bumps into them and knocks them to the floor. After eight weeks they are finally disposed of by having maintenance bring a dumpster to the cubical.

Twenty-three minutes after disposal one of the meeting participants calls and informs the leader of some errors in a few of the pages. Let's review the easel charts and correct the document. What do you mean you threw them out? It has only been a few weeks. Well, the document has too many errors to be useful. We will just have to call the group together again and redo it. In some organizations this is grounds for justified homicide!

Pitfall 8: Lack of Capable Processes

We often find that when the strategic intent is deployed, the lower-level processes are not capable of delivering the operational results required to fund the future needs of the organization. Too often these lower-level processes have been neglected for years and lack the appropriate infrastructure, equipment, people skills, aligned systems, and core competencies to develop and deliver the right product and services to the market when required. This inability to deliver on time and when needed to a customer base results in a slowing of the revenue stream to fund the future. This revenue slowdown usually results in further cuts in the lower-level processes, which continues the erosion of their ability to deliver the needed results. It is a vicious circle that can be stopped only by focusing an organization on a redesign of its core business systems so they are aligned internally and externally to customer needs and expectations.

In order to do a redesign of an organization's core business systems there is a need to have the strategic intent detailed sufficiently so the redesign can be planned against it. An organization must clearly state what market it is going to be a player in, the stream of proposed products and services it envisions to be delivering, the timing of those deliveries, and the technology and people skills base that will be required to support the development and manufacturing efforts. Paul Epstein, et al., translate this requirement into an excellent public health example in Chapter 17 of this text.

Just redesigning core business systems without the benefit and alignment of the strategic intent is a waste of time and resources. Organizations that start redesign efforts in a vacuum soon fail, and the entire approach is given a bad name. It was not the approach that was at fault; it was starting without a concrete direction to align to. If you do not know where you are going, any road will get you there sooner or later. In the early 1990s everyone was jumping on the reengineering bandwagon as the next silver bullet for solving an organization's problems. This reengineering fad did far more damage to organizations than previous management fads since this one tinkered with or changed the major operating systems of the organization. Far-reaching changes were made in organizations' infrastructure without the benefit of a clear focus or direction. Some of these organizations cut their core competencies by mistake and some used reengineering as a cover for layoffs. The reengineering process is a sound one, however, when it is applied in conjunction with a clear strategic intent to refocus core business competencies.

Pitfall 9: Lack of Aligned Measures

Measurement is rarely considered or mentioned as an essential ingredient of strategy development, deployment, or review. Organizations introduce new strategies and goals to achieve breakthrough performance but continue to use the same old measures to track progress. Seldom do they check and evaluate whether the old measures are relevant to the new strategies and goals.

To an observer of the strategic plan, measures should be transparent to the strategic intent. Measures should encapsulate the strategic intent and provide for clarity and reduced confusion at lower organizational levels. This will facilitate alignment of operational plans to support and achieve the strategic intent. Aligned measures will also assist in the review process since they make the operational planning and attainment of results obvious. Aligned measures also focus an organization's continuous improvement efforts at the operational level so that they are aimed at those things that can help the strategy and the goals to be achieved, and not focused on extraneous issues. More is available on measures and alignment in Chapter 6, "Measures for Public Health," Chapter 7, "Leading and Lagging Indicators of Public Health and Public Health Assessment and Accreditation," Chapter 17, "Community-Focused Performance Management," and Chapter 18, "Community Balanced Scorecards for Strategic Public Health Improvement."

Measurement is sometimes feared since it promotes accountability. Accountability equates to responsibility for actions taken. Responsibility can have both positive and negative consequences associated with it. In the review process there must be a built-in mechanism to reduce the fear associated with measurements. The review process must seek to build up individuals' ability to react quickly to measurement results and put action plans in place to correct any obvious deviations or undesirable trends.

Too frequently we measure things because they are easy to measure rather than because they are important to measure. It is easy to measure the number of clients visiting the clinic but more difficult to measure the effectiveness of those visits. Which of these two measures is more important to an organization? We must develop the discipline in managers and employees to seek and use quantitative measures that support the outcomes of the organization, not just count the output of activities.

Measurement makes things concrete, visible, and difficult to ignore. We must keep reminding ourselves that what gets measured gets managed effectively and efficiently. To manage effectively and efficiently we must measure!

Pitfall 10: Casual Consensus

Consensus is defined as general agreement or accords that are a compromise of conflicting opinions. Consensus is difficult to achieve at times but the investment in the time and energy to achieve it is well worth it in strategic planning. Consensus does not mean everyone agrees with every single point. Rather it means we can live with and clearly support the decision since it is best for the organization as a whole.

Many organizations never achieve real consensus but only casual consensus. Casual consensus, or no real buy-in, happens when the senior executives just give lip service to the strategic goals and objectives that they participated in developing. They pretend to agree at the meeting but communicate a different message when speaking to others in the organization or their functional areas of control. This type of senior executive behavior tends to project the image of a rudderless organization—not going anywhere fast. In addition, other employees see it as a norm of operation—agree to anything at a meeting then do as you please afterward. This type of behavior, if not challenged by senior executives, tends to lead to a clubby, paternalistic culture that avoids making tough decisions. This type of culture leads to a slow pace of change at best. Nothing ever seems to happen in this casual consensus atmosphere; the status quo is the norm and we seek to maintain it. Sure, we may challenge one another occasionally but we do not have any teeth in the challenge; it's for show only.

It is extremely important that the top few senior executives totally agree on and support any strategic goals or statements before they are communicated to the rest of the organization. Buy-in must be obtained at the top before any meaningful deployment activities can begin. Invest the time and energy to ensure that the top few senior executives internalize and totally buy in to the future direction of the organization.

Pitfall 11: The Slick Brochure

Every year top management pronounces seven major strategic statements with eight goals and objectives under each of them. The statements are combined into a slick brochure. The brochure is written in flowery, obtuse language that can be broadly interpreted. The strategies, goals, and objectives are motherhood, God, country, and apple pie pronouncements. They are difficult to disagree with but almost impossible to understand and implement. The brochure is distributed to everyone in the organization under the guise of a communication and deployment strategy.

Those who receive the slick brochure either are confused and throw it away or leap to action and use pitfall 7 (Wallpapering) as their process to make action happen. Meetings are held throughout the organization by the professional wallpapering meeting leaders, involving hundreds of employees trying to figure out what should be done with the message delivered in this exquisite brochure from corporate. To-do lists are developed, committees are formed, and the allegiance memos begin to flow. Some enterprising senior professional wallpapering leaders even have wall posters made up and hung in strategic locations for all to see and gaze upon in wonder.

You have probably attended a meeting or two in your career that a slick brochure caused to happen. The slick brochure is received in the mail, sometimes without a letter of explanation. It may be entitled "The XYZ Corporate Direction, Strategy, and Goals for 20XX." Some in the organization discard it but others have questions. Surely they would not have spent so much money if there were not a message for us to learn from. What do they expect from us? What should I do?

How should I show support? Should I mobilize my department? What to do is the key question. The real message is do not do anything—we are not doing anything at the top other than sending out the slick brochure; we fulfilled our planning to-do list.

The slick brochure does not constitute deployment by itself. It is a way to market the strategies to the organization. However, effective deployment of the strategies requires management *involvement* and *action*, a topic detailed in other pitfalls.

Pitfall 12: Keywords

Every organization has "songwriters" who love to attach as many modifiers to a goal statement as possible. These modifiers or jargon blunt any action statements of substance. A strategic goal statement should have an obvious clear intent as to the action that is required to accomplish it. The addition of paraphrases intended to pacify influential parts of the organization usually makes the statement a disconnected group of paragraphs that no one in the organization can understand. There are usually contradictory statements buried within the paragraphs, and in the beginning management spends a lot of time and effort trying to explain what they meant.

The following is a list of keywords that must be eliminated from any strategic intent, goal, or objective statements since they tend to make them not actionable:

• Alert	• Introduce
• Boundaryless	• Leverage
• Create	• Maintain
• Communicate	• Manage
• Delayering	• Partner
• Effective	• Position
• Efficient	• Presence
• Encourage	• Promoting
• Engage	• Reach
• Enhance	• Recognize
• Establish	• Reliable
• Impact	• Respect
• Increase	• Scoping
• Independence	• Support
• Initiatives	• Sustain

Strategic statements must be clear, bold, inspiring, and above all short and to the point. Strategic statements need to inspire the desired action with no confusion or misinterpretation as to what is wanted.

Keywords tend to make weak statements that at best inspire the maintenance of the status quo instead of the desired revolution.

Keywords are a natural ally to pitfall 11 (The Slick Brochure). They enhance the slick brochure's confusion factor.

Pitfall 13: Failure to Blend Resources into Core Competencies

The blending of an organization's technology, people, skills, and other resources into a unique combination of market-differentiated products and services is a feat that many organizations do not perform well. This blending, when linked and aligned to the strategic intent, is a key ingredient for long-term growth, profitability, and market leadership.

A business grows and prospers by having core competencies that are hard for the competition to imitate. These core competencies must not be isolated within one single function of the organization but must extend throughout the entire organization to provide maximum benefit. Core competencies are cross-functional in nature since they transcend individual functions. Core competencies usually are made up of a group of functional specialties that have many handoffs to each other. Which core competencies to invest in and develop internally and which to outsource is a question with which organizations constantly struggle. We should invest in those that develop a proprietary capability in the organization and outsource those that are generic in the marketplace. In the virtual world of the next century, organizations need to invest in proprietary capabilities to maintain their competitive edge but outsource generic competencies to maintain profitability.

Given that customer expectations are constantly shifting, an organization must be able to identify future customer requirements and align its resources and competencies to meet those needs. It is critical for the strategic plan to identify the gap between future requirements and current capabilities and to determine action steps to fill that gap. As customer needs and expectations shift, so must an organization's core competencies. One such identification and alignment approach is the MAPP process (Mobilizing for Action through Planning and Partnerships) of the National Association of County and City Health Officials (NACCHO) as explained in Chapter 10 of this text.

An organization must be constantly monitoring, assessing, and measuring the efficiency, performance, and impact on the bottom line of its core competencies. Core competencies, like customer needs and expectations, must change over time to meet the needs of the marketplace, and successful organizations will be the ones that have appropriate monitors in place to detect the need to change ahead of the competition in the marketplace. The assessment and monitoring process keeps an organization alert to the shifts in the marketplace and protects it from marketplace insensitivity.

Pitfall 14: Lack of Review

The word "review" in most organizations is equated to fear—fear of punishment for results not achieved. Reviews are usually not pleasant experiences. Think of the many reviews you may have been subjected to over the years. The annual medical review, a tax review, a performance review, a fitness for duty review, a midterm school review, and so on. We felt fear in each one of them since we knew something would be said or discovered that would indicate we were headed for trouble or a discomforting experience. What we feared in these reviews as individual participants was reprisal for action taken or not taken. Usually the reviewer or senior management does not find the review process pleasant either since they chastise often and recognize seldom.

The purpose of review should be to develop mutual agreement between management and process owners around objectives, goals, action, alignment, and timing. The current review process must be reengineered so it is one that is constantly providing clarity from the top to the bottom of the organization on:

- Expectations

- Objectives

- Achievements

This process of continuous clarity has an end result of developing a clear and concrete contract between management and process owners for the achievement of substantial bottom-line results.

An effective review process allows senior management the opportunity to display the following exceptional traits of a great leader:

- Coaching

- Teaching

- Encouraging

- Empowering

- Role modeling

- Following through

- Mentoring

- Challenging

Review is an integral part of ensuring that aligned goals and objectives are achieved as rapidly as possible so that their benefit can be realized quickly.

Pitfall 15: No Way to Achieve It

Many organizations lack a disciplined deployment process to ensure that operational goals are aligned to the strategic goals and deliver the agreed-to results. The lack of a disciplined deployment process leaves a void in an organization in which operational units attempt to determine how they can contribute to the strategic intent of the organization. A disciplined deployment and review process helps build commitment to direction and results.

The following four scenarios show what can happen when the strategic intent and deployment processes interact:

- If the strategic intent of the organization is focused and clear but the organization has an ineffective deployment, process paralysis sets in and no action results.

- If the strategic intent is unfocused and the deployment process is ineffective there is a lot of wandering and drifting at lower levels. There are a lot of unanswered questions, and each operating unit will take a different direction to further compound the misalignment.

- If the strategic intent is unfocused but the deployment process is effective there tends to be a lot of functional focus and a lot of the "same old, same old" plans. This scenario tends to promote the status quo and functional stovepipes.

- If the strategic intent is focused and the deployment process is effective then an organization will experience focused and aligned change. The organization as a whole will experience acceleration in its attainment of its goals and objectives.

In order to reduce the confusion in lower levels of an organization and speed up the acceleration of goal attainment it is imperative that an effective deployment process be supported by a focused strategic intent. An effective deployment process is one that has a few well-thought-out process steps that guide an organization's actions to goal alignment. It must make provisions for corporate goal translation into local language and structure appropriate process improvement actions to achieve the goal.

Pitfall 16: Amnesia

Amnesia infects an organization when the top executives develop a short or long-term case of memory loss. These executives become clueless as to the core competencies of their business. They forget what business they are in and expand into areas in which they have no expertise or experience. There are many examples over the past 10 years of organizations expanding into businesses foreign to their core competencies and then closing or selling these ventures at a loss a few years later.

Sony's heartaches in Hollywood[4] is a good example of putting dreams in charge of the bank account and throwing money at something and hoping it will grow into a core competency. Usually the Amnesia pitfall has one overarching cause, aside from patently inept management: it is the nearly incredible reality that senior executives too often do not understand the fundamentals of their business.[5] "They neglect to ask central questions, such as what precisely is their company's core expertise, what are reasonable long- and short-term goals, what are key drivers of profitability in their competitive situation. A lot of senior people at very large companies have no idea what made their organization successful."[6]

The Amnesia pitfall is not usually a one-time phenomenon but can be repeated many times in an organization that does not have the discipline to learn from its mistakes. Too often senior management jumps from one disaster to another. Until an organization takes the time and energy to uncover its core competencies it will never know where the gold is buried in the organization. Once we understand our strengths it is time to set the direction for the future. We must constantly monitor the assumptions on which the future direction is based to catch any fundamental change that would cause us to make a midcourse correction. We can not be complacent after we set the future strategic intent. We must monitor, communicate, and update that intent to our employees on a regular basis and not at the last minute when the bottom falls out of the plan.

Employees assume management has Amnesia when the only time they hear from them is as a disaster is unfolding and they're all asked to participate in a lifeboat drill.

Pitfall 17: Details First

Agreeing on details before deciding the main points happens occasionally when there is no strategic thinking involved. We tend to focus on the fix for a problem before we truly understand the root cause of it. We constantly come across organizations that have implemented hundreds of team-based improvements that really did nothing to enhance the long-term competitive position of the organization. These team-based improvements just made today a little more tolerable.

Before any organization begins to tinker with improvement it must set a clear direction from which criteria for success can be drawn. Individuals and teams in an organization need criteria for success to decide which of the many actions they could take to make daily work improvements are the best suited and aligned to achieve the strategic direction of the organization.

Letting everyone figure out the details in the absence of a strategic direction is a recipe for disaster. There will be many conflicting improvements, some of which may even cost more than they save. Most of the improvements that come in a details-first atmosphere are ones that are suboptimum. They maximize a gain in one area at the expense of the organization as a whole.

In addition, in a details-first atmosphere many of the team-based or individual improvements recommended to management never get acted on since management does not know which are the right ones to approve. Employees never hearing back on recommendations become disillusioned and resist any further attempts to involve them in making improvements. Management should not expect great strides in making an organization better at every level if they don't walk the talk of quickly finding a solution for every problem.

Management must set the direction clearly for the future and then carefully craft a set of evaluation criteria that everyone in the organization can use to judge the worthiness of a proposed improvement. Improvement areas selected with criteria that tie them to the long-range needs of the organization will be readily received by all levels of management. Implementation of these types of improvement projects is easier since there is a benefit to the whole and not just one part of the organization.

Pitfall 18: Lack of Due Diligence

Lack of due diligence occurs when we try to rush through the necessary steps of the strategic planning process. Leaders rush and skip steps and people's inputs in order to quickly craft a plan for a high-level meeting. Under the guise of urgency we rush to develop a plan that usually leaves its audience bewildered and trying to unravel all of the inconsistencies and contradictions.

Lack of due diligence happens when an organization does not view the strategic planning process as a core business process. By not viewing it as a core business process it tends to ignore the fact that the strategy drives the organization. Treating strategic business planning as a core business process requires an investment in time and resources to operate and fund the activity correctly. The strategic business planning process must be seen as a core process that has critical process levers focused on driving the organization to achieve competitive advantages.

By viewing strategic business planning as a critical core process we must subject it to the same measurement and standards that we impose on other critical processes. The strategic business planning process must be performed efficiently and effectively. There must be a process of continuous improvement in place that constantly makes the process more responsive to the organization's needs. The strategic business planning process can be a value-added support process if it has a clear, defined process that all can view and input to at the appropriate time.

One of the first improvements in an existing strategic business planning process is to ensure that input and comments are gathered throughout the organization in an efficient manner. The strategic business planning process owners should focus on developing a simple process of communication, input, and feedback for the organization to use. They should communicate the first draft of the plan and the supporting assumptions to a series of focus groups at the next level and ask for input. The input should be consolidated and reviewed by senior management and decisions should then be made regarding modification of the draft plan. Then feedback sessions should be held with the original input groups to show the modifications and why certain suggestions were or were not used. Then the process can be repeated at other levels as required. This will ensure that due diligence has been achieved. This process also has a side benefit in that it develops ownership of the plan early on.

Pitfall 19: Hobby

Every year we go off to a one-week retreat in a really nice conference center, play golf and tennis, discuss the previous year, and agonize over making and setting goals that we will never keep for the next year. "I have been here 10 years and it is a yearly event and I would not miss it." We have a staff of three people almost full-time to coordinate the golf and tennis games and of course disseminate the important strategic information we generate and analyze. We do it every year and get no real return on the effort, but I have taken two strokes off my handicap over the past two planning meetings. By the time I retire I will be ready for the senior tour.

If this type of yearly planning meeting scenario seems familiar it means you are not treating your strategic business planning process as a critical component in your organization. It has become more of a hobby and recreation process than an integrated planning effort that provides real value to the organization. Goals and objectives are set but no one really believes in them and no one is going to do anything about them.

Organizations spend a small fortune every year going through such a process in the name of planning. The hobby pitfall is a natural breeding ground for pitfall 4 (The Meeting with No Purpose), pitfall 6 (Involvement), pitfall 10 (Casual Consensus), and pitfall 18 (Lack of Due Diligence). The hobby mentality approach to strategic business planning sends a powerful message to the organization that the senior executives are not serious about any real change taking place.

Employees in an organization with the hobby approach to strategic business planning soon learn to recognize the yearly signs that the annual rite has begun. Plane reservations for exotic places are made; questions abound, such as "Can we take our spouses this year?" Hurried meetings are called to develop a show-and-tell slide presentation to be used at the annual planning meeting. Pronouncements such as "We are limited to five slides—how will we tell them about all our accomplishments?" are commonplace. In reality they are glad they are limited to five slides since it will be a stretch to fill them anyway. All these presentations are put into a giant binder for each participant. Unfortunately these binders only wind up gathering dust and do very little to inspire action of any type.

Pitfall 20: Falling in Love

Some organizations fall in love with the planning process and make it a year-round event. We can never gather enough environmental data, or enough customer feedback, or too much employee input. We mail out surveys daily and agonize over the response rates. Some customers receive two to three surveys a week from us on a whole range of topics from many different functions in the company. Organizations that keep gathering data usually do not want to make a decision. We put off the tough decisions with the false excuse that we need more information. Organizations like this become mesmerized with information. The result is that the strategic business planning process never concludes.

Organizations that use this type of approach have great data gathering systems but lack a processing system for the data to go through. Assumptions must be drawn, goals must be set, and decisions must be made in a robust strategic business planning process. There must be a logical outcome to the yearly process. If an organization has a weak data processing system then it must build that capability to analyze data or they will bury themselves in reams of information that will not help them. If your current planning department keeps asking for more space, this is a sure sign that pitfall 20 is alive and well in your organization.

We have all heard the old expression "Data rich and information poor." Robust strategic business planning processes have an advanced analytical process to digest all the information that comes in so meaningful conclusions can be drawn and acted upon. These conclusions need to be communicated to top management on a regular basis with an analysis of trends and summaries of key findings. This type of analytical process makes the planning function a value-added part of the core business process.

We must treat information as a critical organizational asset. We should demand that we receive a return on our investment and be assured that the information process is bottom-line oriented. The top executives of any organization must take information management very seriously since it can help reduce risk associated with major decisions, support decisions at all levels in the organization, guide the improvement of core work processes, and help accomplish the strategic plan of the organization. If their current information systems are not providing useful and actionable information then it is time to reengineer the process.

Pitfall 21: Nightmare on Elm Street

We are all familiar with Freddy Kruger and how he always appeared in someone's dream to cause havoc and destruction. This can also happen when Freddy takes on the role of middle managers in the deployment process and the dream set forth in the strategic intent turns to horror as the deployment process begins. Pitfall 21 is supported and enhanced by pitfall 22 (Rhythm and Blues).

We find in most organizations that there are many enemies within that have severe hostility toward any process that will upset the status quo. They go out of their way to wreck any good planning and deployment process because it tends to upset the natural order of things that they have established and enjoy. Most deployment processes are designed to question each aspect of an operation against the established corporate goals. This questioning process may show up weaknesses that some operational managers would rather overlook. To overcome the questioning process they search for any possible way to derail the deployment process.

The Freddy Kruger syndrome is one that the implementers of the deployment process must constantly be on guard for. The early warning signs are:

- No immediate action starts at the operational level once the deployment process is announced.

- Operational managers always have an excuse why they can not get around to it this week.

- Complaints about the forms, format, and lack of time abound.

- The constant pushback to those who have responsibility to accomplish the deployment. "We are ready when you can send us a trained facilitator to guide us through the process" is a popular pushback.

One way around the Freddy Kruger syndrome is to publish a complete deployment schedule with the review dates already set. This sends a strong message to those who would attempt to derail the process. If we know we are going to be reviewed by top management and held accountable then we'd better follow the timetable and formats. Top management must use the review process to instill in the operational managers the importance and benefits of the entire strategic business planning and deployment process. The review session should be utilized to continually clarify the strategic intent, the reasons for the goals, what has already been achieved, and how far we have left to go.

Pitfall 22: Rhythm and Blues

General Eisenhower once said, "Planning is great until the shooting starts." The transformation of the strategic business plan into operational plans is where the shooting starts in most organizations. We expect the operational plans to have a process focus, achievable and aligned goals, and help to establish accountability.

Unfortunately, smooth deployment of the strategic business plan into aligned operational plans that are focused on achieving the goals of the organization is a rarity in most organizations today. Deployment is the dissemination of the strategic business plan throughout an organization. This needs to be a critical subprocess of the strategic business planning process. We have seen too many organizations leave this vital subprocess to chance. A vague memo is written as to how to deploy strategic business plans into operational plans. Little follow-up happens, and then everyone at corporate level is surprised when they receive a hundred different formats. The different formats do not allow any meaningful roll-up of the various operational plans to see if the corporate goals will be achievable. Usually a second request is initiated to do them over again in a common format. This constant doing over process develops stress and confusion at the operational level as well as a lack of respect for the executive team who keep making the same requests over and over. A common refrain from operational managers is "Why didn't they say that the first time?"

A simple and concrete deployment process with clear linkages is a necessity in every organization. The managers at the operational level need guidance on what is wanted, how it is wanted, when it is wanted, and where it is wanted. It is very easy in the operational level of an organization to get so caught up in the day-to-day reactive process that you never have time to plan properly. Operational managers have even less time to plan if they spend half of their available time trying to figure out the "what and how" of the deployment process.

We must remember that operational planning is just one more add-on to the already overburdened operational manager. If we can make the deployment process clean and efficient, then we will obtain the commitment and buy-in that is needed from operational managers to ensure success.

Pitfall 23: Static Cling

The static cling pitfall is a phenomenon often seen in an organization that has a heavy dose of tradition as its guiding principal. This type of organization has not made an improvement to its business planning process for the past 10 to 20 years. Its top management sees little need to invest in new technology or to upgrade the business planning process. They will always say, "This is the process that got me to where I am today and it is still a good sound process." The question you never hear them ask or entertain is "Will this process be robust enough to keep me here in the future?"

Senior executives in organizations like the one described above have moved beyond the hobby pitfall and have become so tradition bound that they can not change. The business planning process that was so successful for them in the past is now spreading a disease throughout the organization that will lead to their failure. We have all seen the failures of big organizations using a tradition-bound business planning process in the newspapers over the past few years. General Motors and Chrysler executives have been in front of the U.S. Congress in very visible hearings concerning their slowness to redesign ineffective major business processes.

As this process of tradition-bound planning heads into its final stage on the road to complete failure, the employees wonder whether "anyone is out there." The organization begins to lose touch with its customers, competitors, shareholders, and worse, their employees. Employees are put in the position of watching the foundations of the business unravel around them while top management ignores the signs until it is too late. The first round of cutbacks that takes place in the early stages of collapse usually does not affect those who brought the organization to the edge of the cliff but rather those who were trying to get the message out that it was indeed headed for the precipice.

Unfortunately, tradition-bound planning does not provide much of a base to build on. Organizations coming out of this type of complete planning failure need to restart the business planning function as a critical process and focus attention and resources on it until it's again functioning smoothly. Usually this means a good hard shake-up of the entire business planning and deployment function to get the juices going again. The bloat and complacency need to be cut out of the old process before any reconstitution is attempted.

Pitfall 24: O.K. Corral

Every planning meeting is like the gunfight at the O.K. Corral. We all stake out our territory and shoot from the hip with no real data to back up our accusations or assertions. We wear any attacker down with a constant barrage of meaningless opinions, and when we are challenged we attempt to table it until we can get more ammunition.

The classic description of this pitfall is "ready, fire, aim." We keep shooting until our opponent capitulates or it is past 5 PM and everyone agrees to a cease-fire.

What is interesting in this pitfall is how fast the sides change during the shoot-out. As soon as my turf is violated I quickly look for an ally and it could be the person I was just ganging up on. One minute I am backing up "Doc" Holliday and the next minute I have him in my gun sight.

This process also helps provide a sound foundation for pitfalls 4 (Meeting with No Purpose) and 10 (Casual Consensus) to flourish.

This meeting has some resemblance to pitfall 7 (Wallpapering) except that there is nothing to type up. No one had time to write anything down since they were too busy reloading their gun, firing, and ducking for cover.

The gunfight at O.K. Corral usually ends with each participant making up a to-do list of who to get even with and possible areas to look for data to discredit someone with. Unfortunately, this type of a meeting does nothing to build unity toward any common goals or purpose within the organization. Bitter resentment on the part of some participants can result in hostile internal power struggles that are destructive to an organization. The 1947 Dr. Seuss children's book "McElligot's Pool" contains an appropriate quote for the results of this process—"I am an elephant, I am faithful, and I never forget."

Both of the authors have experienced the aftermath of this type of meeting process. If it is allowed to exist in an organization, this type of meeting gets quickly deployed throughout the organization and becomes the norm for conducting business. As a result, it has a paralyzing effect on the decision making, teaming, and consensus process.

Pitfall 25: The "If I's"

If I had only done "x" instead of "y"—senior management has a tendency to second-guess decisions that are made or goals that are set and then change direction, targets, or measures. This is a sure sign that pitfall 10 (Casual Consensus) is working in conjunction with this pitfall. This is a very disruptive process to line and staff managers since they usually have just finished communicating the decisions or goals to their direct reports when they are changed. This process also makes senior management look like they are not clear on what they want accomplished or where the business is headed.

Constantly second-guessing the decisions or goals that are set sends a strong message to the organization that it is all right to change the goal if the results do not match the needs. To have an effective deployment process, an organization needs clear and consistent goal statements that can be deployed with certainty throughout the organization early in the planning cycle. Divisions and departments need to have confidence that the time and energy they are investing in making aligned plans will not be wasted by constant change.

In organizations where constant goal changing is common very little deployment ever happens. Lower-level managers just do the process once and watch for the change signals but do not respond to them since they will change again. In one organization we are familiar with managers have told us that in some instances they just resubmit the same plan year after year and nobody ever questions them. The one caution they gave us was to correct the dates to the current year—do not make it too obvious.

This type of behavior causes the organization not to have capable processes (pitfall 8), resources not being blended into core competencies (pitfall 13), and no way for the organization to achieve its desired goals and objectives (pitfall 15). Constantly changing the goals and direction sets the stage for disastrous operating results, missed market opportunities, and employees who become disillusioned and satisfied with the status quo. Employees who become satisfied with the status quo become unable to cope with rapid change and tend to be rigid when flexibility is needed to meet a competitor's threat head-on.

Pitfall 26: The Train to "Knowhere"

Too many strategic plans detail how many teams should be established and when they should be formed, but they do not indicate what these teams will be doing. Too many strategic plans call for inflicting hours of training on unsuspecting managers and employees without first answering, "What is all this training going to do for us and how will we know if it is working."[7] How many organizations have been duped into setting up elaborate training programs that never returned anything on their investments? Many thousands of dollars have been spent and everyone is trained but nothing productive is happening. It is a sad commentary on many organizations' approach to starting a teaming process.

In too many organizations the fact that there was never any management commitment, no alignment to the strategic initiatives, and no initial employee input somehow never stopped a major training effort from being undertaken. The rallying cry seemed to be "everyone else is doing it," "our customers require it," or "our competition is doing it," and that was all the justification it took for a major outlay of funds that resulted in some slick notebooks and DVDs being purchased. These notebooks and DVDs were distributed and shown throughout the organization in three- and five-day programs and doubtful questions were given the answer, "We have to let the process work—it may take a while."

These training programs provided the organization with knowledge but it was not aligned and directed to get a real return on the investment. No one ever knew if a return on the training investment dollars was ever achieved because no one wanted to put real measures in place since they were equated with responsibility and accountability. So instead, soft measures like number of employees trained, number of teams started, number of classes conducted, and so on, were used. Today we have to demand quantitative measures of training dollars spent since we are in a resource-limited environment and every dollar should be invested wisely.

Training is a necessary ingredient for any successful organization's long-term success. Training must be focused on and supportive of achieving the organization's goals and initiatives both short- and long-term. Training is an investment in changing behavior, and the change must be directed at the future needs and expectations of the organization

Pitfall 27: The Victory Celebration

At the first sign of even a slight improvement management quickly declares a huge victory and that the war is won. They celebrate by rewarding each of the top executives with bonuses. But three months later they realize that the victory celebration was premature and the slight improvement has now turned into a major embarrassing variance. Soon the rank and file realizes that last month the free lunch and cake was really not deserved and that the pink slips are not colored paper for the next celebration but rather the result of management's poor judgment.

Management in most organizations does not have the patience necessary to wait for real change to take place. They are so used to a short-term focus and reward structure that the long term is not something very far in the future. The lack of patience usually leads them to look for any opportunistic sign of success, and this sign does not have to be a very bright sign. What they do not realize is that a declaration of victory is a sign to the employees that they can relax, and that this is an opportunity for the resistors to regroup their forces. During this victory time frame the resistors quickly look for any possible weakness to point out that this change effort was wrong and the old status quo was right for the corporation. The resistors quickly gain back lost ground, and when the victory celebration turns into a defeat it is hard to get the employees motivated to return to the effort. The resistors point out that we have been misled before and why should you believe them now.

Short-term gains should be used to motivate employees to tackle large improvement goals and change issues that can move the organization closer to its vision and desired state.

Pitfall 28: Musical Chairs

We have all seen the major announcements from corporate how this year's strategic planning process will be more efficient, streamlined, and focused on the business we need to be in for the future. With this major announcement come the names of those on the new team to lead this strategic planning effort. We always notice that this new team is part of the reorganization that was just completed to give the organization a leaner look. But what is new is the titles of the players, nothing more. The same old lead weights that brought us last year's new strategic planning fiasco have just played musical chairs. The same old crew is still there. Once again they have shown their resiliency to survive in the worst of times. Like pitfall 21 (Nightmare on Elm Street) they are back in our lives ready to do it again. The worst part is they are more experienced at screwing things up so the results this year should be spectacular. We can hardly wait for the first draft of the new process.

Leaders in organizations have never learned the lesson that to expect something different out of the same old gang is insanity. You can mix them up, slice and dice, and rotate them but the result is always the same. I wonder why?

We need to bring fresh blood and ideas into the strategic planning and deployment process each year. Leaders have to constantly evaluate their executive team to ensure that they are functioning effectively and not just surviving.

Giving a person a new title does not change the way they think, act, and behave. This has to be done through a thorough performance management and planning system. Leaders must identify the shortfalls in their executive team and address them through training, experience, and coaching. Leaders need to prevent ineffective executives from polluting the planning process and detracting from its effectiveness.

Pitfall 29: "Say What?"

Many organizations today are having severe difficulty in deploying their strategic plans effectively and in a timely manner. Through large-scale downsizing and rightsizing, many organizations have eliminated the core of the middle management team that used to serve as translators of the strategic plan. They could talk "operational speakese." They made sense out of the grand strategic language. These translators played a vital role in the organization, which has now been lost in the rush to slash and burn. Unfortunately, nothing was developed to fill the void left by these individuals.

Many organizations that the authors deal with are feeling this void as they attempt to roll out their strategic plan. The glossy brochures have been sent out but nothing is happening. One client recently stated, "I never realized how much grease those middle managers put on the strategic plan. They helped get it into our day-to-day language and made it real to the troops."

To overcome this void it is imperative that *strategic realization workshops* be held in the organizational units to help translate the strategic plan into operational plans with defined outcomes and timelines. A conscious effort needs to be made today to support the organization in taking a set of strategic goals and translating them into ongoing aligned operational plans. If top management does not take the initiative to translate their thoughts and desires into "operational speakese," then the void will continue to widen and operational execution mistakes will increase, dragging down the whole organization. We do not want our organization playing the time-consuming game of "What do you think they want?" This is a waste of resources and ultimately leads to pitfalls 4 (Meeting with No Purpose), pitfall 7 (Wallpapering), and pitfall 12 (Keywords).

Just like in the foreign movies, we need to add the subtitles.

Pitfall 30: Tombstone

This is the last pitfall and by far the most classic. Recently I was with a client reviewing the strategic plan when we uncovered an assumption and a corresponding goal that had changed due to the changing business landscape. As we were discussing how to make the change, one of the musical chair executives, who had been recently rotated left to right, piped up and said, "We can not change it, the glossy brochures (pitfall 11) have just arrived from the printers and are being distributed." Just like a tombstone, we etch the strategic plan in stone and can not change it except once per year. Then we wonder why the rest of the organization is not taking the strategic plan and its objectives to heart.

When the Tombstone pitfall hits an organization it is time to begin to plan the wake and the funeral. When we become so solidified, resistant, and blind to changing conditions that we feel we can wait a year to update our goals and objectives then the end is nearer than we are willing to believe.

The Tombstone pitfall is the capstone to all the other pitfalls since it will be the place to inscribe the epitaph, "Here was the company that could have been. It just did not change fast enough or quick enough."

If organizations are going to survive in the future they must become more fluid and less structured. They need to have the ability to change on a dime. Flexible, fluid, and dynamic are the words that will describe organizations that survive. We will use an Etch A Sketch to write our strategic plans in the more agile planning environment of the near future.

The strategic planning self-analysis tool in Figure 3.6 was developed to help gauge the behaviors supporting an organization's strategic planning process. Take this self-assessment either as an individual or as a strategic planning team. Once you have a score, use your results to generate a discussion with the strategic planning team to improve the organization's planning outcomes.

Hopefully your score is a high one and your organization is doing a good job of strategic planning and deployment. If it is not, identify the areas of weakness and develop an improvement plan for the next time the strategic planning process takes place.

Instructions: After each of the pitfalls check the appropriate column as it applies to your organization—it is *always* there, *sometimes* we have the problem, or *never* in this organization. Multiply the *always* column number of checkmarks by 1, the *sometimes* number of check marks by 3, and the *never* number of check marks by 5. The highest score is 150, which indicates a world-class strategic planning organization.

Pitfalls:	Always	Sometimes	Never
1. Mix-Up			
2. No Linkage			
3. Data Gathering			
4. Meeting with No Purpose			
5. Roles and Responsibilities			
6. Involvement			
7. Wallpapering			
8. Lack of Capable Processes			
9. Lack of Aligned Measures			
10. Casual Consensus			
11. The Slick Brochure			
12. Keywords			
13. Failure to Blend Resources into Core Competencies			
14. Lack of Review			
15. No Way to Achieve It			
16. Amnesia			
17. Details First			
18. Lack of Due Diligence			
19. Hobby			
20. Falling in Love			
21. Nightmare on Elm Street			
22. Rhythm and Blues			
23. Static Cling			
24. O. K. Corral			
25. The "If I's"			
26. The Train to "Knowwhere"			
27. The Victory Celebration			
28. Musical Chairs			
29. "Say What?"			
30. Tombstone			
Total number of check marks:			
Multiply by:	1	3	5
Total score:			

Figure 3.6   Strategic planning self–analysis.

Chapter 4

Public Health Program Design and Deployment

Helen Parsons, MPH, and William Riley, PhD

T he Public Health Foundation projects that more than two million excess deaths will occur over the next decade if communities fail to achieve nine of the major Healthy People 2010 mortality objectives.[1] State, local, and tribal public health departments play an important role in achieving these objectives, as their performance accounts for an important portion (up to 26 percent) of the variation in county health within the United States.[2] One of the challenges in public health is focusing scarce resources on producing the best possible health outcomes for the population. Creating an approach to prioritize public health activities and emphasize common goals will continue to be an important component of ensuring the health of the population over the next decade. One of the most prominent approaches to raising public health performance has been the development of a voluntary public health accreditation system for state, local, and territorial public health departments.

ACCREDITATION

Voluntary public health accreditation has become one of the major initiatives in contemporary public health. The accreditation process is dedicated to improving performance by helping public health departments assess their current capacity and guide them to improve outcomes, thus promoting a healthier population. Studies over the past two decades have found substantial gaps in the performance of public health providers.[3] While several states have embarked on mandatory accreditation at the state level as a means to enhance the quality of local public health,[4] the vast majority of health departments do not have accreditation programs available.

In 2003, the Institute of Medicine recommended that the public health profession explore the feasibility and desirability of accreditation for all governmental health departments.[5] Concurrently, the Centers for Disease Control and Prevention (CDC) Futures Initiative identified accreditation as a key strategy for strengthening the public health infrastructure in the United States.[6] In response, the Robert Wood Johnson Foundation (RWJF) convened stakeholders and launched the Exploring Accreditation Project (EAP) to determine the feasibility of developing a national accreditation program for state, local, territorial, and tribal public health departments. This project brought together a planning committee from the American Public Health Association (APHA), the Association of State and Territorial Health Officials (ASTHO), the National Association of City and County Health Officials (NACCHO), and the National Association of Local Boards of Health (NALBOH). A steering committee comprising representatives from numerous public health practice settings at the local, state, and federal levels convened to examine all aspects of the viability of voluntary accreditation. The final recommendations from the EAP committee indicated that it is feasible and desirable to pursue voluntary national accreditation that builds upon the momentum established by individual state accreditation and performance improvement programs.[7] Further, the EAP committee concluded that accreditation provides the opportunity to advance the quality, accountability, and credibility of governmental public health departments.

The Public Health Accreditation Board (PHAB) was created in 2007 to oversee the accreditation of state and local governmental public health departments by adopting standards and developing an accreditation program.[8] The accreditation program comprises three core components: domains, standards, and measurements. *Domains* are the competencies and broad areas of responsibility for a health department and are based on a large body of work including the 10 essential public health services,[9] National Public Health Performance Standards System,[10] and the NACCHO Operational Definition,[11] to name a few. *Standards* are expected levels of performance that reflect a specific responsibility within a domain. For example, the NPHPSP (local level) has 32 model standards for its 10 domains. Figure 4.1 shows the standards that are associated with each domain at the local level. A *measure* consists of a metric to assess the extent to which a standard is met. Each standard can have one or more measures that reflect a specific level of performance achievement and skill competency.[12]

The foundations for the accreditation process evolved from a groundbreaking report, *The Future of Public Health*,[13] which identified three core functions for public health: assessment, policy development, and assurance. *Assessment* is the regular collection and analyzing of community health information, including statistics, on health status and community needs. *Policy development* is the process by which society makes decisions about problems, chooses goals and the proper means to reach them, handles conflicting views about what should be done, and allocates resources. Finally, *assurance* provides that public health agencies offer the services necessary to achieve the agreed-upon goals.[14] Evolving out of these three core functions of public health were the 10 essential public health services, which provided a framework for the provision of standardized services by public health departments around the country. Figure 4.1 shows a brief overview of these 10 essential public health services.

Incentives for Accreditation

There are costs and organizational commitments associated with agency accreditation. First, an accreditation self-survey allows the local health department to assess how well it meets established standards. Corrective action is taken when an organization detects deficiencies in its performance. This self-survey requires

Assessment

    1. Monitor health status to identify community health problems

    2. Diagnose and investigate health problems and health hazards in the community

Policy Development

    3. Inform, educate, and empower people about health issues

    4. Mobilize community partnerships to identify and solve health problems

    5. Develop policies and plans that support individual and community health efforts

Assurance

    6. Enforce laws and regulations that protect health and ensure safety

    7. Link people to needed personal health services and assure the provision of healthcare when otherwise unavailable

    8. Assure a competent public health and personal healthcare workforce

    9. Evaluate effectiveness, accessibility, and quality of personal and population-based health services

Serving All Functions

    10. Research for new insights and innovative solutions to health problems

Figure 4.1   The 10 essential public health services.
Source: Public Health Functions Steering Committee, 1994.

resources and time from the organization. Second, there is typically a fee associated with an accreditation application. Monetary and other resource costs must be seriously considered before conducting the self-study and committing funding for the accreditation survey.

There are several ways to achieve an affordable accreditation system for a public health department. First and most important, meeting accreditation standards is not an activity that only occurs just prior to an accreditation site visit. High-performing organizations meet and exceed performance benchmarks by continuous attention to performance improvement; standards are constantly monitored to achieve organizational excellence. In this respect, accreditation preparation is not an occasional activity that only precedes visits by external surveyors. Rather, there is relentless pursuit of excellence. Second, quality improvement to meet standards is an ongoing responsibility built into all position descriptions. Performance improvement is not an accountability that resides in a support staff position; it is an accountability for all staff. In other words, when continuous quality improvement becomes the dominant paradigm of a public health department, and meeting accreditation standards becomes a routine part of the agency operations. Third, several states that instituted accreditation have found ways to make the costs of site surveys affordable utilizing a system of volunteers from other health departments in exchange for a low-cost site visit.

What are the incentives for a local public health department to become engaged in the accreditation process? Since accreditation is voluntary, there must be strong incentives for a public health department to undergo the accreditation process. The benefits of accreditation are many: improved quality and performance, enhanced

- Provides a set of clear benchmarks and a straightforward way to identify organizational strengths and weaknesses.

- Encourages continuous quality improvement and provides opportunities for public recognition of the important role of public health.

- Unites communities across the country

- Promotes improved outcomes

- Provides funding opportunities to those who adopt recommendations[15]

- Makes progress visible and easier to track over time

- Keeps all stakeholders in the loop

- Provides the capability to capture and share lessons

- Improves communication

- Helps to identify individual strengths and weaknesses

Figure 4.2   Strengths of standardized methods and goals.

Source: PHAB (2008); B. L. Joiner, *Fourth Generation Management: The New Business Consciousness* (New York: McGraw-Hill, 1994).

credibility and visibility, improved health of the community, and ultimately, greater resources available for implementing the mission of public health. Figure 4.2 provides an overview of several key benefits of standardized methods and goals for the provision of public health services and the process of accreditation.

While there are many benefits of standardized methods and goals, the overarching benefit of a standardized process is the improvement of efficiency and population outcomes on a national scale. Several quality improvement projects are beginning to be reported that have measured the ability of local public health agencies to collaborate in order to improve outcomes and share lessons with minimal technical facilitation.[16] The results have shown that given a shared vision and a set of committed individuals, local public health departments can achieve real change and improved outcomes.

With this knowledge, where then should individual local health departments begin in order to facilitate these changes within their own organizations?

GETTING THE PROCESS OF ACCREDITATION STARTED

Preparing for accreditation does not need to be a daunting process; it is essentially a process of continuous improvement. The key to improving the efficiency and capacity of local public health departments is organizational leadership. Exceptional leadership converts vision into realities, allowing local public health agencies to get extraordinary things accomplished.

The basic components of successful leadership in organizations have been much studied.[17] Kouzes and Posner[18] have developed a set of practices that embody these ideas and set a framework for exemplary leadership practices in local public health. These practices are listed in Figure 4.3.

Modeling the way is an important first practice for exemplary leadership. In other words, leaders must model the behavior they expect to see in others within

- Model the way
- Inspire a shared vision
- Challenge the process
- Enable others to act
- Encourage the heart

Figure 4.3   Five practices of exemplary leadership.
Source: J. Kouzes and B. Posner, *The Leadership Challenge* (San Francisco: Jossey-Bass, 2002).

their organization. Leaders set the example through daily actions that demonstrate that they are deeply committed to their beliefs. Support for shared visions and goals in local public health must be incorporated from the top down, with local leaders showing support for the change as a key to improvement.

Second, exemplary leadership requires a shared vision, a key element of the process of voluntary accreditation and a first step toward improving outcomes and efficiency within public health organizations. In this respect, leaders must have knowledge of their organization's aspirations, visions, and values, and help align these aspects with the shared goals for improvement.

Third, leaders must challenge the process and be willing to step out into the unknown. They must search for opportunities to innovate and improve. The leader's primary contribution to this process is the recognition of good ideas, support of those ideas, and willingness to challenge the system. Using the recommendations of the Institute of Medicine and the Exploring Accreditation Project, local public health leaders can begin to align their current situation with their future goals, identifying the gaps between the status quo and what they want to accomplish.

Fourth, leaders must enable others to act by fostering collaboration and building trust. Quality improvement is not a one-time goal for improvement. It is a continuous process of building on past achievements to consistently improve outcomes and efficiency within public health. Exemplary leaders foster this continuous improvement by enabling others to exceed their own expectations by making individuals feel strong and capable of instituting change.

Finally, leaders encourage the heart. The road to improvement in public health will be challenging. At times, members of the public health agencies will become frustrated and disenchanted. Leaders must show appreciation for the dedication and hard work of their organizations by celebrating the small successes on the road to improvement.

Embodying these practices can help to prepare the public health leadership as they work toward the process of achieving shared goals and improving outcomes in public health.

DEVELOPING A PLAN AND GATHERING THE TOOLS

A fundamental characteristic of public health accreditation is to incorporate the methods and techniques of continuous quality improvement (QI) into governmental public health agencies. Quality improvement is a management technique used extensively in the private sector as well as in acute hospital care to continually improve the quality of products and services produced by an organization.[19]

The purpose of QI is to:

- Understand processes and pinpoint critical problems

- Establish control and reduce variation

- Determine process capability

- Design experiments to improve outcomes and processes

- Assess product reliability

The ten essential services and public health performance standards provide the ideal method to focus quality improvement projects in a public health department. It is not possible or feasible to improve every process that falls within these domains and standards. While accreditation requires meeting standards at specified levels, QI is a methodology used by leadership to create a management vision and approach throughout the entire health department (QI with capital letters), as well as a set of specific techniques to identify and improve specific processes (qi with small letters).

Once public health department leadership commitment to quality improvement has been established, the next step for creating improved outcomes is deciding which area to address first.

A growing body of evidence indicates that public health professionals can be trained to be competent in using QI techniques, resulting in breakthrough improvements in outcomes within their organizations.[20]

While improving public health outcomes using QI methods is attainable, the focus established through public health accreditation provides a standardized method to track progress against a national standard. By having shared methods and goals, we place ourselves in a better position to evaluate the effects of change because there is a benchmark for performance. We can achieve consistently high levels of performance by performing critical aspects of public health using best practices rather than common practices. Once best practices are identified and implemented, the potential to improve health status outcomes will continue.

LEVERAGE POINTS

Most processes have one or two *leverage points*, places where a little change has a great impact.[21] High-leverage points can be found within a public health department, which when standardized help drive consistently high performance. Likewise, low-leverage points where efficiency can be improved can be identified where low-value-added steps are found in a process. As discussed previously, QI methods and techniques are best implemented in repetitive processes in public health. The best application of small QI is to find processes where variable methods seriously detract from our ability to provide high-quality services to consumers of public health services.

There are many opportunities to identify leverage points in public health departments. First of all, start small. Using the 10 essential health services, pick one area that you would like to improve. For example, it was recently shown that quality improvement methods and techniques can be successfully applied to improve the wait time and satisfaction of Women, Infant, and Children (WIC) nutrition service clinics.[22] Using a series of tools that will be presented throughout the remainder of this book, the local public health department was able to improve the efficiency of one of their essential public health services.

There are many QI models that can be applied to public health, including Six Sigma[23] and lean management.[24] However, the model that may be most relevant for public health purposes is the Model for Improvement developed by the Institute for Healthcare Improvement.[25] The Model for Improvement consists of four components: 1) establish the aim, 2) create measures, 3) test changes, and 4) use the plan–do–check–act (PDCA) cycle.

CONCLUSIONS

Our nation spends more per person on healthcare than any other country, yet has one of the lowest health statuses of all industrialized nations. The preponderance of healthcare expenditures are focused on acute care, with less than five percent of all healthcare dollars committed to governmental public health departments. Voluntary public health accreditation is the foremost way to enhance population health status by achieving benchmark standards and deploying proven QI methods.

Many local public health departments operate with a small number of staff who are charged with meeting all of the public health needs of their communities from immunizations to nutrition counseling. It is oftentimes difficult to prioritize quality improvement in the midst of competing interests that are dictated by legislative mandate or grant requirements. However, standardized methods and goals using quality improvement methods and techniques provide an important first step toward improving the efficiency and outcomes of public health using many of the resources already available to local health departments.[26]

Voluntary accreditation can help provide positive change in local public health departments around the nation. Two important reasons for this change include:

1. *High performance and quality improvement.* Among state and local public health departments there is a high value placed on performance improvement and continuous quality improvement. A successful accreditation program should provide a transforming process that supports these goals. A successful accreditation program should result in improved health outcomes.

2. *Recognition and validation of the public health department's work.* A successful accreditation program should be credible among governing bodies and recognized by the general public, providing accountability to the public, funders, and governing bodies (legislatures and governors at the state/territorial level, tribal governments, and boards of health, county commissions, city councils, and officials at the local level).

The importance of local control is an important feature of the public health system in this nation. Local control can be fostered in the voluntary accreditation process by recognizing that each public health department's particular combination of population characteristics, professionals, and processes creates patterns that reflect ways of serving the community. The concept of the "five P's"[27] is useful for public health departments in using QI to design the most effective population-based services. This discussion adopts the concept of the "five P's" to a public health department setting:

Purpose. Be clear about the aims of the QI project and the relationship between the work processes and population outcomes.

Population. Know the community that is served, the needs of the community, and other organizations that support the community needs.

Professionals. Who are the personnel within the organization that provide the public health services, and who supports them? Does everyone see their work as interdependent, and how is the morale?

Processes. Public health professionals are adept at understanding systems, but are often not versed in process design and analysis.

Patterns. What are the health outcomes or the services provided by the public health department? How does the health department interact internally and externally with partners and collaborators? How does the organization stay mindful of both its successes and shortcomings?

The process under way by the Public Health Accreditation Board has an established information program that promotes the value of accreditation to the public and provides documentation, promotional materials for customized use, and specialized support to pursue public health department accreditation. In addition, the PHAB maintains an active program promoting the value of quality and performance improvement in public health and the role of accreditation in encouraging and documenting continuous improvement in public health departments.

The following chapters will focus on specific tools for identifying these key leverage points for change and their application in public health settings.

For more information on voluntary national accreditation, please visit www.phaboard.org.

Chapter 5

The Baldrige Criteria for Performance Excellence As a Framework to Improve Public Health

Carlton Berger, MPA

The Malcolm Baldrige National Quality Award program has entered its third decade and for many good reasons. For one, the Baldrige Criteria for Performance Excellence, often imitated, never duplicated, aren't just for the private sector anymore. Over the past 20 years, the Award Criteria have indeed evolved to include public sector, education, healthcare, and nonprofit organizations. And the rapidly accelerating demands on government for outcomes and accountability to the ultimate customer base, the taxpayers, have only served to make performance improvement a priority.

Many states model the Baldrige Criteria and Award in designing their own programs, often copying documents and structure verbatim. The fact is that the Criteria for Performance Excellence (CPE) are a time-proven, systematic framework for any organization to manage their daily operations. The Criteria's seven categories, described in detail at the Baldrige program Web site, www.baldrige. gov, are: Leadership; Strategic Planning; Customer and Market Focus; Measurement, Analysis and Knowledge Management; Workforce Focus; Process Management; and Results. The Web site provides extensive background on the origin, history, and evolution of the Baldrige program.

This chapter seeks to provide practical advice and encourage the reader to apply constructs from each of the seven CPE categories to improve public health. The audience of this book is primarily public health leaders looking to improve organizational performance, some of whom may one day apply for a local, state, or even the national quality award. But whether or not the readers and their organizations ever go through the rigorous process of application and examination, all can learn from the Baldrige Criteria body of knowledge.

USING THE SEVEN CPE CATEGORIES TO IMPROVE PUBLIC HEALTH ORGANIZATIONS

The Baldrige Criteria Scoring System is based on a total of 1000 points divided among 18 items across seven categories. The Organizational Profile required for the application requests an Organizational Description and Organizational Challenges. And as the instructions mention, this can help you to self-assess and identify potential gaps and focus on requirements and results. Even if your organization does not have a performance improvement initiative, this can provide a reality check as to what needs to be done. If you do choose to address the questions in the Profile, it is important to first read the entire Criteria, to best understand the totality of performance improvement. Before you begin to draft the Organizational Profile, consider reviewing and using these documents, each available via links on the Baldrige homepage: *Are We Making Progress? Are We Making Progress As Leaders?* and *Getting Started with the Criteria for Performance Excellence: A Guide to Self-Assessment and Action.*

Leadership

Leadership accounts for 12 percent of the total point score for the Baldrige application, and the CPE evaluates both senior leadership and an organization's accountability and community support. To summarize, this category is concerned with how senior leaders guide and sustain the organization, set organizational vision, values, and performance expectations, communicate with staff, develop future leaders, measure performance, and create an environment that encourages ethical behavior and high performance.

From the inception of the Baldrige Criteria, Leadership has always been category number one and that is not coincidental. The commitment of senior organization leaders is absolutely essential to the success or failure of any performance improvement effort. And that commitment must be visible at all times. Senior management must walk the talk to reinforce it.

The type of leadership approach necessary can be summarized as: changing the organizational culture to encourage trust between workforce and management, providing a strategic vision of the organization and communicating that vision throughout the organization, and making performance improvement part of the organization's long-term plan.

In 1991 Jack Grayson, founder of the American Quality Center, summed up the critical importance of leadership. "Only the leaders of the organization can ensure the permanent cultural change that develops and maintains trust between workforce and management. Successful improvement is eminently strategic, and the leaders are finally the keepers of the strategy. Only they can affirm the importance of adding value for the customer and employee empowerment."

To capture the necessary elements of organizational culture and management style, focus on the right column of the comparative chart in Figure 5.1.

For the purpose of relating Leadership and the six remaining categories of the Criteria to your public health organization, let's assume you have the time and flexibility to assemble a task force to brainstorm critical components to improve your organization, regardless of the size, scope, or delivery method of the services your public health organization offers. For the Leadership category, your task force might consider:

- Establishing appropriate measures or indicators that senior leaders track in their performance reviews. Role model organizations look for opportunities to exceed requirements and to excel in areas of legal and ethical behavior.

Old	New
Old	New
Authoritarian	Participative
Hierarchical	Decentralized
Managers	Leaders
Individualistic/competitive	Teamwork/collaborative
Control	Support
Quota/quantity based	Quality based
Detection/inspection	Prevention
One-way communication	Two-way communication
Market oriented	Customer oriented
Vendor tolerance	Vendor partnering
Risk avoidance	Innovation
Quality specialists	Train entire workforce in basic tools
Policy variation	Policy consistency
Business as usual	Continuously improve

Figure 5.1   Two styles of management/organizational culture.

- Developing a performance evaluation system that monitors your senior management performance.

- Creating activities for future leaders that might include personal mentoring or participation in leadership development courses.

- How committed senior leaders are to developing future leaders and to recognizing and rewarding contributions by members of the workforce.

Strategic Planning

Comprising 85 points of the Criteria, this category focuses on development and deployment of the organization's strategic objectives and action plans. The Strategic Planning category examines how an organization determines its key strengths, weaknesses, opportunities, and threats (SWOT), and ability to execute its strategy.

It has often been said that "Quality begins with a vision." A strategic vision:

- Outlines the desired state of the organization at some point in time

- Details how the organization will work after a performance improvement program is in place

- Outlines roles and responsibilities

- Considers elements such as service quality and organizational mission and culture (including values)

Strategic visions tend to be expressed in words—not numbers—clear and understandable, positive and inspiring. Major areas a strategic vision should address are: quality, employee empowerment, education and training, and reward and recognition systems. After developing a strategic vision, senior management needs to communicate the vision throughout the workplace using all available methods of communication.

One example of a strategic vision statement is:

By ongoing training of all levels of our workforce, we will develop an internal capacity to prevent and solve quality problems at the source in a timely fashion.

The *Take Care New York* annual report by the New York City Department of Health and Mental Hygiene is a good example of a strategic plan for a local public health organization. Available by searching the four word title at http://www.nyc.gov/html/doh/, the plan sets down 10 or so agenda items, performance indicators, goals, status (across several years), and progress. Each agenda item is summarized on one page: objectives, current activities and accomplishments, and strategic directions for the next year.

To develop objectives consider the SMART approach. SMART = *specific, measurable, achievable, relevant,* and *time-bound*. The Centers for Disease Control and Prevention encourage and often require public health leaders to use the SMART objectives format as part of their grant applications. Figure 5.2 shows an example of a SMART objective.

In County X, increase the percentage of adult patients with non-resistant TB who complete treatment within 12 months (as measured by cohort review) from 80 percent to 90 percent (the national goal) by 2008.

The objective is *specific* because it identifies a defined event: adult TB patients will complete treatment in less than 12 months. The objective is *measurable* because it specifies a baseline value and the quantity of change the intervention is designed

Objective	Increase the percentage of adult patients with non-resistant TB who complete treatment within 12 months from 80 percent to 90 percent by 2008.						
Breakdown	**Verb**	**Metric**	**Population**	**Objective**	**Baseline measure**	**Goal measure**	**Time frame**
	Increase	Percent	Adult patients with nonresistant TB	Completion of treatment within 12 months	80%	90%	By 2008
Indicator	Percent of adult patients with non-resistant TB who complete treatment within 12 months in 2008.						

Figure 5.2   Example of a SMART objective.

Source: Pages 13 and 23–24 of the CDC Web site's 2006 *TB Program Evaluation Handbook: Introduction to Program Evaluation* at http://www.cdc.gov/tb/.

to achieve: from 80 percent to 90 percent. As in the example, it is worthwhile to note whether there is an existing data source for the objective. The objective is *achievable* because it is realistic given the 10-year time frame. The objective is also *relevant* because it relates to the elimination of exposure to TB. Finally, the objective is *time-bound* because it provides a specified time frame by which the objective will be achieved (from 2004 to 2008).

In working to achieve the elements of the Baldrige Criteria Strategic Planning category, your task force might consider:

- Converting strategic objectives into short- and longer-term action plans to accomplish objectives

- Using software such as Microsoft Access and Visio to track progress on action plans

- Education and training initiatives, such as developmental programs for future leaders, partnerships to help ensure an educated and skilled workforce, and the establishment of training programs on new technologies important to the future success of your workforce

- Modifying compensation and recognition systems to recognize team, organizational, customer, or other performance attributes.

Customer and Market Focus

As with Strategic Planning, this category accounts for 85 points and is concerned with identifying customer groups and using the voice of the customer (feedback) to determine key requirements, needs, and changing expectations. Figure 5.3 captures the mind-set an organization needs to truly be customer focused.

It is important to identify both your organization's *internal* and *external* customers. For internal customers, who include all employees, consider the following questions:

- What do you really need from me?

- What do you do with what I give you?

- How am I doing?

For external customers, the vital questions are:

- Whose interests do we serve (all stakeholders)?

- Whose expectations must we satisfy?

- Who sets the requirements that govern our operation?

- Who can best provide feedback to help us improve?

Customer satisfaction surveys, either at point of service or as follow-up shortly thereafter, are a great way to capture information. Your task force might consider:

- Ways to determine how to use relevant information and feedback from customers for purposes of planning and making work process improvements

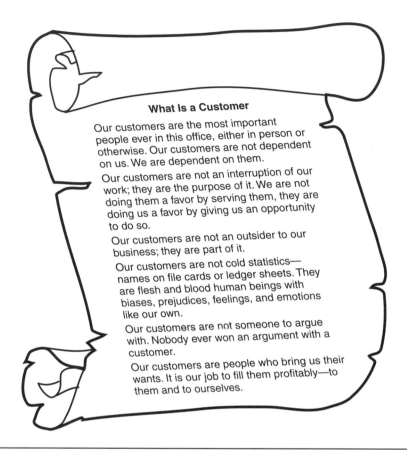

What Is a Customer

Our customers are the most important people ever in this office, either in person or otherwise. Our customers are not dependent on us. We are dependent on them.

Our customers are not an interruption of our work; they are the purpose of it. We are not doing them a favor by serving them, they are doing us a favor by giving us an opportunity to do so.

Our customers are not an outsider to our business; they are part of it.

Our customers are not cold statistics—names on file cards or ledger sheets. They are flesh and blood human beings with biases, prejudices, feelings, and emotions like our own.

Our customers are not someone to argue with. Nobody ever won an argument with a customer.

Our customers are people who bring us their wants. It is our job to fill them profitably—to them and to ourselves.

Figure 5.3   What is a customer?

- Developing customer feedback instruments such as the use of the customer complaint process to understand key product and service attributes, and survey or feedback information, including information collected via the Internet

- Listening to the voices of internal customers to identify training opportunities and methods to retain staff through employee empowerment and to innovate forms of recognition for staff excellence

Measurement, Analysis and Knowledge Management

This category represents nine percent of the Criteria's point total and is about how you measure, analyze, and then improve organizational performance. The saying "In God we trust, all others bring data" captures the essence of managing by facts/data.

The approach to managing by facts/data must be driven from the highest level of the organization. Data replaces opinions, hearsay, and conjecture. Relying on opinion and word-of-mouth reports of variation only increases the chances of making decisions based on subjective information. Managing by fact improves workforce morale and trust between workforce and management since both sides are integral to the data collection and analysis process.

Achieving consistent results is a core tenet of continuous performance improvement. Understanding variation and using the tools of the scientific method to reduce variation can allow senior management to take the lead to use facts to identify, analyze, and solve problems.

Montgomery Measures Up! is an annual report by the Montgomery County, Maryland, Department of Health and Human Services available at http://www.montgomerycountymd.gov/ombtmpl.asp?url=/content/omb/FY08/mmurec/index.asp. It is an excellent example of a page-at-a-glance summary of each of its dozens of programs with the focus being program measures. It uses a logic model format by beginning with outcomes measures and working backward to input measures. The report then rolls up selected measures into several departmental outcomes that reflect the organization's priorities.

Potential task force considerations with respect to Measurement, Analysis and Knowledge Management might include:

- Addressing how performance measurement requirements are deployed by senior leaders to track process-level performance on key measures targeted for improvement (this would include the selection of key performance indicators for all parts of your organization)

- Reviewing the use of data and information systems to improve areas most critical to effectiveness

- Considering the relationship between knowledge management and innovation, that is, how the ability to identify and meet workforce capability and capacity needs correlates with retention, motivation, and productivity

- Researching (benchmarking) where your organization stands relative to other health departments, and best practices to adopt, since comparing performance information may lead to a better understanding of our own processes and performance

Workforce Focus

This category comprises 85 points of the Criteria and focuses on workforce engagement in the improvement process and the organizational environment. Workforce engagement is characterized by performing meaningful work, having organizational direction and performance accountability, and having a safe, trusting, and cooperative environment. High-performance work is characterized by flexibility, innovation, knowledge and skill sharing, good communication and information flow, alignment with organizational objectives, and customer focus.

With respect to employees—the organization's *greatest* asset—the mind-set must be one of employee empowerment. That means:

- Bringing the workforce into the decision-making process

- Respecting people and their ability to contribute to improvement

- Understanding that improvement includes everyone in all parts of the organization

- Recognizing the untapped potential in all employees

- Encouraging innovation and entrepreneurialism among the workforce

- Empowering workers to halt the work process when errors are detected

- Empowering them to prevent errors before they happen, as in participative management

Potential task force considerations with respect to Workforce Focus are:

- Addressing barriers to workforce engagement identified via a survey or session with managers and senior leadership.

- Developing workforce surveys similar to the two assessments that are found on the Baldrige Criteria Web site (one version for the organization's leaders and another for all employees).

- Identifying workforce development needs including gaining skills for knowledge sharing, communication, teamwork, and problem solving, and interpreting and using data. Education and training delivery might occur inside or outside the organization and may involve on-the-job, classroom, computer-based, or distance learning, as well as other types of delivery.

- Developing recognition systems tied to demonstrated skills and rewards for exemplary team or unit performance, linkage to customer satisfaction measures, and achievement of organizational objectives.

Process Management

This 85-point category is concerned with how an organization manages and improves key work processes. Process management examines core competencies, work systems, and design of work processes, with the aim of creating value for customers and achieving organizational success.

There are several overarching tenets that govern process improvement:

- Every activity is a process to be improved.

- Improvement occurs project by project. Organizations that have successfully implemented quality improvement efforts generally undertook project-by-project improvement at a revolutionary pace.

- Many organizations find it wise to have both short-term and long-term projects going on at the same time.

- It is popular to rhapsodize about "no quick fix," but most management secretly (or overtly) expects some short-term effect, too.

- A little short-term improvement sustains the patience required for the larger and more significant long-term result.

Table 5.1 Potential actions to reduce avoidable costs.

Problem	Possible action
Duplication	Eliminate activity
Fragmentation	Combine activities
Misplaced Work	Transfer activities
Complexity	Simplify flow and methods
Bottlenecks	Change methods/add resources
Review/approval	Self-inspection
Rework/errors	Eliminate causes
Delays	Change flow/balance loads
Low-importance outputs	Do less frequently

An easy way to start to identify opportunities for process improvement is to begin at the personal level. Ask each employee to complete the two-part statement:

- I wish I could spend *less* time working on _____

- So that I could spend *more* time working on _____

Process improvement actions to reduce what are termed *avoidable costs* are noted in the matrix in Table 5.1.

Potential task force roles with respect to Process Management might be:

- Considering your organization's core competencies, that is, your areas of greatest expertise and how they relate to your mission, key performance indicators, and action plans

- Examining work systems involving your workforce, key vendors, contractors, and partners needed to produce and deliver your products and services (the group might perform process mapping and use information from customers of processes—within and outside your organization)

- Brainstorming ways to ensure the continuity of your operations in an emergency, as organizations whose mission includes responding to emergencies will have a high need for service readiness

- Evaluating and sharing successful strategies across your organization to drive learning and innovation

Results

The seventh and final category of the Baldrige Criteria accounts for 450 of the total 1000 points. This category is concerned with examining organizational performance and improvement in all key areas—product and service outcomes, customer-focused outcomes, workforce-focused outcomes, process effectiveness outcomes, and leadership outcomes.

Adapting the formats described earlier: SMART objectives, *Take Care New York,* and Montgomery Measures Up! can help you capture the information necessary to determine results.

Potential task force roles with respect to Results could include:

- Developing unique and innovative measures to track key processes and operational improvement. All key areas of organizational and operational performance should be evaluated by measures that are relevant and important to your organization.

- Considering measures and indicators of process effectiveness and efficiency, including work system performance that demonstrates internal responsiveness. Examples of such indicators may be improved performance of administrative and other support functions.

- Tracking workforce-focused performance results with the aim of demonstrating how well your organization is creating and maintaining a productive, engaging, and caring work environment for all staff. An outcome measure might be increased workforce retention resulting from establishing a peer recognition program.

- Acknowledging and communicating awards, ratings, and recognition from customers and independent rating organizations, including site visits.

ADDITIONAL RESOURCES FOR IMPROVING PUBLIC HEALTH ORGANIZATIONS

As mentioned at the beginning of the chapter, many national, state, and local performance improvement organizations and awards exist. The Public Health Foundation Web site at www.phf.org contains a tremendous amount of background material, tools, case studies, and resources specifically targeted to their customers and members—public health organizations.

Also at the national level, the American Society for Quality (www.asq.org) is the largest membership organization in the world devoted to performance improvement for all organizations. Their Web site offers tools and information on training and certifications. There are over 250 local sections that can provide access to a network of experts willing to share advice.

States with active groups that encourage organizations, including public health, to apply for recognition or tap into resources include:

Florida Sterling Council: www.floridasterling.com

South Carolina Quality Forum: www.scquality.com

Tennessee Center for Performance Excellence: www.tncpe.org

Local health organization information can be found at the Florida Department of Health's Office of Performance Improvement Web site: www.doh.state.fl.us/hpi/. They have a five-step performance improvement process model that allows all 67 of Florida's county health departments to systematically assess, plan, manage, and evaluate their own performance improvement.

FINAL CONSIDERATIONS FOR PUBLIC HEALTH PERFORMANCE IMPROVEMENT

A former state health commissioner stated emphatically that public health organizations are among the most resistant to change, partly because of the methodical nature of the sector and also due to a "that's the way we've always done it" mindset. That doesn't mean that efforts at public health performance improvement are destined to fail; however, leaders must anticipate resistance to change, and one of the best ways to lessen this is through a dual strategy of leadership and empowerment. These are two mutually complementary concepts and, as already described, necessary throughout all stages of performance improvement implementation.

Consistency of data is vital to measuring progress toward your objectives and outcomes. Consider your methods and systems for collecting data, and whenever possible develop standardized forms or templates. Remember that improvement applies to both programs/service delivery and administrative functions. All work is a process to be improved constantly and forever.

Performance improvement is about:

- Never allowing the status quo to suffice

- Working SMARTer (as in SMART objectives)

- Adding value to products, services, and processes for the customers—the final determiner of quality—and delighting customers by providing unexpected quality

- Benchmarking other organizations to determine what they do best and adapting their best into your organization

Performance improvement for public health organizations is not just a trend or fad, but a strategy for survival in an era of flat or decreasing funding and increasing customer expectations. The ultimate outcome is to create an organization that relies on the talents of its workforce to provide the best possible levels of service. Best of all, it is a proven method for improving organizations, their employees, and public health outcomes.

Chapter 6

Measures for Public Health

Fredia S. Wadley, MD

In public health our challenge is to make major changes in the health of a city or state with only a fraction of the resources needed for the problem. We are hesitant about allocating limited resources for evaluation of our efforts. Our justification is that a strong evaluation of a population intervention can cost more than the intervention itself. A frequent approach is to adopt an evidence-based strategy, modify it to conserve costs, but never evaluate to determine if the modifications decreased the effectiveness of the strategy. The lack of accountability that results is a major reason for the lack of support and funding for public health operations and initiatives.

CRITICAL CONCEPTS CONCERNING MEASURES

- A commitment to measure must be sustained at all levels of the organization.

- Outcome measures are the ultimate proof of success.

Commitment to measure progress must have the support of leadership as well as the frontline workers of a health department to assure that resources are available to build the systems that will support the function. This commitment will be stronger when all levels of the organization recognize that planning and decisions rely on the data generated. When no one uses the data, commitment to measuring is nonexistent, or rapidly declines.

The second critical measuring concept is "It is all about outcomes." For any one quality improvement project, you may need multiple measures, but ultimately the proof of success lies in the amount of improvement in the outcome measure(s).

In 1966 Avedis Donabedian gave us the framework for thinking of measures by categorizing them as structural, process, and outcome.[1] To facilitate understanding of the following concepts concerning measures, examples will relate to the public health problem of childhood obesity.

Structural Measure

Assesses your infrastructure or capacity. Many states and communities are working to decrease the prevalence of obesity in children and adolescents. An example of a structural measure is to create a community counseling program for families of children with a body mass index (BMI) at or above the 85th percentile for age. Another measure might be to recruit nutritionists for all the counselor positions. The assumption is that the program and the counselors' skill level will result in a decrease in the prevalence of obesity in children. Structural measures are static, but licensing and accreditation programs rely heavily on them by including the requirement for equipment, protocols, or a process. The protocols may be present, but the information within them is not assessed for correctness. This is the weakness of structural indicators.

Process Measure

Provides feedback on how well you are performing a process designed to impact the outcome. Once you have created your community counseling program for childhood obesity, you will want measures that give you an indication of how well things are working:

- The number of families enrolled within 12 months

- The percent of families enrolled in the program completing at least five of six sessions

These are only two examples of process measures that you could select for your counseling program.

Outcome Measure

Shows whether you made progress in reaching your ultimate goal. Your goal is to decrease childhood obesity. You created the counseling program (structural measure), recruited and counseled 100 families (process measure)—but did behavior change as a result of the program, producing a lower prevalence of obesity in the study group (outcome measure)? The outcome measure is the ultimate assessment for the effectiveness of your strategy. An additional cost outcome measure can be beneficial to assist decision making relative to the use of limited resources. For example, 90 percent of the 100 children in the counseling program lost weight (an unusually high rate), but the cost per child was $10,000 per year. The program is effective but not efficient enough to be practical for the community.

A comprehensive community initiative with a variety of interventions to prevent or decrease childhood obesity may require a mixture of structural, process, and outcome measures to adequately track progress and guide necessary changes. The ultimate goal is to decrease the community prevalence of childhood obesity, but a community approach may be to:

1. Create a counseling program for families to help children decrease their BMI.

2. Increase the percentage of children with one hour of exercise five days a week by increasing the requirement for physical education, developing after-school athletic programs, and building recreational opportunities for children across the community.

3. Improve nutrition by changing school lunch menus and removing vending machines from schools. Multiple interventions are more likely to produce a significant impact on complex population health problems, but the more comprehensive the community effort, the more critical it is to have a good system for measuring and tracking progress for each intervention.

Baseline Measurement

For some improvement projects the baseline measurement already exists and is the motivating factor for change. However, for other projects, allocating time and resources to determine the baseline measurement is an important part of the plan. Implementing the intervention without a baseline measurement and waiting six weeks to six months to obtain the first measurement does not allow an assessment of progress over this time period. The team can not assess progress and complete the PDSA (plan–do–study–act) cycle until two measurements are available for comparison. The best way to avoid wasted time and resources is to begin with a baseline measurement and continue with frequent and ongoing measurements that are carefully analyzed for planning purposes.

Sometimes a baseline measurement may not seem obvious. For example, a community school wants to promote healthy lunches for middle school children. They substitute healthy fruits and vegetables for the high-calorie, high-fat items routinely appearing on the menu, and claim victory for nutrition. However, with a baseline measurement they would know that 95 percent of students were purchasing lunches before the menu change, but six weeks later only 75 percent were purchasing lunches. And complicating the issue was the fact that the purchase of ice cream had almost doubled. Can these data be used to improve the nutrition intervention? Yes, the school nutritionist should seek more appealing healthy foods for this age group and track the number of lunches and amount of ice cream sold over the next six weeks.

Rapid Cycle Measurement

Integrate an early measurement, six to eight weeks after starting implementation, into your plan to provide critical feedback about the progress of your intervention. Many times this measure has to be a process measure because it is too early to have a good outcome measure. For example, the outcome measure of your counseling program is to have the participating children decrease their BMI. However, rapid weight loss can be unhealthy in children. The preferred approach for managing the exercise and diet of many young children is to let them "grow into their weight" and slowly decrease their BMI. For this reason, the rapid cycle measurement(s) for the counseling program might be:

- The number of counseling sessions/sites available (structural)
- The number of families enrolled in the program (process)
- The rate of attendance after enrollment (progress)

The intent of the rapid cycle measurement is to provide data that can be analyzed to determine if changes might make the intervention more effective. For example, if the enrollment were far less than expected, you should consider all possible reasons. If families find it difficult to take off of work to attend these sessions during the afternoon, then consider holding this service at night. After six to eight weeks of the night sessions, obtain another rapid cycle measurement to determine if enrollment has increased. Each intervention in your childhood obesity initiative will need this type of measurement and feedback to avoid wasting resources and time.

Proxy Measures

Process measures that are highly predictive of the outcome measures are sometimes referred to as *proxy measures*. They are never as reliable as outcome measures but may be acceptable when it is not feasible or possible to collect data for the outcome measure. For example, the goal is to prevent/decrease vaccine-preventable illnesses in children. When the immunization rate in children begins to climb, herd immunity increases, and some of these diseases may be relatively uncommon. However, we are aware that outbreaks can occur when pockets of susceptible children come in contact with the organism. Therefore, we now measure the rate of children immunized with each vaccine to determine our progress in preventing these diseases. Immunizations are the purest preventive technology we have, and immunization rates are very acceptable proxy measures.

However, the predictive value of process measures in other scenarios is rarely this good. In our childhood obesity initiative, enrolling 100 families in a counseling program is not a good proxy indicator for decreasing childhood obesity. Weight control is difficult to accomplish even with evidence-based interventions and may be achieved only in a minority of your participants. Even if research has shown that a specific counseling program resulted in 50 percent of children losing weight, it is still dangerous to assume that 50 percent of your participants will do the same. Evidence-based interventions are often implemented in a different environment using modifications that can affect the outcome. Public health is notorious (due to limited funds) for adopting an evidence-based strategy requiring $5000/child/year and modifying it to cost $500/child/year without measuring the outcome to see if the modifications decreased the effectiveness of the intervention.

Being suspicious of proxy measures is healthy for a good evaluation. Just keep reminding your team that "it is all about outcomes."

SELECTING OR DEVELOPING YOUR MEASURES

Selecting measures for any community initiative requires a great deal of consideration because measures must satisfy both *accountability* and *program management* requirements while being calculated with data that is already existing or feasible to collect. Accountability involves demonstrating not only effective but also efficient use of public resources. The private business sector created the term "return on investment" for calculating the gain that could be realized with an established amount of expenditures. Public health and population interventions are frequently more complicated than business interventions and have the potential for producing social, health, and economic benefits across the public and private sectors in the near and distant future, but this complexity does not negate the need to prove efficiency. This is a challenge preventive medicine strategies also face in the healthcare industry.

The key principles to remember when selecting measures are:

- Use standardized measures whenever possible. When not possible, carefully define the numerator and denominator of your new measure.

- Use existing data if available and applicable. If existing data are not suitable, understand the resources that will be required to collect the data for your measures.

- Understand the processes to be used for your intervention to select the best measures to guide you in program management.

- Understand the issue you are trying to improve well enough to define success in a realistic manner and select the best measures.

Why Use Standardized Measures?

Public health uses many measures that have been defined and refined over the years to represent reliable and valid data. The broad use of these measures across the nation stimulates comparison of outcomes, and this can be a strong motivating factor for states and communities to undertake quality improvement projects.

When a standardized measure does not work for your intervention, or if you need additional measures for program management or accountability, then carefully define the numerator and denominator for each new measure chosen. Here are two examples of the same measure with the second being more specific about how to determine the numerator and denominator:

1. The number of families completing weight control counseling sessions

2. The number of families completing at least five of six counseling sessions, divided by the number of families that enrolled in the program and attended at least one session

Often the first definition is used until the intervention gets under way and someone asks for a clarification or definition of the word "completing." Does it mean every session or a certain percent of the sessions? Clearly defining the measure before implementation of the intervention can also help you determine if collection of the data is possible.

Why Use Existing Data?

One of the biggest challenges for performance management and quality improvement projects is having good data to make decisions. Public health collects a great deal of data, but too often these data are housed in program areas and are not readily accessible even to other public health professionals at the state and community level. Valuable resources might be saved if existing data can be used in your quality improvement efforts. Learn what data are being collected in the community or state relative to your project. For example, the Youth Behavior Risk Factor Survey includes questions that could apply to your childhood obesity project. However, in some states the data sample size may not be sufficient to yield reliable and valid data for each county. Even if there are existing data being collected, you must verify how they are collected and determine whether they can meet the needs of your community project. If you determine that the data are not reliable and valid for the county level, a potential opportunity exists for your county or community to pay for a larger sample size as a way to obtain the data you need. The Behavior Risk Factor Surveillance System has optional modules that can be added to the basic questions, such as the module for diabetes. Investing in additions to existing surveys with standardized measures offers many advantages.

Understanding the Processes of the Intervention Can Lead to Better Measures for Program Management

In the previous example, we used a measure to tell us how many enrolled families completed at least five of six counseling sessions of our weight management program. But what if the number enrolling was far less than you expected? Then you would want to know why more families were not getting to your program. You have several processes to facilitate recruitment and enrollment: 1) public awareness with media announcements, 2) school nurses referring families, and 3) physicians referring families. Having physician offices and school nurses send a referral notice to the counseling program for each child referred to the program will require communication and planning among the stakeholders. The effort to collect data always sounds easier if the responsibility lies with another party. Working with the school nurses and physician offices to understand their work processes can lead to the development of new office processes or tools that can facilitate the generation of referral notices to the counseling program staff.

Will these data be of significant value for program management? If you learn that the schools have referred 25 children and 15 have enrolled, while physician offices referred only two children over the six-month time period, you should be concerned. Research has shown that individuals and families are more likely to make lifestyle changes that are recommended and supported by their physician. Determining why the physicians are not supporting the community initiative and the weight counseling program can be critical for the success of this intervention.

Understanding the Problem to Define and Measure Success

Private and public health sectors have a tendency to adopt an "all or none" philosophy about what constitutes success in a performance or quality improvement project. One of the reasons pay for performance in healthcare has progressed slowly is because paying providers only when the ultimate outcome goal is achieved can negate a great deal of improvement in the chronic condition of patients. An individual with diabetes that decreases their hemoglobin A1C from 9.5 to 7.2 has made a great deal of progress and is healthier even though he has not reached his goal of having the level below 7.0. The challenge for pay for performance programs is defining sufficient progress for individual patient success, developing measures for tracking all patients with the condition, and assigning a reimbursement amount that represents an adequate incentive for the provider to spend additional office resources to support patients in changing their behavior.

A similar challenge in defining success exists for many public health quality improvement efforts. Childhood obesity is a good example of why public health professionals need to do a little research and become familiar with the latest research and studies on the issue or condition they are addressing. A little "Googling" can help you locate standard measures and lessons learned in measuring progress of childhood obesity interventions.

Key points relevant to childhood obesity success and measures:

1. BMI used instead of weight to track success.

2. BMI must be plotted on growth chart for children.

3. Achieving and measuring success with weight management programs is not for the faint hearted.

BMI and Not Pounds

Most health professionals now recognize that the BMI is a far better measure for tracking success with weight management interventions than the weight of individuals. Weight is a one-dimensional measure and does not tell you the other important variable, which is height. A child at four years of age is usually around 40 inches and 40 pounds. If a four-year-old weighed 60 pounds at four years of age, he would be overweight, but the same weight after growing several inches would be normal. This is why we often use the phrase, "children can grow into their weight." Unfortunately, not all public or private clinicians calculate the BMI and include it in the health or medical record for monitoring patients. The effort to get providers to use the BMI as a standard measure has been more successful than implementing the metric system in the United States, but we have miles (or kilometers) to go before we can rest assured that the BMI is routinely used in all settings.

Growth Chart for BMI

Children pass through developmental stages in which the percent of body fat normally changes. Growth charts for plotting height and weight are routinely used with children to account for the growth differences in these developmental stages, and the Centers for Disease Control and Prevention has developed such a chart for plotting the BMI of children. In adults, a BMI of 25 indicates the person is overweight and one of 28 denotes obesity. A child is said to be overweight when the

BMI is at or above the 85th percentile for age and obese when the BMI is at the 95th percentile or greater. Figure 6.1 is a CDC growth chart with the BMI plotted for a ten-year-old male. Note that a BMI of 23 is above the 95th percentile for age and indicates obesity for this child.

We find the term "childhood obesity" frequently in the media, but the public and policy makers who hold public health accountable do not have a clear understanding of how we measure and track progress with this problem. Part of the challenge with any public health quality improvement project is to clearly define the measures and state how we will calculate them. Although this chapter has used childhood obesity as an example to demonstrate critical points to consider in selecting and defining measures for a quality improvement project, many other topics will offer similar challenges. Researching your subject during the planning phase will help you select better measures to monitor progress.

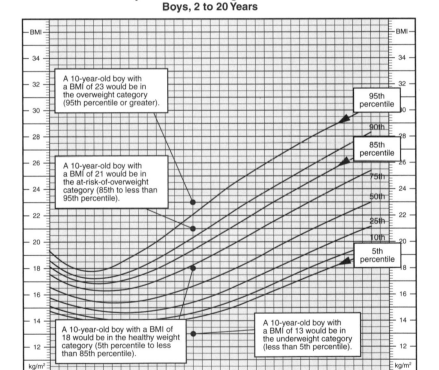

**Body Mass Index-for-Age Percentiles:
Boys, 2 to 20 Years**

Figure 6.1   CDC growth chart plotting 10-year-old male BMI.

Defining and Measuring Success

Selecting a goal to define success for a quality improvement project is another step in the quality improvement process, and another chapter of this handbook. However, continuing with a few words of caution may be beneficial to the many states and communities addressing this problem because with childhood obesity this process is so dependent on understanding your measure and your topic.

A simplistic view of success could be lowering the BMI. However, keep in mind that:

- Even the most successful weight management (or BMI management) programs don't have a high rate of success.

- Children are still growing and developing, and the BMI level for one age may indicate obesity but be normal at a later age.

- Progress is not "all or none"—like cost containment in healthcare, you may not decrease your measure (the cost), but you may slow the rate of increase.

Unfortunately, many health officials have found themselves before a city council or state legislative committee trying to explain the progress of a program even though the initial goal for their project has not been met. Credibility can be questioned when you change the definition of success after failing to meet the original goal. Reaching consensus on a realistic definition of progress and success before implementation of the intervention can help preserve credibility and support for the effort.

Here are some examples of goals representing progress for a child obesity program:

1. *X percent* of the children in the program will *have no increase* in BMI percentile rating.

2. *X percent* of the children in the program will *decrease* their BMI percentile rating.

3. Of the children in the program who have an increase in their BMI percentile rating, *X percent* of these children will *increase their BMI percentile rating at a lower rate than the previous year.*

4. The percent of children in the program with a *BMI above the 85th* percentile for age (all entering the program are at or above this percentile) will *decrease by X percent.*

Some of these goals require more data and analysis. Health or medical records may not be available to compute the third example. The point is to know the measure and topic well enough to recognize that progress and success may be defined and measured differently. Once these potential definitions of progress are identified, the likelihood of selecting a realistic goal for which data collection is feasible becomes greater.

SUMMARY

If evaluating our work were easy, public health would be getting more than a mere three percent of health expenditures. Selecting measures for quality improvement projects or performance management requires an understanding of the issue or problem being addressed, the processes involved, and the environment. Many measures may be needed for accountability and program management of a comprehensive and complex project, but at the end of the day, *it is all about outcome measures.*

Chapter 7

Leading and Lagging Indicators of Public Health and Public Health Assessment and Accreditation

Alina Simone and Paul D. Epstein

The public health field is ripe with data, including countless health outcome indicators. These are mostly lagging indicators that, at the local level, describe the health status of the community. Health status outcomes result from numerous influences, some of which have been at play in the community for many years. So, as important as these indicators are, they are often only of limited use for telling public officials and community leaders what to do to improve community health.

NEED FOR BOTH LEADING AND LAGGING INDICATORS OF PUBLIC HEALTH IMPROVEMENT

Lagging indicators provide the kinds of data that drive public health agendas. They indicate which diseases are most prevalent among children, what kinds of diseases and accidents yield the highest mortality rates, which demographic groups are most susceptible to infectious diseases, which neighborhoods exhibit higher rates of illness associated with pollution, and so on. This kind of information shapes budgets and informs public health policy makers about how communities need to be mobilized to address both current health problems and growing health risks. However, the path toward achieving public health goals is fraught with myriad decisions and actions. It is the sum of many safety, health, economic, social, and environmental choices spread across the many sectors that impact public health that combine to "move the needle" on major health outcomes.

In one community, progress in lowering infectious disease rates, which are lagging indicators, may be hampered because the local hospital has not provided doctors with adequate supplies of antibacterial soap, sterile masks, and disposable gloves. Local health officials must first recognize that problem in order to take action. Then they should also recognize that for their community *the hospital's line infection rate*, a measure of service quality, is one of the key "leading indicators" they should track to see if they are making progress toward their long-term goal of lower infectious disease rates in the community as a whole. If a nursing shortage is keeping the hospital and community clinics from adequately providing treatment and preventive services, then *the percentage of nursing positions vacant* in the community health system can be another important leading indicator. In addition to indicators of quality medical practices or adequate medical personnel, leading indicators in a community might include *the number of hours per week community clinics are open,* or *the number of clinics with adequate multilingual staff* to serve the non–English speaking residents in their local service area.

Leading indicators provide the crucial signposts on the road map toward improving community health. Leading indicators can include:

- Indicators of the short-term implementation of health-related services and initiatives (for example, measures of inputs such as resources dedicated, and outputs such as people served)

- Indicators of service quality or timeliness (for example, line infection rates, waiting time to receive treatment)

- The short-term or medium-term results of services and initiatives (for example, outcomes for people directly served, such as the number or percentage who changed behaviors or experienced improvement in their health)

As the above examples suggest, appropriate leading indicators can vary from community to community depending on the particular public health challenges faced in each community. Leading indicators should be carefully chosen to tell community health leaders whether their strategy for improving public health is being implemented as intended and whether it is starting to succeed based on short-term or medium-term results. Eventually, if the community health improvement strategy is working, improvements should start to show up in lagging indicators. Before waiting that long, leading indicators give managers and leaders an early warning of whether midcourse corrections are needed in their strategy. For a more comprehensive approach to developing and managing a community public health strategy, including the use of leading and lagging indicators, see Chapter 18, "Community Balanced Scorecards for Strategic Public Health Improvement."

PUBLIC HEALTH ASSESSMENT AND ACCREDITATION: LOCAL CAPACITY AND BEST PRACTICES

There are several recognized structured processes for public health assessment, such as the National Public Health Performance Standards (NPHPS) with assessment instruments for state public health systems, local public health systems, and local public health governance. The National Association of County and City Health Officials (NACCHO) provides an assessment instrument for local health departments based on NACCHO's "Operational Definition of a Functional Local Health Department." The NPHPS and NACCHO assessment instruments all use the "10 essential services of public health" as their main organizing framework. Also, several states have their own systems for local public health assessment. These approaches are all being considered in development of a national public health accreditation system, targeted to begin on a voluntary basis by 2011. In the meantime, more than 50 local health departments across the country are already piloting a variation of accreditation based on assessment against the standards in NACCHO's Operational Definition.

Essentially, all these assessment tools work by providing sets of public health standards, and for each "standard" specifying a list of recognized best practices for comparison against existing practices at the organization or health system level. By providing a source of best practice benchmarking, these assessments can be a valuable source of "leading indicators" of public health improvement. The degree of progress health departments or systems make in achieving strategically-chosen standards can become leading indicators of later changes in community indicators of health outcomes. The rest of this chapter uses NACCHO's Operational Definition as an example, but the idea of using assessment standards as a source of leading indicators can also work for the other public health assessment approaches.

NACCHO's Operational Definition breaks down each essential service of public health into several "focus standards," and then to "operational definition indicators." In all, there are 225 operational definition indicators, each representing a "best practice" for achieving one of the standards. The five-point scale shown in Figure 7.1 is used in NACCHO's pilot accreditation assessment process to rate each operational definition indicator. As described on the scale, a score from 0 to 4 is determined based on the assessed capacity of the local health department to achieve the best practice represented by the indicator.

A local health department uses the assessment process to identify strengths and weaknesses in its capacity to perform important public health practices and improve performance. Thus, key operational definition indicators can be selected as *leading indicators of the department's ability to make progress* on improving health outcomes that require adequate capacity to perform those practices effectively. Building capacity to perform critical practices better, and following through to make strategic improvements in practice, can eventually lead to improvements in health outcomes. Thus, tracking capacity to perform key practices can be seen as tracking leading indicators to measure progress toward achieving lagging community health outcome indicators

For example, a community's approach to lowering the incidence of HIV may include saturating high-risk demographic groups or neighborhoods with information concerning how the disease is transmitted and safety precautions people can take. However, if the targeted groups do not speak English as a first

---

0: *No capacity:* There is no capacity, planning, staff, resources, activities, or documentation to fulfill the indicator

1: *Minimal capacity:* There is minimal planning and staffing capacity to fulfill the indicator but no implementation activity or documentation

2: *Moderate capacity:* There is moderate planning, staffing, and other resources to fulfill the indicator but only minimal activity and/or documentation

3: *Significant capacity:* There is significant planning, staffing, and other resources and a moderate amount of activity and/or documentation

4: *Optimal capacity:* There is significant planning, staffing, and resources and significant to optimal activity and/or documentation to fulfill the indicator

---

Figure 7.1   Operational Definition assessment scoring scale.
Source: Local Health Department Self-Assessment Tool, NACCHO.

language, and the local health department does not have funding for translation or the expertise necessary to conduct a culturally-appropriate public education campaign, then the long-term goal may remain out of reach. The health department can track its progress toward addressing its capacity shortcomings in this area by using the indicators outlined under Standard III–C of NACCHO's Operational Definition: "Provide targeted, culturally appropriate information to help individuals understand what decisions they can make to be healthy." Progress toward meeting the standard can also be seen as progress made toward achieving larger public health objectives, such as lowering HIV rates.

CAVEATS FOR USING ASSESSMENTS OF CAPACITY AS LEADING INDICATORS

Assessment of capacity using NACCHO's Operational Definition and scoring scale necessarily involves many judgment calls by the people making the assessment. Those judgments make these capacity indicators soft measures compared with more objective indicators such as the number of people served by a program, the number of people served whose health clinically improves, and the total incidence of a particular disease in the community. So, one caveat, especially as NACCHO's pilot accreditation system has started as a self-assessment process, is that the people doing the assessment be as careful and objective as possible in a process that necessarily involves some subjectivity.

Another caveat is that local health officials seeking to improve their department's scores on reassessment do not simply do the easiest things they can to "check off the box" and increase their capacity scores for various Operational Definition indicators. Instead, health department managers must consider what specific best practices will enhance their specific community strategy to improve public health. So, rather than translating existing HIV informational flyers into Spanish and checking off that they have become more culturally competent, the department might, for example, try to improve its capacity to fulfill Operational Indicator III-C-5, which calls for "members of the target population [to] participate in the development and distribution of health education materials." If department managers believe the participation of people from high-risk groups in developing and delivering materials to be crucial for effective outreach and public education on HIV, then they will target increasing their capacity to perform that practice. In that case, the department's capacity rating for Operational Indicator III-C-5 can be one of several leading indicators of the eventual lagging outcome measured by the rate of new HIV infections.

USING A COMBINATION OF MEASURES FOR A VALUABLE MIX OF LEADING INDICATORS

Using a mix of different kinds of measures is the best way to create a powerful system of leading indicators. As suggested by the earlier examples, leading indicator measures may include:

- Measures of services provided and results (for example, inputs, outputs, service timeliness, service quality, short-term or medium-term outcomes)

- Measures of special projects or initiatives (also could be inputs, outputs, short-term or medium-term outcomes, as well as timeliness of implementation)

- Measures of assessment or accreditation progress—"soft measures" of:

  - How local practices measure up to recognized best practices

  - Local capacity to implement best practices

The important thing is to identify a set of leading indicators that best reflect how the public health practices attempted in the community are expected to address particular community health conditions and the causes of those conditions. For some public health practices, such as "health promotion," simply totaling outputs (for example, number of smokers reached, number of community organizations participating in neighborhoods with high rates of smoking-related illnesses) may not say enough about the effectiveness of local efforts. Combining further measures of capacity and comparisons with best practices better suggests whether the health promotion effort is likely to make a difference.

Also, while the output measures may indicate whether the health department is reaching enough of the targeted population, they may not say enough about whether the target population is actually altering its behavior based on the interventions. To continue with the smoking example, it may also be necessary to collect data for short-term or medium-term outcome measures that help determine whether the health promotion effort is indeed influencing people to change their behaviors and break their smoking habits. Eventually, this should lead to change in relevant lagging indicators, such as the incidence of deaths from smoking-related diseases.

By incorporating a strategically-determined mix of leading indicators in their performance management systems, public health leaders will have access to data to alert them in real time about whether needed progress is being made toward major goals, and to help explain why or why not. This kind of data will no doubt test the assumptions of public health practitioners regarding the sources of health problems and the best path toward solving them, but by doing so, will raise the probability of eventual success as gaps in their logic chain are identified and bridged.

For example, the simple logic chain detailed below outlines several different kinds of leading indicators that management can use to determine how to improve public health outcomes without waiting years to see how lagging health status indicators change.

The *assumed logic in the chain* proceeds as follows:

Improving capacity for best practices and increasing the use of those practices (as determined in accreditation or another assessment process) reflects the ability to provide better services, projects, and initiatives

which leads to:

Better implementation of services, projects, and initiatives (inputs, outputs, timeliness, service quality)

which leads to:

Short-term or medium-term better outcomes for people served or targeted parts of the community

which leads to:

Long-term outcomes for the larger population (lagging indicators): improved health status indicators over time.

For more on using logic chains with performance indicators for strategic planning and strategy management, see Chapter 18, "Community Balanced Scorecards for Strategic Public Health Improvement."

A DASHBOARD OF LEADING INDICATORS AND TARGETS

Drawing out the smoking reduction example into a full scenario can provide a more complete picture of the use of a strategic mix of leading indicators. For example, a community partnership may be convened by the local health department to address smoking and its primary and secondary impacts. The partnership may select "deaths from diseases related to tobacco smoke exposure (for example, lung cancer, emphysema, heart disease)" as the lagging indicator of health status it most wants to improve. The goal would be to move the needle down for this indicator, and see a reduction in total deaths from smoking-related disease in the community as a whole. The partnership may also aim for the largest reductions in populations with the highest smoking-related death rates, both as the fastest way to reach the communitywide goal and to reduce health outcome disparities.

From there, the partnership could implement a number of different methods to improve that long-term outcome. Smoking cessation efforts could be launched, with key efforts focused on target populations with high smoking rates. To reduce peoples' exposure to secondhand smoke, business groups in the partnership could promote smoke-free workplaces, and laws could be proposed to restrict smoking in public spaces. Another tactic could be to target youth smoking prevention as a means of reducing the size of the problem in the future. Initiatives could include, for example, public education campaigns, promotion of healthier alternatives to tobacco, and provision of free or subsidized behavior modification programs and products to reduce nicotine addiction for those who want to quit. Of course, these and other methods to reduce smoking and exposure to secondhand smoke are used in many parts of the country with reasonable expectations for success. Leading indicators and what is known of those expectations can be used to target and monitor performance and sharpen the community's strategy over time.

Indicators related to these various efforts, as well as to the desired long-term outcome, can provide the partnership and the health department with a customized and adjustable dashboard capable of providing useful readings regarding how quickly and effectively progress is being made. For example:

- A target for the long-term outcome, such as "a 20 percent reduction in deaths from smoke-related illness by 2012," is the communitywide lagging indicator and provides the *destination*.

- More detailed lagging indicators and targets, such as "25 percent to 40 percent reductions in smoking-related deaths in specific targeted populations by 2012," allow health leaders to *zoom in for a closer look at the destination*.

- Strategically chosen capacity measures, such as the "ability to provide culturally appropriate information regarding smoking health risks," is one leading indicator of *how fast the partnership can accelerate* toward its goal, given enough resources.

- Measures of resources, or inputs, such as "dollars allocated to smoking cessation programs" and "increase in health code inspectors" to enable enforcement of smoking bans provide a *gauge of the amount of fuel* in the system.

- Output measures such as the "number of people who join smoking cessation programs" suggest how well various programs *have gotten into gear*, versus programs that are just spinning their wheels.

- Outcome measures targeted for short-term and medium-term results, such as "number of people in funded programs who stop smoking," "cigarette sales," or "new incidences of smoking-related pulmonary disease" will tell *whether the right course has indeed been charted*.

All of the above types of indicators, leading and lagging, *can be targeted* using the logic chain progression as a guide, and assumptions of what various types of programs and initiatives can accomplish. In some cases there can be fairly good evidence for setting a target. For example:

- If there are well-established unit costs for each person served by particular types of smoking cessation programs, those can be used to help establish output targets for those programs for given levels of funding.

- If those types of programs have a track record of the percentage of success with particular target populations, those past records can be used as evidence to set outcome targets by applying those percentages to the number of people expected to be served.

In deciding initially which programs to fund, a combination of unit costs and past track record can provide a projection of the unit cost per outcome, such as the cost per person who stops smoking. However, care must be taken not to simply fund only the programs that are apparently most cost-effective based on unit costs if other evidence suggests that a variety of interventions, whose unit costs vary, are needed for different target populations, whether those target populations are defined clinically, behaviorally, culturally, economically, or geographically. If some programs are experimental, or there is not enough known about their effect on a given target population, then one approach is not to target the programs for an initial "experimental" period (for example, the first year), then set targets based on what is learned in that period. Alternatively, targets may be set for these programs based on best assumptions, but managers and policy makers should be informed that there is less confidence in those targets, which will be revised when more evidence is known.

Reported data on a variety of leading indicators aimed at a key lagging indicator, targets for the indicators, past evidence, and the logic chain add up to a performance monitoring system. This kind of comprehensive approach helps public health managers and policy makers use their dashboard both to track the success of the overall strategy and its various parts, and to make midcourse corrections that improve the likelihood of long-term success. Viewing the entire dashboard of leading indicators in the logic chain, rather than just individual program-by-program results, can help public health leaders make better judgments about the reasons for strong or weak performance. For example, were certain smoking cessation programs aimed at key population groups underperforming because they were ineffective, or because health promotion and outreach efforts failed to convince key target populations to participate?

By using such a variety of leading indicators, public health leaders can analyze progress and results of the various parts of the community strategy to reduce long-term mortality. As less successful approaches are weeded out, more resources can be channeled into activities with proven results, and gaps in the community strategy can be identified and filled. Public health leaders don't have to wait until a significant reduction in the mortality rate is registered years later to determine whether progress is being made toward the community's strategic public health goals, and to sharpen the strategy to increase the community's effectiveness in achieving those goals.

Chapter 8

Reporting: Telling Your Story— The Saginaw County Department of Public Health

Natasha Coulouris, Christina Harrington, Cheryl Plettenberg, Patricia Ritter, and Tamara Theisen

INTRODUCTION

The Saginaw County Department of Public Health (SCDPH) has been asked to tell the story of our continuous quality improvement (CQI) journey, which we hope to offer as just one example of how several local health departments (LHDs) throughout the nation are using innovative approaches to achieving our common goal of improving the public's health. We still feel like beginners who have committed to a long journey, learning at each step of the way. In this spirit we have included "Traps and Tips" throughout the chapter, which we hope will provide practical advice to LHDs interested in initiating their own CQI processes.

The SCDPH is a single-county health department that serves 210,039 residents in the central portion of Michigan's lower peninsula, adjacent to both the agricultural and industrial centers of the state. Saginaw County reflects a diverse mix of urban and rural health issues and is currently experiencing an economic transformation with the decline of the automotive industry and the rise of the healthcare and alternative energy fields.

As Saginaw County and the state of Michigan have been hit hard by the deterioration of its economy and housing market, concepts such as CQI provide a tool for LHDs to clearly demonstrate the value of public health to the public and policymakers. CQI can help guide LHDs through a process that builds upon business practice to improve efficiency and effectiveness, and provide measurable outcomes that build the case for public health. Faced with stagnant county funds for 20 years, state cuts to essential programs such as community assessment, and the loss of nearly 20 percent of its workforce over the past 15 years, SCDPH has begun to see this process as a survival strategy. "A QI philosophy recognizes there are costs to everything we do and costs to everything we do not do, but should. Until we are completely satisfied with our public health funding levels and accomplishments, we should continually seek quality improvements that reduce costs and improve outcomes."[1]

Trap. Getting fooled into thinking CQI is just another new trend that takes you away from your core work and adds burden onto an already stretched staff.

Tip. CQI should be seen as essential, not superfluous, to public health. LHDs are in peril if they can not demonstrate their relevance. In tough economic times, CQI can provide evidence of the value of public health. CQI requires buy-in starting from the top and extending through various levels of staff and management.

A variety of factors led SCDPH to begin the CQI journey. First and foremost, SCDPH initiated "MOD (Moving in One Direction) Squad" in 2004, an ongoing, comprehensive, agency-focused strategic planning initiative. A multidisciplinary team representing frontline staff, managers, and a governing body representative developed a framework for the department's operation, including the mission, vision, vision priorities, and guiding principles and values (see Figure 8.1). In each cycle, a new group learns strategic planning skills, reviews our vision priorities and develops goals to support them, monitors progress on the action plan, and makes changes as necessary. MOD Squad embodies many of the same principles and elements found in the CQI process, and laid a foundation for SCDPH to begin incorporating formal CQI tools. Further, it encouraged a philosophy focused on breaking down programmatic silos to improve agency performance, and big-picture thinking focused on anticipating future trends.

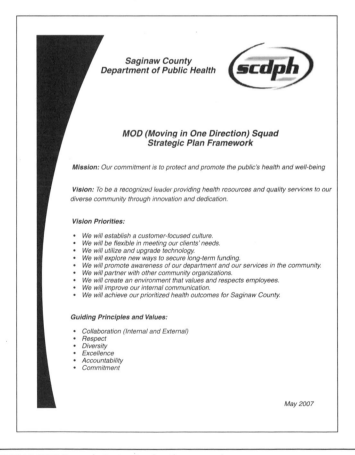

Figure 8.1   SCDPH MOD Squad strategic plan framework.

Trap. Feeling overwhelmed by CQI and not knowing where to start.

Tip. If you have a comprehensive strategic planning process, this is a great foundation to build upon. If not, start with people both interested and proficient in big-picture thinking. We recognized that the MOD Squad was *essential* to our ability to incorporate CQI concepts. In essence, it had built an infrastructure and organizational culture that provided a natural extension into the CQI world.

Second, in 2007, SCDPH became aware of the National Association of County and City Health Officials (NACCHO) accreditation preparation and quality improvement demonstration site grant, and was attracted to its strong CQI focus. As a successful grantee, SCDPH completed an agency self-assessment tool measuring capacity to meet the NACCHO metrics identified in the Operational Definition of a Functional Local Health Department, determined strengths and weaknesses, selected a CQI project focus, and completed the plan–do–study–act (PDSA) cycle. Working with CQI experts through the Public Health Foundation provided an opportunity to learn CQI tools and apply them in our practice.

Trap. Anticipating an overnight CQI revolution!

Tip. Start small, and incrementally build success toward the long-term goal of incorporating CQI into the organizational culture of your organization.

Last, as the chapter title suggests, "telling the story" is critical to providing evidence of the value of public health. It's not enough to achieve internal success; the outcomes must be shared with others to have an impact.

Trap. Getting so wrapped up in the CQI process itself that you forget to document your process and tell your story to others.

Tip. Be sure you maintain detailed documentation that helps capture history and project outcomes, provides a road map for the future, and assures sustainability. Answer the "so what?" question by telling your story to your stakeholders: the public, policymakers, funders, community partners, and so on.

HOW TO DO IT

SCDPH utilized the plan–do–study–act (PDSA) cycle for our CQI project. The following steps will walk you through our entire CQI journey and what we feel is essential in considering CQI for public health.

Prepare to Plan

1. Educate Staff on CQI Concepts and Processes. Before SCDPH could begin our project we had to learn the CQI language and tools, and how they could be applied to public health. The executive team received eight hours of training facilitated by Grace Duffy, a Public Health Foundation (PHF) consultant. A copy of the *Public Health Memory Jogger II,* a pocket guide of CQI methods, was provided to each participant as a "tool box" that assisted in identifying and determining the scope of our grant project.

> *Trap.* Lingo and acronym confusion! Public health, CQI, and strategic planning all have their own distinct languages. Terminology can be confusing at times!

> *Tip.* The *Public Health Memory Jogger II* is a helpful resource. However, substantial training on these tools is essential.

2. Build Support and Mobilize a Team. Because the department already had a strong strategic planning process in place, the groundwork for building support had already been established. By completing the CQI training exercises, the SCDPH executive team was able to recognize the importance of improving department performance to remain relevant in a challenging political climate and in the face of dwindling resources.

At the conclusion of the executive team training session a core CQI pilot team was selected. The CQI pilot team was charged with developing a team charter, which identified a few critical roles, for example, a team sponsor/champion of the process, a team leader to keep the group focused, organized, and on track, and core team members to offer expertise, ideas, opinions, and to share the workload. Our team included the health officer, emergency preparedness director, former community health assessment coordinator (currently the substance abuse director), and our strategic planning team facilitators, the regional laboratory director, and environmental health office manager.

> *Trap.* Letting the perception of a time-intensive process inhibit getting started.

> *Tip.* Secure broad buy-in early on. Identify staff who are committed and enabled to dedicate time to the process.

Plan the Project/Process [Plan]

3. Getting Started in Planning/Identify the Performance Gaps. We identified gaps in performance based on the executive team's completion of an agency self-assessment tool based on the metric from the NACCHO Operational Definition of a Functional Local Health Department. We utilized an electronic survey tool to tabulate and graph results. The areas found in greatest need of improvement based on low scores were:

- Essential Service I—Monitor health status and understand health issues facing the community
- Essential Service IX—Evaluate and improve programs
- Essential Service X—Contribute to and apply the evidence base of public health

4. Prioritize Based on Established Criteria. Since more than one performance gap was identified, we used the following criteria to determine which essential service would reap the most benefits of our pilot project:

- What area needs the most improvement?

- What area has the greatest potential impact in the organization?

- What is the most feasible gap to address?

Another major consideration in our selection was alignment of our activities with goals and actions already established in the department's strategic plan.

5. Select a Manageable Project Scope. As a beginner in the CQI process, SCDPH initially selected a project of conducting a community health assessment. Community assessment has been a core historical activity within SCDPH. In the past, however, the approach had been strictly strength-based, with close involvement of community partners.

During the past 12 years our community partners came out to assist in the development of a continuing project from the identification of the issues (problems) to the strengths needed to eliminate the issues by playing a major role in the development and implementation of the Community Health Assessment Initiative (CHAI). The commitment and the overall concern for the community of Saginaw were and continue to be evident.

One of the most ambitious projects was within the urban community. The Urban Regional Committee felt that the most important issue was the future of their neighborhoods and the condition of the families that dwelt within. The group identified urban blight and health concerns throughout the city, and as the process continued to evolve it became evident that they had their fingers on the pulse of the urban community.

The rural community, with a composition similar to the urban project, included stakeholders from the southern part of Saginaw County with representation from teachers, physicians, the board of commissioners, high school students, educators, faith-based organizations, farmers, and other civic leaders from the surrounding communities. These individuals were just as committed to identifying the rural issues and developing a plan to eliminate/reduce these concerns.

The CHAI process was primitive in nature but truly worked from within the community and drew the identification of the community issues from the "grass roots." Community leaders who were concerned about their families, friends, and neighborhoods developed into the leaders of the community (from the grass roots up) and, though different in approach, proceeded with the utmost commitment.

Using brainstorming, affinity diagrams, and fishbone diagrams in the CQI training session, the team quickly realized that embarking on a new, full communitywide assessment was too ambitious a project given the time constraints of the grant. These tools enabled the team to drill down to specific barriers to successfully completing a community health assessment. By identifying root causes for assessment challenges we were able to easily select a pilot project for improvement.

The team crafted a SMART (specific, measurable, attainable, realistic, timebound) aim statement for the project: *By May 15, 2008, we will conduct staff training on assessment methods to increase appropriate knowledge of standards and processes for conducting a community health assessment.*

> *Trap.* Don't try to do it all! Avoid making your first CQI effort a large-scale project that you always wanted to implement.

Tip. Be *realistic!* Remember to start at the beginning rather than rush to the end. Select a manageable project.

6. Develop Goals and Objectives. The core CQI pilot team met to complete the team charter, which identified objectives, success measures, and barriers to implementation of the project. See Figure 8.2.

2. Team name: CQI core team	3. Version: 1.0	4. Subject: Standard 1-C
5. Problem/opportunity statement:		
We are not currently conducting or contributing expertise to community health assessments.		We will implement PDCA for standard 1-C to meet the NACCHO pilot grant objectives.
6. Team sponsor: Natasha Coulouris, MPH, Health Officer, SCDPH		**7. Team leader and scribe:** Chris Harrington
8. Team members		**Area of expertise:**
1. Cheryl Plettenberg		Previous community health assessment experience
2. Tammy Theisen		Strategic planning
3. Pat Ritter		Strategic planning

9. Process improvement AIM (mission)

By May 15, 2008, we will conduct staff training on assessment methods to increase appropriate knowledge of standards and processes for conducting a community health assessment.

10. Scope (boundaries):

Key SCDPH staff as a subset of the broader public health system.

11. Customers (primary and other):	Customer needs addressed:
SCDPH executive team	Knowledge of assessment methods and tools to conduct community health assessments
SCDPH key staff	Knowledge of assessment methods and tools to conduct community health assessments

12. Objectives:

- Develop training module (curriculum) and guide
- Conduct training with knowledgeable instructor(s)
- Measure training conducted through pre- and post-test scores
- Identify the PDCA cycle to be used as the basis for our report

13. Success metrics (measures):	
Comparing pre- and post-test scores resulting in an increase in knowledge of assessment methods.	Posting the assessment guide/tools on the intranet for all staff access.
The training was conducted and completed within the given time frame.	A PDCA cycle is completed and a report/storyboard is generated

Figure 8.2   SCDPH CQI team charter.

14. Considerations (assumptions/constraints/obstacles/risks):

Severe time constraints that allow for less than six weeks to accomplish the grant objectives. No dedicated staff to accomplish the pilot project, thus adding additional workloads for already overloaded staff.

The infrastructure for conducting community health assessments has eroded due to loss of funding.

We assume that our training will increase the department's ability to conduct community health assessments.

15. Available resources	**16. Additional resources required:**
Cheryl Plettenberg—previous CHA experience. The core pilot team is committed to this project/grant. Grace Duffy—CQI consultant NACCHO tools MLC-2 guidebook and piloted health departments University of Michigan, SPH	University of Michigan, SPH—Prevention Research Center SVSU/Delta National and state experts United Way and Community Foundation assessments Saginaw Health Plan assessment

17. Key milestones:	**Date:**
A developed training module and guide to utilize	Mid-April
Training is conducted	End of April
Report is complete and turned into NACCHO	May 31, 2008

18. Communication plan (who, how, and when):

E-team and staff have already received an introduction to CQI processes and the language shift in December 2007.

E-team received training via CQI consultant from the PHF in March 2008.

Governing entities (BOC, BOH, advisory boards) will receive updates via the health officer's report monthly.

Other stakeholders (MALPH, MLC-3) will receive the report after 05/31/08.

MOD Squad involvement and updates will continue through facilitators and the strategic planning process monthly.

NACCHO and the PHF will receive the final report by 05/31/08.

The community will be informed of the results when a community health assessment is completed after May 2008.

19. Key stakeholders:	**Area of concern (as it relates to the charter):**
Board of health	The potential money and time spent for the process; how this will affect the overall operations of the department.
Board of commissioners	The potential money and time spent for the process; how this will affect the overall operations of the department.
SCDPH staff	This will generate more work and additional procedures to be followed.
Assessment partners	How this will integrate with our work/processes.
Community	The validity of this project and how it will affect services.

Figure 8.2   Continued.

7. Manage Your Progress. Many components of the process can occur simultaneously. Therefore, it is critical that the process be tracked through a tool such as a Gantt chart. This will help the team clearly understand individual roles and deadlines, stay focused, and progress throughout the process. Throughout the process, detailed documentation of meetings and CQI tools used as well as action registers and communication items is helpful in repeating the process. See Figure 8.3 for an example of the SCDPH Gantt project management worksheets.

8. Examine the Current Approach. A common CQI tool utilized for this step is to flowchart the current process. Since we did not have a current approach to providing assessment training, we completed a flowchart of the steps necessary to conducting assessment training.

Note in Figure 8.4 the innovative circular representation of the improvement process flow. This format reflects the iterative nature of the communitywide assessment learning process for a public health department. This is one of the brainstorming outcomes of the SCDPH leadership team project activities.

9. Identify Potential Solutions. Brainstorming during our CQI training session revealed several potential solutions to our performance gaps in monitoring health status. We achieved agreement on one solution through the development of our AIM statement to conduct staff assessment training. From there we brainstormed

Saginaw County Department of Public Health Gantt Chart
NACCHO Accreditation Pilot Grant 2008

Task: Saginaw County HD	29-Feb	7-Mar	14-Mar	21-Mar	28-Mar	1-Apr	10-Apr	15-Apr	21-Apr	1-May	8-May	13-May	19-May	27-May	28-May	6-Jun	13-Jun
Finalize self-assessment analysis	X																
Align with SCPHD Mod Squad	X																
Identify priority project	X																
Plan PHF consultant visit		X															
Set agenda and travel schedule		X															
Saginaw/PHF PI meeting			X														
Plan pilot PI project and milestones			X	X													
Validate PHF hours remaining			X		X			X		X		X	X		X		
Teleconference consultant update							X	X	X		X	X	X		X		
Decide team meeting schedule					X	1:30	2:30	1:30	10:00	10:30	10:00	10:00	9:00	9:00	10:00		
Hold formal team meetings					X	X	X	X	X	TRG	X	X	X	X	X		
Complete team charter					X												
Flowchart desired staff training proc							X										
Analyze causes of staff exp issues			X														
Select solutions as appropriate			X														
Design training		X	X	X	X	X	X	X									
Establish measures and outcomes							X	X				X	X				
Conduct training										X							
Gather measures and analyze											X	X				X	X
Analyze and modify process as needed												X	X	X	X	X	
Monitor competency levels (6 wk eval)																X	X
Measure pilot											X	X					
Create report of improved outcomes												X	X	X	X	X	X
Final report and storyboard														X	X		
Final NACCHO/PHF report by 5/30/08															X		

Legend: Complete ▭   Watch ▭   In progress ▭   Late or at risk ▮   Updated: 5/27/08

Figure 8.3   SCDPH CQI team project management Gantt chart.

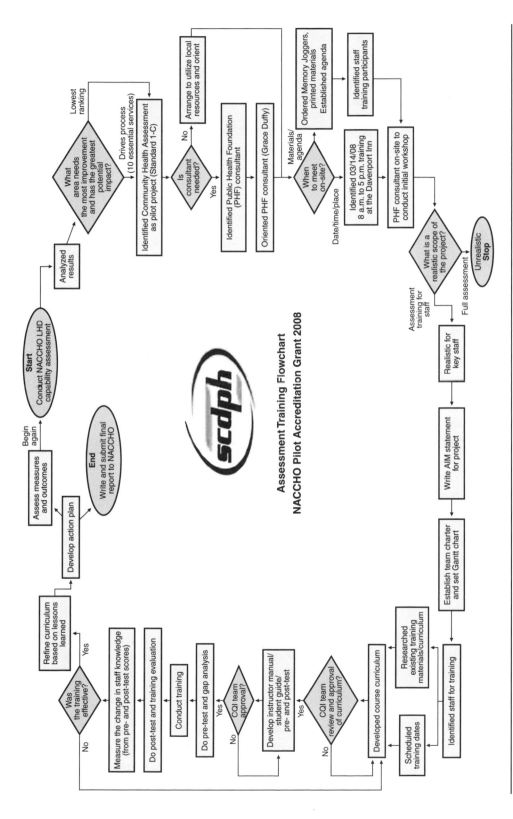

Figure 8.4 CQI team process flowchart for communitywide assessment training.

options for carrying out the project, including selecting the assessment model, the curriculum, and initial target audience.

A significant outcome of the brainstorming and improvement activities was the choice of the comprehensive *Mobilizing for Action through Planning and Partnerships* (MAPP) assessment model supported through the National Association of County and City Health Officials (NACCHO). This assessment model views the community through four perspectives:

1. Community themes and strengths assessments

2. Local public health system assessment

3. Community health status assessment

4. Forces of change assessment

Our previous strength-based community assessment model closely parallels the first MAPP perspective, including the additional three perspectives provided for internal operations, national comparison of data and trends, and a forward looking/visionary view as well.

Trap. Assuming you have to follow a cookie-cutter process for each step.

Tip. Some steps may occur simultaneously or at different points in the process. Be flexible.

10. Develop an Improvement Theory. To develop an improvement theory of *If . . . then . . .* the team charter can be useful to consider the objectives and success measures to formulate multiple improvement theories. Our improvement theories included:

- *If* we conduct training, *then* we will begin to increase knowledge and capacity in community health assessments.

- *If* a curriculum was developed to train staff on community health assessment, *then* the process could be sustained if key staff members left the agency.

- *If* a pre- and post-test were administered, *then* success of the training could be measured.

Implement the Plan [Do]

11. Test the Theory. This is the stage where implementation begins. Within the flowchart we included check points to evaluate the efficacy of our project. This helped keep the team focused on where we were in the PDSA cycle and offered opportunities to make midcourse adjustments. This also determined measures of success along the way.

Trap. It's easy to hand over this step to the "experts" or others outside the process.

Tip. Make sure the core team stays connected throughout the whole process to assure relevance and overall success.

Review the Process, Revise the Plan [Study]

12. Study the Results. After implementation of the project, results should be analyzed. You should ask yourselves—did we accomplish the success metrics? If not, why? Did we accomplish our objectives with this approach? If not, why?

Pre- and post-test content questions were administered during the pilot workshop to assess learner knowledge. The histogram in Figure 8.5 shows a varied response across the five questions administered. Three of the five questions showed an increase in learner ability. Two of the questions showed a slight decrease in performance. Analysis of the teaching methods suggests a better balance of content coverage when the workshop is rolled out on a permanent basis.

> *Trap.* A failure of one component of the process does not constitute a failure of the entire improvement effort.

> *Tip.* Celebrate your successes, and evaluate your failures.

Standardize the Improvement or Develop a New Theory [Act]

13. Act. The act phase is one in which you essentially begin again. A determination will need to be made on either standardizing the improvement to become operational, or developing a new theory. At this point the process will lead to the development of future plans.

> *Trap.* Don't drop the ball after studying the results, refine it!

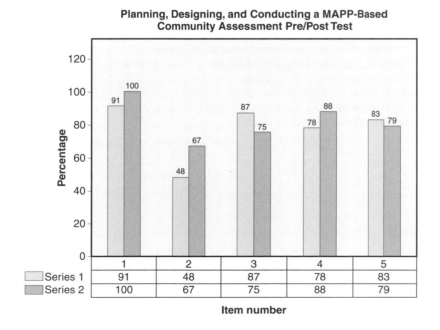

Figure 8.5   Histogram of pilot training pre- and post-test results.

Tip. Aligning the CQI process with the organization's strategic planning allows for the continuation of CQI in future plans.

14. Report Results. This is your opportunity to build further buy-in within your organization as well as external stakeholders and policy makers. A CQI success can provide evidence of the value of public health. *Tell your story . . .*

LESSONS LEARNED

The CQI pilot conducted as part of the NACCHO grant helped increase SCDPH awareness of CQI processes and tools. Furthermore, it moved us toward more fully integrating CQI with our daily operations. Some specific lessons learned of our process:

- The process initially appeared to be incredibly time-intensive to implement. However, upon completion of the CQI project we realized that the benefits outweighed the investment of time.

- Current mandates, performance standards, and reporting requirements may not directly reflect CQI processes; however, they often align with demonstrating performance outcomes. With the new focus on performance measurement, LHDs using CQI processes will have a competitive advantage.

- The first training for an expanded communitywide assessment is done, the worksheets are completed, the issues have been identified, plans have been initiated, and leaders and/or stakeholders who can make the difference have been assembled. CHAI was the catalyst to a beginning. The next few years, with the implementation of the four-phase MAPP approach as an enhancement to our historical strength-based assessment results, will make a difference in our ability to support the community.

- Everyone involved in this process had to accept that there is a learning curve in regard to CQI, strategic planning, and public health terminology.

- This grant project exposed staff to the CQI process, terminology, and concepts but did not necessarily fully prepare us for implementing CQI in other areas of work. We realize that each renewed cycle of CQI will bring us toward integration of CQI throughout our department.

WEB LINKS

- SCDPH—www.saginawpublichealth.org
- NACCHO—www.naccho.org
- MPHI-MLC-2—www.accreditation.localhealth.net
- Public Health Foundation—www.phf.org

Chapter 9

Creating Lasting Change

Kathleen F. (Kay) Edwards

INTRODUCTION

Though most people talk about the ubiquitous nature of change, there also is talk about the rapidity of change. We lament that things are "always changing," that there is no time to catch up and just think about and plan for the future, much less decide what is worthwhile from earlier and ongoing efforts.

This seems to be the case for most industries, and public health, as part of the rapidly changing healthcare industry, is no exception: public health agencies are often asked to make numerous changes such that it can be difficult to implement the changes decided on in such a way that they become a part of the fabric of the agency. What is new today quickly becomes old and forgotten, while the public health agency is required to move on to new and ever expanding areas of growth. Managing change becomes a critical skill for all public health workers, not just those in top leadership roles.

Quality improvement (QI) has many things to offer public health. One of them is to help workers deal effectively with change, and to help make effective change last. And another concept that QI has taught us is that improvement usually involves change, learning from one's experiences, and a need to understand the social context of the change—times, places, and situations.[1]

A final thought by way of introduction to this chapter is that those who work in governmental systems often find that their roles seem more complex than those same roles in private industry. The reasons that are given for this assessment include that public sector organizations tend to focus on predictability and stability. Those who study governmental organizations believe that public sector organizations are governed by more complicated relationships, with entry into the organization limited to those with firmly set qualifications, that tasks are narrowly defined and controlled by rules, and that power is "distributed in a clear hierarchy."[2]

To the extent that these findings are accurate, QI efforts in public health may need very creative handling to assure that when improvements are reached, the continuous nature of QI's concept is supported in an ongoing way.

CHANGE MANAGEMENT THEORIES, FOCUSING ON STAGES OF CHANGE AND CHANGE MANAGEMENT STYLE

Change in public health is sometimes likened by those who work in the field to being in "white water"—the surging, foaming, turbulent movement of water that can toss boats and people away from their desired destinations. Public health is thought to be in white water because its timelines are often set by others, because there are priorities that compete for the same resources, and because challenges to the health of the community can change from day to day, while the most recent challenge still demands full attention. There are other reasons why public health workers feel pressure; some of these perceptions relate to the political realities of the jurisdictions served. Some perceptions relate to how the community views a particular health department or other public health agency. And some perceptions have no basis in fact, dinosaurs that are remnants of earlier times.

The people who write about change tell us that change can come about in a patterned way, moving from an identification of a need for change, to putting something different—a change—in place, followed by the settling in of the change, leading eventually to a need for another change.[3] The concept of the cyclical nature of change forms the basis for some of our thinking about change, implying that it should actually be expected, not considered unnatural or unhealthy. Lewin described a three-step model of change involving unfreezing of the status quo, movement toward a desired end or state, and refreezing of the new change to make it "permanent."

There are downsides to change, and when these occur it is difficult to create effective, lasting change. One downside of change management happens when people resist the change, for a variety of reasons. Fear of the unknown, or of discomfort, or of someone believing that she or he may be found lacking in some way are some of the reasons that people demonstrate a resistance to change. Fear of a potential loss of status or power can be another reason for resisting change, as can also be a perceived threat to one's values and ideals, or even just resentment of interference with what one is doing.

In order to deal with change resistance, we're told that knowing why the change is coming is key. People want to trust that those who are telling them about the change have their interests at heart, somewhere in the planning. The people who will be asked, for instance, in a public health department, to implement a change will have a much higher success rate in working with that change and making it last if they are involved in the planning phase for the change. Though this goal may not always be possible, public health workers tell us that when their opinions are sought before the decision about how to go about making the change is put in place they are much more likely to participate wholeheartedly in the change process. I've often heard public health, and other, workers say, " . . . why didn't they ask what I thought? I work with that problem every day and I have some good ideas on how it might be fixed. . . . " The latter statement of the worker also links with quality improvement since part of the QI approach emphasizes that those closest to an identified problem or concern are usually the ones who know the solutions to those problems.

Some authors have actually described situations where there is movement toward workers in organizations *embracing* change. What was found in these authors' research is that when respondents described change situations, they made positive statements in a ratio of 1.9 positive statements to every 1.0 negative statement. The authors suggest that not only is resistance to change undergoing change but that the term "resistance to change" needs further clarification, since resistance can include " . . . willful opposition, valuable passion, or energy and paradox."[4]

And this input raises another link to quality and creating lasting change, which is that quality links to creating lasting change when public health workers appreciate that their attitudes toward change have an effect on how well they carry out their public health roles: that when they plan for change, the time needed to move back to former levels of productivity will be shorter and that the loss of productivity will be less.

Quality also is linked with change management when public health workers value that though they may not always be able to plan for change in the orderly and meaningful way they would like, they can control their response to change by using effective change management strategies.

Effective change management strategies are those that lead to the desired change and those that contribute to creating lasting change.

A part of an effective change management strategy can include an awareness of one's own way of dealing with change. Musselwhite discusses three main preferences that people may have for responding to change in a certain way and tells us that all three of the change style preferences are needed.[5] Though each of us may show a preference for one of these three categories of change response, we also may embody preferences of the other two categories, as well.

The first of the change management style preferences, mentioned in this chapter in no particular order, is a conservative, or traditional, approach where the person likes to keep things as they are, believing that stance to be best for preserving best practices in a public health agency. Others may label this tendency to conserve the past as inflexible or overly cautious.

The second preference leans toward a more middle-of-the-road position, sometimes referred to as a pragmatist. The person who often sees both sides of an issue fairly equally and may appear flexible when viewed complimentarily, or unwilling or unable to commit when viewed negatively.

The third preference is toward the creative, free-flowing, sometimes called innovative or quixotic, preference in dealing with change. Innovators often come up with new ideas but prefer that others work them through and implement them.

When a person chooses or uses a change style preference, she or he is offering an opportunity for quality to enter into the process. I say this because if people have choices as to how they will deal with a given situation, the combined effect of each person's change style preference may enrich a decision. It's said that creativity and innovation are heightened with diversity of views and backgrounds of the people involved. To the extent that this is true, then having on a public health team the innovative, the conservative, and the pragmatist approaches to change could lead to more effective change outcomes. Yes, it also is said that such diversity on a team can mean that more time will be needed to assure common definitions and goals, but when the time is available, using the strength of each type of change style preference should lead to a higher-quality outcome.

CHANGE MANAGEMENT THEORIES AND PRINCIPLES FOUNDATIONAL TO QUALITY IMPROVEMENT

One of the key components of change management related to quality improvement in public health is setting the stage for motivation to change. We've learned that when people are prepared for change, they seem to do better with it. And motivation for anything includes how hard a person moves toward an identified goal. So if change as a part of a QI process in a public health setting is desired, the workforce in that public health setting will need motivation in order to move toward that goal.

What has been found is that in order for a goal to be met, the challenge associated with it must be attainable and needs to be presented in such a way that we realize it's possible to be reached. Also, if people participate in setting their own goals, they may be more accepting of difficult goals, even if they are arbitrarily assigned a task.[6] It also may be helpful to consider that when implementing quality improvement efforts in public health settings, a small number of "key influencers" may be able to move the QI agenda forward in the whole organization.

What also has been found is that though employees are generally expected to keep the health of their organization as their key focus, at the same time they may be asked to make changes that produce short-term results. The balance that workers need to achieve—of keeping the long-term renewing change in mind, while at the same time producing short-term results—is one that calls for managing balance.[7]

Another aspect of understanding lasting change is that many employees feel pressured to let go of the "old" and to adopt new methods and procedures. There is wisdom to sometimes retaining what are called "embedded business practices." These are the tried and true methods, the successful things that represent " . . . the way we do business . . ." These can be considered a strength, since without such embedded constructs, organizations would probably be in chaos and paralyzed by not knowing what to do. The key—as with the balance needed to manage short- and long-term organizational needs—is to know that sometimes when times change, companies also need to; and this is when things can be more of a challenge, since constructs are difficult to change.

Those making basic change can look to research that suggests that there are some tips to making tactical changes:

- Analyze reasons for the disconnect between "the way we used to" and "what today needs" and discuss the need for change.

- Make business relationships *before* they're needed, and develop them in other than structured business meetings.

- Involve a broad range of people in designing basic but major change.

- Showcase, rather than pilot, the change.

- Look for winnable opportunities and choose your timing.

- Have more than one project going on for the same underlying problem.

CHANGE MANAGEMENT CONSIDERATIONS IN QI ACTIVITIES

In thinking about how best to carry out QI activities, knowing that change will be a part of those activities, there needs to be a focus on the stakeholders: who, and what, may be helped by this change and who may perceive that they may be harmed by it? An analysis can be carried out at the agency level to determine this balance and to try to resolve any conflicts that are detected. One way to prevent negative reaction to QI activities can be the inclusion of as many as possible of the key stakeholders in the planning of the activity prior to implementation. In that way, reservations about the activity can begin to be addressed early on, and later implementation and feedback parts of the QI process can be strengthened.

Another thing to consider as part of QI planning relates to the thought that public health leaders have many additional duties besides assuring that quality improvement efforts are in place and ongoing. To the extent that there are in a public health agency, it's hoped that able, willing, and interested others can assist the public health leader(s) to design, implement, and evaluate QI activities. The public health leader may want to delegate this role and still demonstrate that the QI aspect of the agency is seen as crucial.

An objection that is sometimes heard in relation to QI activities is that finding the time to carry out regular duties while also taking on something new can be troublesome. If one of the basic tenets of QI work is that in order for QI to be done well it should be thought of as part of everything that a public health agency does, then the public health agency's leader(s) sharing that philosophy will be crucial to the acceptance of the philosophy.

In order to move ahead of this criticism of QI, communicating within, and without, the public health setting about the change that QI may bring about is wise. These are some tips toward effective communication about change:

- Don't rely on one, loud, obvious announcement to persuade.

- Specify the nature of the change in the form of tangible goals.

- Discuss the need for the change.

- Let everyone know the scope of the change, even if it includes what some may perceive as "bad news."

- Those involved with the QI effort will want to ensure buy-in to the change by using consistent words and actions.

- Training may be needed to enable public health workers to obtain the necessary knowledge and skills.

- If the progress of work toward the goal is charted, the change process will be seen as more than rhetoric.[8]

In designing successful approaches to QI linked to change management, public health workers can benefit by thoughtful planning and implementation on the part of the organization and its leaders and managers. Here are some suggestions drawn from general management literature to assist public health settings to make and keep needed change:

- Set the stage for change.

- Decide what to do.

- Make it happen.

- Make it stick.

- Create a sense of urgency.

- Help others see the need for change and the importance of acting quickly.

- Pull together the guiding team. Develop the change, vision, and strategy.

- Clarify how the future will be different from the past.

- Clarify how the future can be made real.

- Communicate for understanding and buy-in.

- Ensure that others understand and accept the vision and strategy.

- Empower others to act.

- Make sure there is in place a powerful group, with necessary skills, to guide the change.

- Remove as many barriers as possible.

- Produce short-term wins.

- Don't let up: press harder and faster after first successes, and if first efforts produce "failure," still press on, to help determine what may have gone wrong.

- Create a new culture.

- Hold on to the new ways of behaving and make sure they succeed until they become strong enough to replace old traditions.

FACILITATING SUSTAINABLE CHANGE MANAGEMENT IN PUBLIC HEALTH SETTINGS

In order to make it easier to sustain change in a public health setting, one of the things that leaders can do is to consider that when making change and wanting it to "stick," the willingness of top management to provide for planning, allocation of resources, and compensation are all important.

Other considerations to help you know if what is planned may take hold in the organization:

- Try to always start by determining whether the change that is needed for the QI effort requires a change in attitude or behavior, since the QI tools and methods to be used will vary depending on which it may be.

- It is good to develop a vision for the QI effort, and to have a chance to talk about what the future of the organization may look like once the change is in place, including posing possible scenarios of the results of the change.

- It is easier to create lasting QI change if you know early on what the possible barriers to the identified changes will be.

- Some assessment of the particular situation would be good, along with creating a sense of urgency that this is a significant issue in the life of the public health setting.

When things change in the public health setting, there will be possible stress and trauma. If those who are impacted by the QI changes can be helped to deal with any resulting pain, and have time to grieve, if such should occur, the better the lasting change can be solidified.

THINGS TO AVOID

Here are some things that public health settings can do to help prevent failure when developing, designing, implementing, and evaluating QI changes:

- Make the agency's QI rationale, plan, evaluation tools, and QI practices as explicit as possible, just in case the change wasn't communicated clearly, and as a result the change seems to be perceived by workers as a loss of personal control. Other reasons for making sure the components of the QI activities are clear include maintaining honesty in the organization.

- Involve other persons in planning and implementing QI changes.

- Use logic and appeals to knowledge and facts and avoid fallacious logic and that which may use false or misleading information, including deception and errors in reasoning.

- Avoid using position power to reward and punish since it may not garner the support for QI efforts that a public health setting would want.

EVALUATION OF QI ACTIVITIES AND CHANGE

In order to evaluate whether change will be lasting, one of the first things to consider is whether what is being planned and implemented is on sure footing ethically. QI activities are linked to several ethics principles, as are discussed more fully in Chapter 28 of this handbook. Here is a brief review of ethics principles involved in change. By knowing ethics principles that relate to change management, public health leaders can reinforce the strong ethics roots of public health's history, as well as public health's continuing involvement in social issues that affect the health and well-being of the entire community of interest:

- Honesty

- Truth telling, sometimes including speaking *truth to power*, which can relate to public servants giving unbiased advice about the policies they wish to pursue

- Fairness

- Respect for persons

- Justice

- Equity

Those working in QI activities in public health, for instance, will want to show honesty and truth telling in all aspects of the QI process, not simply because the truth will eventually emerge but to show respect—another ethics principle—for those involved in QI activities. If there is a disconnect between what public health workers have heard about QI initiatives and what the reality is, the QI efforts could be stymied or doomed.

Fairness must be exercised in choosing communities to engage in the QI process; workers to participate in planning, implementing, data gathering, evaluating, and redesign will be needed in all phases of the process; and standards to be employed will need to be applied evenhandedly across the full range of QI activities. The demonstrations of justice and equity that these suggestions provide should bring good will and a desire for involvement in QI efforts.

Other considerations beyond ethics, when evaluating whether the change brought about by QI efforts is lasting, can be measured by available QI tools: obtaining baseline data, data along the way, and final data can form the basis for comparisons with identified indicators of progress. Anecdotal data also can be valuable, from employees, the community, and other interested parties, to determine if there is a "sense" that the change is lasting. Given that human perception also can be impacted by subjective inputs, having trend data combined with insights and informed opinion may serve as the richest measure of lasting impact.

CONCLUSION AND DISCUSSION

As those who care about public health move forward to strengthen public health practice in the community, there are some basic concepts from the healthcare literature that can help focus our thinking. These are:

- Individual disciplines/professions in public health must collaborate with others outside of public health agencies in order to solve public health problems.

- Some very key collaborations are needed, for instance with medical care and business communities.

- The current national investment strategy in health needs revision.

- The United States needs to move beyond simply identifying health disparities and risk factors and move toward advocacy and targeting of public health effort.

To the extent that these concepts are true, efforts toward improving quality in public health settings should help strengthen public health practice by encouraging collaborations, by refocusing investment strategies toward initiatives that have been tested, and by providing a results orientation that can help target those most in need of public health services.

Chapter 10

Accreditation As a Means for Quality Improvement

Penney Davis, MPH, Julia Joh Elligers, MPH, and
Jessica Solomon, MCP

HISTORY OF PUBLIC HEALTH DEPARTMENT ACCREDITATION

Over the past 20 years, several large-scale efforts have significantly influenced public health practice and initiated a movement toward national accreditation of public health departments. The 1988 Institute of Medicine (IOM) report, *The Future of Public Health,* declared public health to be in disarray and prompted national discussion about the status of public health and the steps necessary to strengthen its role. With public health defined as "what we as a society do collectively to assure the conditions in which people can be healthy," the report contained proposals for ensuring that public health service programs are efficient and effective enough to deal with relevant public health issues for the present and future.[1]

The three core functions of public health (assessment, assurance, policy development) developed by the IOM's 1988 report were widely accepted among public health's policy and academic community, but they did not explain to legislators or the general public what public health does on a daily basis. In 1994, a Public Health Steering Committee developed the *10 essential public health services* (EPHS) as a means to provide a working definition of public health and a guiding framework for the responsibilities of the local public health system.[2]

In 2003, the IOM reexamined the state of public health in its report, *The Future of the Public's Health in the 21st Century.* Of particular relevance in the updated report was the charge to strengthen "governmental public health infrastructure, which forms the backbone of the public health system."[3] In addition, the report called for establishment of a national steering committee to consider whether an accreditation system would be useful for improving and building state and local health agency capacities.

Within its Futures Initiative, the Centers for Disease Control and Prevention (CDC) identified accreditation as a key strategy for strengthening public health infrastructure.[4] In addition, several states already managed statewide accreditation or related initiatives for local health departments. Within this context, in 2004 the Robert Wood Johnson Foundation (RWJF) convened public health stakeholders

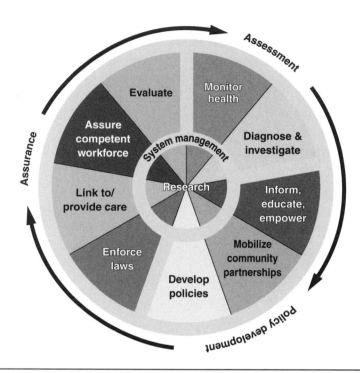

Figure 10.1   Relationship between the three core functions and the 10 essential public
health services.

Source: Public Health Services Steering Committee, *Public Health in America* (1994).
http://www.health.gov/phfunctions/public.htm.

to determine whether a voluntary national accreditation program for state and
local public health departments should be explored further. The consensus was to
proceed, and with support from the RWJF and the CDC, the Exploring Accreditation project was launched.

In 2005, the Exploring Accreditation steering committee and work groups
undertook a year-long investigation into determining the feasibility and desirability of a voluntary national accreditation program for public health departments.
In September 2006, after extensive research and input from the public health field,
the steering committee concluded that a voluntary national accreditation program for state, local, tribal, and territorial public health departments was both
feasible and desirable, and recommended moving forward with implementation.
Chief among the reasons to move ahead was the opportunity to advance the quality, accountability, and credibility of governmental public health departments in
a proactive manner.

ACCREDITATION AS A MEANS FOR QUALITY IMPROVEMENT

The goal of the national accreditation program is to improve and protect the
health of the public by advancing the quality and performance of public health

departments.* Accreditation establishes standards and benchmarks for the provision of essential public health services, engages health departments in ongoing quality improvement, and validates that communities are served by governmental health departments that meet national standards. Accreditation is also a public mechanism to hold health departments accountable to their governing boards, policy makers, and the communities they serve. The national accreditation program will not only recognize high achievers but will also bring national attention and resources to bear on quality and performance improvement for all health departments (HDs) that choose to participate. The Public Health Accreditation Board (PHAB) presents a unique opportunity to improve governmental public health capacity at the state, local, territorial, and tribal levels.

The Exploring Accreditation Final Recommendations report provides the general framework that is guiding the development and describes several features of the program.[5] A key component in this, and other, accreditation programs is a self-assessment based on standards and measures. Health departments will undertake a self-assessment to measure themselves against the standards and measures of PHAB. Along with scores, health departments must provide evidence to illustrate how they meet the standards and measures. Results from the self-assessment will be reviewed during a site visit and will lead to a determination of accreditation status. The process of conducting a self-assessment along with interpreting the results provides a tremendous learning opportunity for health departments. Not only will the assessment show areas of great strength, but it will also illustrate areas where a health department needs to improve capacity.

Since PHAB standards are focused on overall health department capacity, health departments will improve their understanding of where they fall short of meeting the 10 essential public health services. Quality improvement (QI) processes can then be used to work toward meeting the standards. Further, when a health department meets a standard or measure, work need not end there. It was agreed that the bar for national standards should be set at a level that assures public health protection—above the minimum—and that the national program needs to encourage quality improvement, regardless of how a health department is performing. In this way, achieving accreditation status is not only feasible but also identifies opportunities for continuous improvement. It is in this way that health departments can use QI in very discrete ways to focus on areas where there is little capacity, as well as ingrain QI into health department culture. Quality improvement will enable health departments to enhance their performance and their ability to protect, promote, and preserve health.

With the emergence of a voluntary national accreditation program, QI has moved to the forefront of interest in the public health community, with its definitions and applications the subject of much debate. While QI is not a new concept—

---

* Committees and work groups are developing the standards and measures; the procedures to assess health departments; a "substantial equivalency recognition" process to accommodate existing state-based accreditation and related programs that are closely aligned with PHAB's program; fees and incentives for participation; and a research and evaluation plan. Draft standards will be publicly vetted for comment in spring 2009, and a beta testing phase is scheduled to begin in late summer 2009. It is anticipated that the first applications for national accreditation will be accepted in 2011.

having emerged at the end of the 13th century with guilds that developed strict rules for products and services—it is a relatively new idea in the field of public health.[6] One explanation for what constitutes QI is described below:

> *QI activities are conducted using variations on a four-step method: (a) identify (determine what to improve), (b) analyze (understand the problem), (c) develop hypotheses (determine what change[s] will improve the problem), and (d) test and implement, or plan, do, study, act (PDSA). In the fourth step, the solution is tested to see whether it yields an improvement; the results are then used to decide whether to implement, modify, or abandon the proposed solution. If the tested solution does not achieve desired results, the process cycles back to the third step for reiteration. If the results are achieved, the solution is implemented on a larger scale and monitored over time for continuous improvement.[7]*

The notion of defining a problem and working to understand the cause is familiar territory to practitioners. Public health's challenge with QI is to first understand the processes used in public health, then change those processes in order to improve by undertaking the PDSA process. Public health practitioners often want to "do, do, do." Quality improvement requires that the enthusiasm to act be balanced by evaluation to determine just how well the "doing" is working. This is where accreditation fits in.

Achieving accreditation and implementing QI processes can not be accomplished overnight; therefore, many health departments are beginning to prepare for accreditation while the national program is being developed. Although created before the conception of a national accreditation program, a number of tools and processes are in place now that can assist local health departments specifically in preparing to meet accreditation standards and measures. Notably, the application of the Operational Definition, Mobilizing for Action Through Planning and Partnerships (MAPP), National Public Health Performance Standards Program (NPHPSP), and Project Public Health Ready (PPHR) provide experiences, develop competencies, and enhance local public health system and agency capacity, which can be applied to accreditation preparation. These programs are described in more detail in the next section.

ACCREDITATION PREPARATION TOOLS

Operational Definition of a Functional Health Department

The 1988 IOM report specifically acknowledged the difficultly in "defining what constitutes an adequate operational definition of a governmental presence at the local level," and stated that, "No citizen from any community, no matter how small or remote, should be without identifiable and realistic access to the benefits of public health protection, which is possible only through a local component of the public health delivery system."[8]

Operational Definition of a Functional Local Health Department

Regardless of varying capacity, authority, and resources, local health departments (LHDs) have a consistent responsibility to intentionally coordinate all public health activities and lead efforts to meet the 10 essential public health services. With these thoughts in mind, the National Association of County and City Health Officials convened work groups in 2005 and systematically, and iteratively, created the Operational Definition of a Functional Local Health Department. The Operational Definition is a shared understanding of what people in any community, regardless of size, can reasonably expect from their governmental LHD (see Figure 10.2). The standards are framed around the 10 essential public health services and were reworded to more accurately reflect the specific LHD roles and responsibilities related to each category. Moreover, the Operational Definition standards and measures serve as the framework for accreditation standards and measures.

LHDs that assess how well they fulfill the functions outlined in the Operational Definition and engage in capacity-building quality improvement activities will likely be better prepared for accreditation. To that end, the standards and measures from the Operational Definition were developed into a tool titled the *Local Health Department Self-Assessment Tool for Accreditation Preparation.* The Local Health Department self-assessment tool allows LHDs to measure themselves against the Operational Definition and identify areas of strength and areas for improvement.

Using a scale of 0–4, local health departments score each Operational Definition measure based on a self-assessment of the health department's capacity to fulfill each measure. This includes both capacity provided by the health department staff and capacity provided through contracts and/or agreements with other entities. The tool also contains a section labeled "Documents and/or Activities That Demonstrate That the Indicator Has Been Met," which provides examples of documentation and types of activities that be can used as a reference in determining capacity for each indicator. While LHDs may choose not to document this information as part of this self-assessment process, these examples may be useful to

---

The operational definition comprises ten standards:

1. Monitor health status and understand health issues facing the community.

2. Protect people from health problems and health hazards.

3. Give people information they need to make healthy choices.

4. Engage the community to identify and solve health problems.

5. Develop public health policies and plans.

6. Enforce public health laws and regulations.

7. Help people receive health services.

8. Maintain a competent public health workforce.

9. Evaluate and improve programs and interventions.

10. Contribute to and apply the evidence base of public health.

Figure 10.2   The 10 essential public health services as written in the Operational Definition of a Functional Local Health Department.

consider as documentation will be required in the national accreditation program. Many LHDs have used this tool to enhance their understanding of their agency activities, to increase staff interest in quality improvement, and to increase their ability to meet accreditation standards in the future. Once PHAB standards and measures are available in draft form, they will replace the standards in the Operational Definition for the purposes of accreditation preparation, yet the Operational Definition will remain important in defining the work of local public health practice, that is, what everyone has a right to expect from the governmental public health presence at the local level.

Mobilizing for Action through Planning and Partnerships

Mobilizing for Action Through Planning and Partnerships (MAPP) is a communitywide strategic planning process for improving community health and strengthening local public health systems. Facilitated by public health leadership, MAPP provides a framework that helps communities prioritize public health issues, identify resources for addressing them, and develop, implement, and evaluate community health improvement plans. The result of MAPP is not a strategic plan for the LHD; rather, MAPP results in a strategic plan for the entire community (see Figure 10.3).

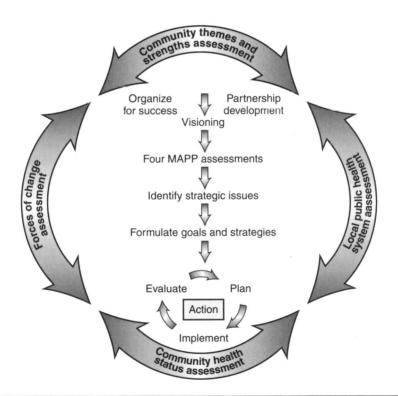

Figure 10.3 Diagram of the MAPP process.

The MAPP process combines a series of six distinct phases designed to facilitate development of a community-derived and community-owned strategic plan. Communities begin by organizing, planning, and developing partnerships (phase one). Following this initial planning phase, community members develop a collective vision of their ideal community (phase two) and, with their vision as a guide, complete the following four complementary assessments (phase three):

- The Local Public Health System Assessment, which is completed using the National Public Health Performance Standards Program (NPHPSP) local instrument,* measures the capacity of a LPHS to deliver the 10 essential public health services.

- The Forces of Change Assessment identifies forces (for example, trends, factors, or events) that are occurring or might occur in the future that influence the health and quality of life in a community.

- The Community Themes and Strengths Assessment collects information about local assets and challenges identified by community residents.

- The Community Health Status Assessment identifies priority community health and quality of life issues.

These four assessments reveal community challenges and strengths and provide a comprehensive picture of public health in a locality. In subsequent phases of the MAPP process, the assessment data are used to identify the strategic issues (phase four) a community should address in order to reach its vision. After identifying strategic issues, communities formulate goals and strategies (phase five) and then enter an action cycle (phase six), which is a continuous quality improvement process involving planning, implementation, and evaluation.

The MAPP process can help local health departments better position themselves for accreditation in several ways. Activities conducted during a MAPP process will make significant contributions toward fulfilling seven of the Operational Definition standards (1, 3, 4, 5, 7, 9, and 10). For instance, the Operational Definition includes conducting a community health assessment, which is one activity completed during the MAPP process. In addition, completing the National Public Health Performance Standards Program local instrument helps local health departments identify which entities provide specific essential services in a community. According to the Operational Definition, if a local health department does not directly provide an essential public health service, it should *assure* that services are being provided by another entity within the community. MAPP helps local health departments establish formal relationships to *assure* that when it can not deliver an essential service, another organization is able to fulfill the needed capacity. Because local health departments are the backbone of public health systems, the MAPP process benefits both the health department and the entire local public health system.[9]

---

* Many local and state health departments and boards of health use the NPHPSP instruments independent of a MAPP process. For more information on NPHPSP, visit http://www.cdc.gov/od/ocphp/nphpsp/.

Project Public Health Ready

Project Public Health Ready (PPHR) is a competency-based training and recognition program that assesses preparedness and helps local health departments or groups of local health departments working collaboratively as a region to respond to emergencies. It builds preparedness capacity and capability through a continuous quality improvement process of planning, training, and exercising. This process both reveals needed improvements and highlights strengths. As a result of completing an exercise or responding to a real event, local health departments must create an After Action Report and/or an Incident Action Plan that includes a plan of correction for gaps in their response, training, and exercise plan. The health departments must then create a future exercise plan that clearly shows a process of continuous quality improvement, with specific and measurable objectives.[10] Each of the three PPHR project goals—all-hazards preparedness planning, workforce capacity development, and demonstration of readiness through exercises or real events—has a comprehensive list of standards that must be met in order to achieve PPHR recognition.

Through PPHR, health departments conduct a readiness assessment, document their ability to meet PPHR standards, participate in a review process, receive feedback on areas of strength and weakness, and await a final determination on whether all criteria have been adequately addressed. While the national accreditation program standards will not focus on program-specific areas like preparation, the PPHR application process is an example of how local health departments experienced with PPHR would be familiar with the similar application process of national accreditation. In addition, PPHR offers a regional model that allows health departments to improve their understanding and capacity to share services. This model supports a collaborative approach between health departments to work together to meet standards, and joint applications will be accepted in the national accreditation program. More than 152 local health departments have already been recognized through PPHR.

ONE STEP AHEAD: STORIES FROM THE FIELD

The following stories provide brief examples of how the use of the Operational Definition, PPHR, MAPP, and NPHPSP can help to position local health departments for accreditation preparation and quality improvement.

Profile 1: Coconino County Health Department, Arizona

Interview with Barbara L. Worgess, MPH, Director
Population served: 130,000 people
Jurisdiction: County includes a mix of urban, rural, suburban, and frontier areas.

Engaging in MAPP, PPHR, and Using the Operational Definition. For Coconino County Health Department (CCHD), engaging in MAPP, PPHR, and using the Operational Definition were all done as a means to improve public health practice. As with all local health departments, CCHD has limited resources and does the best it can; however, it also acknowledges that the health department can do things better and more efficiently. For that reason, Barbara Worgess, Director of CCHD, decided to use MAPP and the NPHPSP, followed by Project Public Health Ready, and finally the Operational Definition.

CCHD took full advantage of the different QI tools and processes available to local health departments. Though MAPP and NPHPSP are processes that focus on the entire public health system, CCHD felt that the information captured through working so closely with system partners would inform an agency strategic plan. Because the MAPP process uses four different assessments, it provides multiple lenses through which the public health system can view itself. Worgess also felt that NPHPSP "brought all of the system partners together, which afforded us the opportunity to educate our partners about what public health is and what falls under the responsibility of the health department as well as the system partners. It was such a success that partners are still talking about it!" PPHR provided a framework to capture and document work that was required by the Centers for Disease Control and Prevention and show that CCHD was "ready." With the Operational Definition, the health department felt that it described what it really ought to be doing, so when NACCHO offered the demonstration sites project,* Worgess felt that it was time to measure CCHD against the standards in the Operational Definition: "The Operational Definition keeps appearing as a relevant model and framework for describing the work that we do in public health departments, particularly as it relates to accreditation."

Improving Practice, Getting Ready for Accreditation. All in all, MAPP, NPHPSP, PPHR, and the Operational Definition helped Coconino County Health Department improve public health practice. "In each case, using the tool or process allowed us to see how we measured up to nationally recognized standards and where we need to focus on improvement," noted Worgess. "We helped our partners recognize that there is a public health system, and that they are important partners in it." The local health department's strategic plan, developed after working with system partners on the MAPP process, allowed CCHD to modify the staffing plan to hire staff that later had the responsibility and authority to undertake the Operational Definition project. Worgess describes one benefit as, "Working through PPHR, to be recognized, allowed us to develop and use an animal evacuation plan during a real-life wildfire evacuation, that otherwise wouldn't have been developed. Thus, undertaking these activities allowed us to do our existing work better and determine where improvement was needed." In Coconino County, all-hazards preparedness planning includes animals!

Looking ahead, Worgess feels that "viewing the health department through different lenses and using QI techniques, as in the case of the Operational Definition project, continues to allow us to build capacity and be ready for accreditation in 2011." While the processes have different focuses and were undertaken for different reasons, they are interrelated. CCHD acknowledged that each process is valuable for what it offers, and they continue to work on improving so as to be ready for accreditation. Worgess noted that, "These tools present frameworks

---

* NACCHO's demonstration sites project provided grants to LHDs to use the LHD Self-Assessment Tool, identify an area for improvement, and either implement a QI process or work collaboratively with neighboring LHDs to develop a mechanism for improvement.

for working through processes that build local health department capacity and allow us to understand—and work within—the public health system in Coconino County. Rather than serving as extra work, we have begun integrating these activities into our daily lives and the culture of Coconino County Health Department, all as a means to become better."

Profile 2: North Central District Health Department, Idaho

Interview with Carol Moehrle, RN, District Director
Population served: 110,000 people
Jurisdiction: The North Central District includes five counties and covers 13,500 square miles.

Project Public Health Ready Recognition and Regionalization. The PPHR process is similar to the process proposed in the national accreditation program. In the North Central District Health Department in Idaho, Carol Moehrle and her fellow district health directors jumped on the opportunity to apply for Project Public Health Ready recognition for one reason: "We knew we could succeed! And if we did, we could be the first state on the map to have full statewide PPHR recognition. It's a big deal to have that recognition; our state loves it and our boards love it." Acknowledging that preparing to meet the large number of PPHR standards could sound daunting to staff, Moehrle framed it as a challenge instead. "We told them that we needed to put our money where our mouths were and prove how good we were. So when the recognition came through, everyone was really excited that it was acknowledged by an external party." Looking ahead, Moehrle acknowledges that PPHR was a great first step in introducing local health department staff to standards so they could experience small successes before taking on accreditation.

Working in a District/Regional Model. Idaho moved from a county-based public health model to seven public health districts, or regions, in the 1970s. Though Moehrle admits it didn't happen overnight, there are a number of advantages to a district approach: "Consistent public health coverage for the entire population is probably the biggest advantage. It took a while to get implemented, but decreases in administrative costs and increases in efficiency have been well noted." Through the district model they have been able to provide more access to public health services, especially to counties with small populations that couldn't otherwise afford to provide services. Moehrle figured that "only 24 of 44 counties would run health departments at the county level if we returned to a county-based structure, so that would mean no family planning, epidemiology, or dietician services in smaller counties." Another big benefit of working in districts for Idaho is that all the health districts in the state collaborated to write one statewide strategic plan for local public health. They agreed on terminology, measurements, and goals, all based on the 10 essential public health services. Moehrle noted, "We feel it is a huge benefit of our district structure that we can make it happen on a statewide level, and not duplicate energies seven times." By increasing the capacity to meet the essential services as districts, and reaching consensus on one strategic plan, the seven districts have created common goals, and are able to share documentation, templates, and plans for meeting accreditation standards in the future.

Practice Makes Perfect. Moerhle believes that PPHR, while undertaken for other reasons, served as "a tease for the staff as we move toward accreditation," adding that, "It introduced them to the fact that meeting standards is doable. And it also helps them see that moving to a bigger scale will require bringing on all staff. If we can do a piece of it, we can do more for national accreditation." The success with PPHR recognition has been positive, and Moerhle noted that it helps accreditation feel less daunting. Specifically, PPHR also forced the districts to document their work: "To prove something in writing was a huge step. We knew in our heads that we do these things but we didn't have it written down so someone else could open it and read it. Proof in a written document has helped us look ahead to accreditation and what we may need to do to show we meet those standards."

The North Central District Health Department is hoping that the combination of a regional model, PPHR recognition, and strategic planning is positioning them for accreditation. As Moerhle framed it, "We're a small state and very strong at the local level. When we do apply for national accreditation, all seven districts will likely do it together."

Profile 3: Northern Kentucky Independent District Health Department

Interview with Alan Kalos, Health Planning Administrator
Population served: 380,000 people
Jurisdiction. The four-county district is located near Cincinnati, Ohio, and includes urban, suburban, and rural communities.

History of Planning. For the past 15 years, the Northern Kentucky Health Department has been diligently working toward improving the quality of public health in its community. The LHD has a history of facilitating community processes starting with the Assessment Protocol for Community Excellence in Public Health (APEX-PH) and the Protocol for Assessing Community Excellence in Environmental Health (PACE-EH). In 2001, the local health department initiated MAPP in an effort to consolidate and apply previous assessment and planning work toward performance and quality improvement (see Figure 10.4). The strategic plan the community created through the MAPP process was consolidated with several other existing community health plans into one *Master Health Plan for Northern Kentucky.* For several years the community worked collectively to implement and evaluate its strategic plan. In 2008, the district initiated a second iteration of the MAPP process because much of the *Master Health Plan* was outdated.

Improving Essential Public Health Service Delivery. The MAPP process has helped elevate the importance of essential services as a framework for quality improvement in Northern Kentucky. As explained by Alan Kalos, Health Planning Administrator at the LHD, "When the health department first facilitated the NPHPSP in 2001, we had a committee of about a dozen participants. Half of the participants were health department division directors and managers while the other half represented community and system partners. They didn't have much knowledge of the 10 essential public health services or the significance of essential services to their jobs as public health professionals. In addition, staff did not have a strong understanding of the local public health system or how the system relates to the

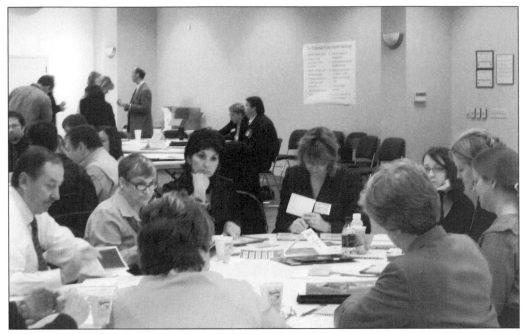

Figure 10.4   Northern Kentucky Health Department work session.

health department. However, by the time we facilitated the NPHPSP again in 2008, the number of participants increased to over 70, and most of the participants understood the concept of the public health system and their roles in it."

The recognition that essential services are crosscutting responsibilities relevant to understanding the effectiveness of both the local health department and public health system resulted in organizational changes at the local health department. As Kalos explains, "Before completing the MAPP process in 2002, the community planning function for the health department was embedded in the health education and planning division. In this capacity, the essential services identified in the Operational Definition standards related to planning functions were viewed as a division function and not as a health department function. The level of community visibility garnered through the facilitation of the MAPP process elevated the planning functions from the intra-division level to the office of the district director. In this capacity, planning functions have been given greater credibility and visibility within the health department, with the board of health, and in the community."

The ability of the health department to assure that all essential services are provided in their community is further enhanced by the relationships developed through the MAPP process. Kalos notes, "As a result of two decades of community processes, the Northern Kentucky community has moved from working as silos to working within a unified public health system where the key system members know each other and communicate on a regular basis. It is not unusual to personally know more than half of the members of a newly formed committee or task force. Given that there are approximately 380,000 residents over four counties and 820 square miles, this is a great accomplishment."

Preparing for Accreditation. As a result of facilitating the MAPP process in its community, the Northern Kentucky Health Department is better positioned for accreditation preparation. Using the NPHPSP instrument, the health department has a comprehensive picture of how well its public health system provides essential public health services and its own role within the system. In addition, as a result of using the NPHPSP instrument, the health department and the system have experience in applying performance standards and measures toward quality improvement. Furthermore, partnerships developed through the process will help the health department assure that services it does not provide will be provided by a public health system partner.

CONCLUSION

For at least the past 20 years, since the IOM published its report on the state of public health, health departments have been working diligently to improve the quality of public health services. Health departments have used different processes, standards, and measures to identify areas for improvement and avenues for advancement. Regardless of whether tools and processes focus on the individual health agency, the public health system, or a particular program area such as emergency preparedness, they all work toward improving the quality of public health practice. Communities and health departments that have used the Operational Definition, PPHR, MAPP, and other improvement tools and processes have already taken steps toward documenting their abilities to provide public health services and demonstrating quality improvement. In preparing for the 2011 launch of national accreditation, all health departments should consider how their previous and current quality improvement efforts can contribute to accreditation preparation.

For more information on accreditation, visit the Public Health Accreditation Board Web site at www.phaboard.org. For information on local health departments, visit the NACCHO Web site at www.naccho.org. For information on state health departments, visit the ASTHO Web site at www.astho.org.

Chapter 11

Improving and Enhancing Community and Client Relationships

Marlene Mason

Public health is entering a new era of accountability. At its core, this shift is exemplified by the increasing demand for reporting and improvement and the movement toward public health accreditation. This renewed focus on improvement and accountability requires that public health agencies increase their capacity to build strong partnerships with community stakeholders and to address the needs and expectations of their clients. Public health leaders must learn to "listen" more often and more acutely in order to target strategic initiatives and program activities based on the needs and priorities of their clients and stakeholders. This is especially important as public health leaders and staff struggle with the thorny dilemma of allocating scarce resources. Increasing stakeholder involvement and client satisfaction through the application of quality improvement methods and tools is no longer just an option for public health. It is one of the major strategies for identifying community champions for public health and for widening the base for strong and progressive health policy.

Many public health practitioners will tell you that their departments do not have customers, as they are focused on population-based health. This is not the case, however. Health departments provide clinical preventive services that are designed based on population-based research or evidence and are delivered to groups or individuals. Business operators seek permits to operate food services or install on-site sewage systems. Some health departments provide primary care services to low-income or uninsured clients. Every public health department—local, state, territorial, or tribal—has stakeholders in the community. All of these are customers that need to be involved in the planning and improvement of public health services. The term "customers" is used throughout the rest of this chapter to refer to all of these types of clients.

This chapter describes some of the methods and tools, with public health examples, used to enhance and improve stakeholder and customer relationships, specifically:

- How to assess customer needs and expectations

- How to analyze customer needs and satisfaction information

- How to use data analysis to identify opportunities for improvement

- How to conduct a rapid cycle improvement project to address the opportunities for improvement

- How to identify and target key stakeholders in different sectors of the public health system

CUSTOMER NEEDS AND/OR SATISFACTION ASSESSMENT

Whether you apply the principles for delivering quality services based on W. Edwards Deming's teachings or any of the many other methods for improving and sustaining quality, one of the fundamental principles is to know and successfully address your customers' needs.

The identification of customers' expectations and needs should always be conducted within the context of the Shewhart or Deming cycle for improvement: the plan–do–study–act cycle. The data-gathering step is part of the *plan* step in the cycle. The data analysis provides the information for developing the plan for establishing or improving public health services (see Figure 11.1).

There are numerous methods for assessing the expectations and needs of community members and those you serve directly, when planning and improving services. One of the easiest is to conduct several focus groups with eight to 10 members of the target population. Focus groups can best be used for gathering two types of information:

- Data about initial expectations and needs before designing a more detailed and focused satisfaction survey

- Specific detailed information about an area of opportunity for improvement that has been identified through another mechanism, such as point-of-service surveys or analysis of complaint data

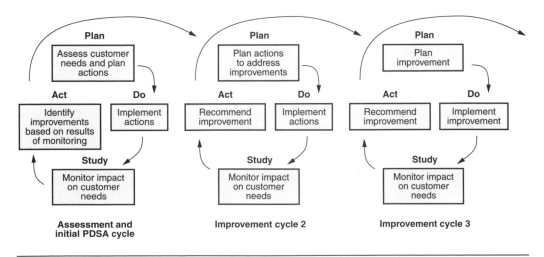

Figure 11.1   Continuous quality improvement related to assessing and taking action on customer needs and expectations.

The questions asked of the focus group members support the different types of information gained from this mechanism.

One of the other most common and frequently used methods for identifying customer needs is to conduct formal satisfaction surveys. Local public health departments around the nation are starting to conduct surveys to quantify and monitor satisfaction. Point-of-service surveys are conducted when a person presents for any type of service, such as family planning, immunizations, treatment for TB, or training in food safety. A minimum number of surveys (usually at least 30) should be conducted and analyzed on a quarterly basis so that early action can be taken on the results. Numerous examples of customer satisfaction surveys exist from local and state health departments.*

Figure 11.2 is an example of a point-of-service survey from a local health department reception area, and Figure 11.3 shows an example of a mailed satisfaction survey for environmental health services with the related analysis and report of results.

All too often, the missing link for creating real improvement is the analysis of these surveys. It is critical that agencies not conduct any focus groups or customer surveys unless there is a plan to analyze and use the results. Without the analysis and application of results, the time and energy expended in developing and conducting the effort will be wasted. Perhaps more importantly, an agency would have misled its customers into thinking that some action or change will be made based on the results. This is also true for any assessment of staff satisfaction. No assessment should be conducted without full leadership and staff commitment to using the results in a valid and effective manner.

ANALYSIS OF SURVEY RESULTS

In Figure 11.3, the feedback from food establishment operators, the local health department mailed 487 surveys, received 194 responses, and tallied the results to identify areas for improvement. Such volume of responses gives food safety programs valid results to determine how satisfied the food operators are with program services.

Food safety program satisfaction survey results based on the mailed survey are shown in Figure 11.4.

Health departments should establish thresholds or benchmarks for results of customer surveys. Surveys that use a four-point scale, like the examples above, could establish the threshold for taking action at more than 25 percent combined fair/poor responses, or less than 75 percent combined good/high responses. Once the threshold for action has been set, a group of public health leadership and staff must regularly review the tallied and trended survey results to identify any items that exceed the thresholds and need to be improved. In Figure 11.4, a group would focus on improving the quality of the materials that are provided, as item 4 was the only area where the good/high responses tallied at less than 75 percent.

---

* Numerous good examples of customer surveys and related reports are available on the Washington State Department of Health Web site (http://www.doh.wa.gov/phip/PerfMgmt) and on many other Web sites for public health model practices (such as http://naccho.org/topics/modelpractices).

The staff and administration of the Health Department would appreciate your taking a few minutes to complete this evaluation and return it to our office. We are very interested in your comments on how we do our job, especially if you can offer suggestions for improvement.

Please provide the following information:

How many times did you need to speak to Health Department staff to get what you needed?

_____ One time   _____ Two to five times   _____ More than five times

Based on your interaction with Health Department staff, please rate your level of satisfaction with our service in the following areas:

1 = Poor   2 = Fair   3 = Good   4 = Excellent   N/A = Not applicable

	1	2	3	4	N/A
1. Friendliness and courtesy of the staff.					
2. Ability of staff to put me at ease.					
3. Timeliness of service.					
4. Staff demonstrated understanding of my situation.					
5. Staff knowledge.					
6. Accurate and useful information was made available to me.					
7. Options and alternatives were offered when possible.					
8. Professional staff treated me with respect and courtesy.					
9. Reliability of services.					
10. The reception staff treated me with respect.					
11. My overall level of satisfaction with the Health Department.					

12.   The phone system for the Department makes it easy to call the Health Department.

_____ Yes   _____ No

13. Do you have suggestions or comments to help improve our services?

Figure 11.2   Point-of-service customer satisfaction survey.

ADDRESSING RESISTANCE TO INVOLVING CUSTOMERS

Often, before public health leaders and staff can successfully identify and address customer needs, they must understand and address areas of resistance to improving the quality of public health practice and services. One of the biggest areas of resistance to improving the quality of services is often the erroneous belief that this means that "the customer gets whatever they want." Providing quality services requires clarity regarding who gets to "call the shots," or make decisions about specific aspects of public health services and activities.

Dear Facility Operator:

The Health Department values your opinion on their services. Please take a moment to fill out the following survey and return it to the health department via any of the following methods. Thank you in advance for taking the time to fill out this survey so that we may continue to improve our quality of service to you our valued customer.

Please fill out the survey and return:

❏ by mail to:

❏ by fax to:

❏ take the survey online at:

Providing quality service to our food establishment customers is a priority to the Health Department. Thank you for your participation!

Please mark the box for each question that reflects your opinion of your experience with the Health Department's service in 2008.	Low	Fair	Good	High
How satisfied were you with the knowledge level of the employees who assisted you and/or inspected your facility?				
How satisfied were you with the courtesy, respectfulness, and professional manner of the employees who assisted you?				
How satisfied were you with our staff's responsiveness and efficiency?				
How satisfied were you with the quality of the materials you received?				
In general, how satisfied were you with the level of service that we provided you in 2008?				
Other comments or suggestions?				

Figure 11.3   Environmental health customer satisfaction survey.

Please mark the box that best reflects your opinion of our services during the previous year.	Low	Fair	Good	High
1. How satisfied were you with the knowledge level of employees who assisted you and/or inspected your facility?	5%	14%	41%	39%
2. How satisfied were you with the courtesy, respectfulness, and professional manner of the employees who assisted you?	6%	13%	20%	58%
3. How satisfied were you with our staff's responsiveness and efficiency?	5%	12%	48%	35%
4. How satisfied were you with the quality of the materials you received?	15%	39%	19%	26%
5. In general, how satisfied were you with the level of service that we provided you in 2008?	7%	10%	49%	34%

Figure 11.4   Food safety program satisfaction survey results.

Figure 11.5 indicates three aspects of services and the primary decision makers for each of these areas.

For the aspects of services that directly relate to customer expectations regarding timeliness and courtesy, the customers get to call the shots and establish the standards and benchmarks. If we use family planning (FP) services as an example here, the FP customers would give the FP manager and staff information about waiting time at the health department, the best time of day to offer FP services, how courteous the FP nurses are, and whether the information provided during their visit met their needs.

For the clinical and evidence-based aspects of services, the public health practitioners get to call the shots by establishing the standards for public health practice. For FP services, this would include the information about birth control methods and requirements for prenatal care if the woman were already pregnant.

Finally, in the arena of public health policy, it is the funders, key community stakeholders, and public health leaders that make the decisions about setting priorities and performance requirements. For the family planning example, this means that the stakeholders and public health leadership in the community would establish that the FP program was a priority for the community based on criteria such as a high teen birth rate, and would allocate funding to establish the program.

By clearly identifying who the decision makers are for each of these basic aspects of public health services and activities, leaders and staff will be more successful in understanding and addressing the expectations and needs of various public health customers.

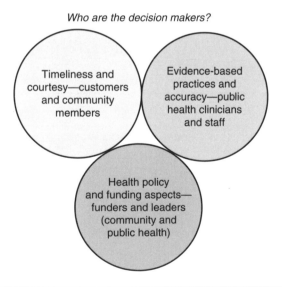

Figure 11.5   Three aspects of services and their primary decision makers.

DESIGNING THE IMPROVEMENT ACTION

In the food safety example (Figure 11.4), all but one of the questions show less than 25 percent low/fair responses and more than 75 percent good/high responses. Question 4, related to the materials the food operator received from the food safety program staff, received 54 percent low/fair responses. This represents an opportunity for improvement that the health department could target with a QI team project. Because the leadership and staff of the food safety program can readily revise the materials they distribute as part of the food establishment inspection or educational sessions, this type of satisfaction issue can be improved by applying the *rapid cycle improvement* (RCI) method described by the Institute for Healthcare Improvement (IHI). This method uses the PDSA cycle preceded by three important questions that the QI team must answer to start the improvement project.

The RCI method is being successfully used in many local and state health departments to quickly create sustainable improvement in work processes and outcomes. Figure 11.6 shows the basic RCI method.

The first three questions are intended to guide the improvement team to 1) establish an aim for improvement that focuses the group effort, 2) identify the quantifiable measures needed to evaluate and understand the impact of changes designed to meet an aim, and 3) identify the who, what, when, and how of designing tests of changes to create improvement.

The plan–do–study–act cycle is a trial and learning method consisting of the following steps: design or plan, test or implement, check or study the results, and act on the conclusions to discover an effective and efficient way to change a

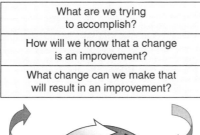

Model for Improvement

| What are we trying to accomplish? |
| How will we know that a change is an improvement? |
| What change can we make that will result in an improvement? |

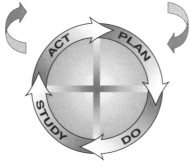

Figure 11.6   Rapid cycle improvement (RCI) method.

process. This cycle is repeated until the desired aim is achieved. The goal may be reached after one cycle, or it may remain elusive even after 10 or more cycles.

If a QI team were to start a rapid cycle improvement project, should they jump right into revising food safety materials? No, they first need more information about what exactly is unsatisfactory about the existing materials.

The first activity in the *plan* step might be to conduct a focus group to gather detailed feedback. The team might also search for materials used by other health departments that could be adapted for use. These pieces of information would help guide materials revision, which should then be tested with another focus group prior to adoption, printing, and distribution.

Much more information is available on the RCI method at the Institute for Healthcare Improvement Web site (http://www.ihi.org/IHI/Topics/Improvement/ImprovementMethods/HowToImprove), a leader in the application of these methods in healthcare.

CONDUCTING THE RAPID CYCLE IMPROVEMENT PROJECT

There are many QI tools and project management tools that can be used during the RCI project to collect and analyze data, to identify the major contributors to the problem, and to design or apply proven interventions to improve the work process (like the process for developing, testing, and distributing materials for food establishment operators) or outcome (like satisfaction of food operators with food inspection visits).

In answering the first question of the RCI process—"What are we trying to accomplish?" —it is important to focus and target the improvement effort on a specific work process or aspect of the work. Often, RCI projects are not as successful as they could be because a team has tackled too large a problem or not described the problem clearly enough to design an improvement action that will directly address the problem.

For the second question of the RCI method—"How will we know that a change is an improvement?"—it is critically important to establish quantifiable measures for monitoring and evaluating the level of improvement created by the improvement action. The data description tool shown in Figure 11.7 has helped many public health QI teams establish valid measures for RCI projects.

Many teams format the information from the data description questions in tables for the several performance or outcome measures used in an improvement project. One example of such a table is shown in Table 11.1.

The third step in the RCI process—"What change can we make that will result in an improvement?"—requires that the QI team brainstorm ideas to test to improve the problem. This is often done through a brainstorming process with the team. If the problem has been tackled by other public health departments, the QI team should search for model practices to adapt for their improvement effort, as this will save time and effort. Using model practices also increases the probability of success as the improvement action has already been tested and proven to create improvement.

The project planning tool example shown in Figure 11.8 can help an RCI team plan and track the specific tasks for each of the improvement actions they are testing.

Performance or Outcome Measure: Description of performance or evaluation measure stating numerator and denominator as well as the source of the data.

Statement of the measure: _____

_____

1. What is the target population?

2. What are the numerator and the denominator for this specific measure?

3. What is the target or goal for performance?

4. Who will collect this information?

5. What form or what tool will be used to collect these data?

6. How often will the data be collected? Reporting period—calendar year or every quarter?

7. Who will conduct the data analysis?

8. Frequency of analysis reports and review by program leadership and staff to make conclusions and take action?

Figure 11.7 Performance and outcome measures data description form.

Table 11.1 Family planning program improvement project example–data description table.

	Measure #1 (example)	Measure #2	Measure #3
Statement of measure	Percent of high-risk pregnant women with prenatal visit in first trimester		
Target population	All pregnant women		
Numerator:	Number of high-risk pregnant women with first trimester prenatal visit		
Denominator:	Number of high-risk pregnant women		
Source of data:	Clinic visit records		
Target or goal:	95%		

Project: Increase the percent of adults receiving influenza vaccine														
Aim:	Increase by 50% the estimated number of eligible persons ages 65 and over who receive an annual influenza vaccination from their primary care physician or in the hospital in _____County, without decreasing vaccinations in other settings.														
Measures (goals):	1. The percent of eligible persons ages 65 and over who receive an annual influenza vaccine (increase)														
	2. The percent of ordered vaccine that is administered (Increase)														
	3. The number of sites offering influenza vaccines to older adults (Increase)														

Cycle number	Change tested	Person(s) responsible	1	2	3	4	5	6	7	8	9	10	11	12
1	Institute a reminder system														
2	Regular feedback														
3	Identify follow-up actions														

Figure 11.8   RCI project planning tool.

An RCI project usually takes 12 to 16 weeks to complete. At the end of the project, the program or health department leadership and staff must monitor the performance measures to determine how much improvement has been achieved. If the improvement meets the goals of the project, then the improvement intervention should be implemented across the program or the health department, as appropriate. Sheila Kessler, in her book *Total Quality Service*[1] shows the logical steps in a QI project, as shown in Figure 11.9.

Excellent resources for the tools used in an RCI process include the *Public Health Memory Jogger* available through the Public Health Foundation (http://phf.org/pmqi/resources.htm#memoryjogger2) and the many tools and methods available at the American Society for Quality's Web site (www.asq.org).

The 2008 *Embracing Quality in Local Public Health* QI guidebook (http://www.accreditation.localhealth.net/MLC-2%20website/Michigans_QI_Guidebook.pdf) developed by the Michigan local public health accreditation program describes the application of RCI in four local health departments with a step-by-step process for conducting the RCI process and detailed storyboards for the four RCI teams.

INVOLVING KEY STAKEHOLDERS IN PLANNING PUBLIC HEALTH SERVICES

One of the long-standing strengths in public health practice has been the skill and mechanisms for involving community members and key stakeholders in setting priorities and planning for public health services. A simple organizational charting tool called *sector mapping* may be used to identify and group the larger

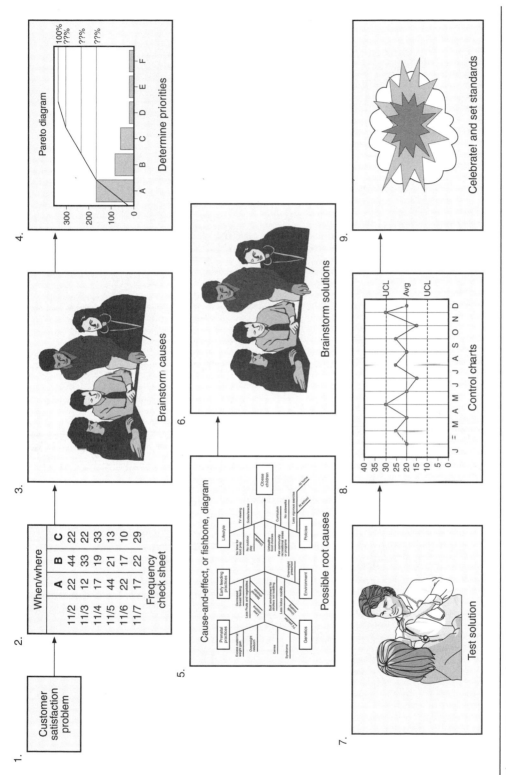

Figure 11.9   Logical steps in a QI project.

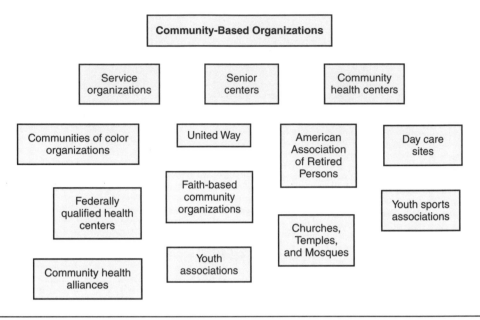

Figure 11.10   Community-based sector map for a statewide system for chronic disease.

public health system for planning and assessment activities. Sector mapping facilitates the identification of partner entities in various sectors, such as public health, private healthcare delivery, community-based, and academic sectors. The sector maps are used to ensure representation from each sector in planning or assessment processes when a broad range of stakeholders is important. The sector maps also assist the many partners in understanding where they fit in the overall system. An example of a community-based sector map for a statewide system for chronic disease is shown in Figure 11.10.

Identifying and addressing customer and community needs for public health services is critical to the effectiveness of public health services and has strong implications for the funding of these services. Public health agencies need to make concerted efforts to assess their customers' needs and expectations and carefully analyze and apply assessment results, using data to identify and monitor opportunities for improvement. Rapid cycle improvement teams offer an excellent method to address opportunities for improvement. Learning and applying improvement methods and tools is not an option, but an essential part of public health practice.

Chapter 12

Already Doing It and Not Knowing It

Stephanie Bailey, MD, MSHSA

In its simplest form, *quality improvement* means learning why something does or does not work and applying the lessons learned to the next strategy or planning session. It causes "trusted" change and enhances cooperation by all for better outcomes. Many are doing this kind of reflective thinking and application and may not be calling it a quality improvement process.

In 1999, metropolitan Nashville and Davidson County, Tennessee, were number one in the country for syphilis. Nashville, according to the study that was eventually done about the epidemic, had actually been in an epidemic state since 1996. The information first came to my attention in the spring of 1998. When asked how this happened, the answer revealed an acceptance of the historical cyclical nature of syphilis epidemics; that is, the pattern of the disease cycles up and down over the years. I declared, "Nashville and syphilis: no more!" It was my intent that when we got it down this time we would keep our vigilance and not allow it to trend upward again. In fact it was my desire to eliminate syphilis from Davidson County: we had the will, political and otherwise—for no Mayor wants his city to be known for this 'number one'—manpower, and strategic focus. As we began our attack, little did we know that "out of the past, we'd find our future."

> 1877: Nashville was the fifth deadliest city in the United States and citizens blamed the Board of Health for ruining the city's image.
>
> 1904: The Division of Disinfection established the first step toward organizing communicable disease control work. Seventy houses were disinfected by this division.
>
> 1914: Department of Health requested that a medical officer be hired to provide more attention to individual cases of communicable disease.
>
> 1918: Men at the jail and workhouse camps were treated for venereal disease and circumcised. Dr. Thompson carried scissors, needle, and thread.
>
> 1919: The city Venereal Disease Program began.

1936: Dr. Lentz, the director of health, reported that there were many unreported syphilis and gonorrhea cases in the county. Dr. Lentz noted that the work loss by syphilitics and inability to support their families were more expensive to the county than the cost of adequate clinics to treat the syphilis.

1938: United States Public Health Services funded venereal disease education in some communities. A syphilis control program for high schools was approved by the Board of Health.

1940: 337 cases of syphilis—approximately one new case of syphilis diagnosed for each two contacts named and investigated. Dr. Lentz further said, "It becomes more and more impressed upon us that the control of syphilis is a result to be attained through a furthering of the program of education."

1941: The development of an army camp 60 miles from Nashville created a syphilis problem.

1942: At the request of the Army, the Board of Health gave Dr. Lentz the power to quarantine prostitutes with infectious diseases.

1943–1945: 300,000 servicemen were stationed near Nashville. Thirty-three out of 100 health department employees worked in VD to prevent transmission among army personnel. 150 men per month were infected with syphilis in the city and over 3000 men had been rejected for military service because they were infected with syphilis.

So, there were core groups of transmitters (prostitutes and the military), the main strategy was education, jailhouses were a major source for transmitting, the cost/benefit ratio for treating was favorable, and there was underreporting or no reporting by community doctors. Nashville, in the late 1900s (1996–2000) has a syphilis epidemic; where do we begin?! At this time in history, less than one percent of U.S. counties accounted for half of the reported syphilis cases. One half of all new syphilis cases were concentrated in 28 counties mainly in the south and selected urban regions. Davidson County was one of the ten counties/cities with the highest number of reported syphilis cases. So we created STDFree!

The key strategies needed for reaching our vision and intent included: expanding surveillance and outbreak response, rapid screening, enhanced community awareness and involvement, and an epidemiological study. One of our community health action teams (CHATs) took the lead for STDFree. This was the business of the city, not just the STD clinic.

Our first study helped guide us in our strategy. A small group of transmitters—those seeking drugs and exchanging sex for drugs—set up an environment for rapid transmission because of the "right" social-sexual network. Nashville was experiencing increasing poverty and crime, rapid growth as a metropolitan statistical area, a high demographic of females, and a 200 percent greater incidence rate in our homeless female population than for Nashville overall. Nashville possibly was becoming the center of a social-sex network favorable for syphilis transmission.

The Tennessee Department of Health loaned personnel to Metro Public Health Department (MPHD) to review all charts from the previous two years in order to recontact and reinvestigate. A weekend "blitz" was conducted in May 1998 in the county jail system, which resulted in nine new cases.

The CHAT team launched STDFree with a community forum in October 1998, the purpose of which was to inform the community of the problem and to solicit their involvement in the solution. Four groups turned out to be key to increasing the awareness of our syphilis problem and being arenas where strategies should stem from: criminal justice, education (primary through college), and faith-based and community organizations. The teams engaged in a focused strategic planning effort to guide their efforts, indicators, and evaluation. STDFree provided a network for accessing particularly those disproportionately affected by syphilis, built the capacity of the community for sustained efforts in addressing the disease, allowed the community to address the problem from within, acknowledging that the community is capable of addressing the problem, and improved the health of the community. Some of the many successful strategies included: STDFree Haunted House developed by over 400 college students, and the February 14th "love sermon."[4] The Haunted House event picked up new cases of syphilis among a population previously thought to be at a significantly lesser risk for the disease, and the love sermon was delivered by over 200 ministers in Nashville. Each has been an annual event.

On October 7, 1999, the Centers for Disease Control and Prevention (CDC) announced a National Plan to Eliminate Syphilis in conjunction with Nashville's Health Department. Nashville, along with Indianapolis and Raleigh, was selected as a short-term demonstration site to evaluate and refine national strategies for elimination efforts. What we were doing was being watched by the field of public health and used to inform national strategy. This was history in the making! We had declared war on syphilis! The CDC-funded Nashville Jail Syphilis Demonstration Project was launched in November 1999 and conducted for 12 months. Mandated rapid screening was instituted for persons arrested with charges related to sex for drugs or anything drug related. Thirty-eight percent of new cases came from this effort.

The community was surveyed regularly regarding their awareness and habits. The Behavior Risk Factor Surveillance Surveying was enhanced, allowing us to survey greater numbers than was usual by the state. The state surveyed annually about 200 persons in Davidson County. We enhanced the number of participants to over 3000. STDFree became a 501(c)3 organization in 2004.

Figures 12.1 through 12.3 depict the national ranking for Nashville going from number one in 2000 to number seven in 2001, out of the top 10 by 2002, and out of the top 40 by 2003. Figure 12.4 shows the control efforts imposed on the number of cases per month. In June 2006, MPHD received a letter from the CDC congratulating us for being on target to be the first county to reach the definition for elimination of syphilis in females.

In medical school you are taught that "he who knows syphilis, knows medicine." I posit that "he who knows syphilis, knows the community."

Being number one did not only strongly suggest a crisis and a need to act, but it strongly suggested a need to do better so that reoccurrence does not happen. If

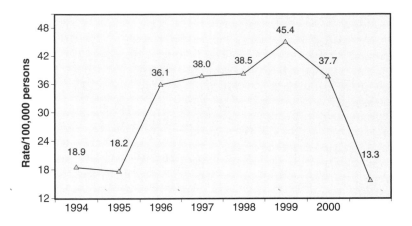

Figure 12.1   Incidence rate of P & S syphilis, Nashville, Tennessee, 1994–2001.

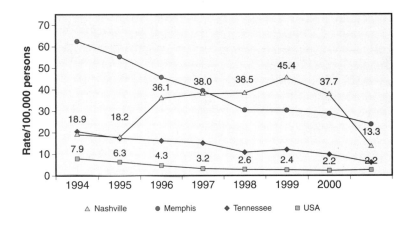

Figure 12.2   Incidence rate of P & S syphilis, Nashville, Tennessee, and USA, 1994–2001.

the default state of being for public health is steeped in a QI process rather than managing in a crisis, like a syphilis epidemic, it is more likely to succeed and be sustained. In quality improvement, this means standardizing improvement processes that would maintain vigilance and cause timelier intervening.

What would be some tips or techniques to make things easier for implementation and for sustainability?

IMPLEMENTATION

Leadership. Every effort must have a voice or champion who can show a way forward and sets the charge. I think "declaring war" and not accepting a cyclical explanation as the Director of Health was important. The situation did not seem hopeless nor something we just had to live with.

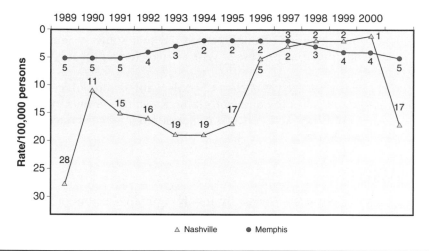

Figure 12.3   P & S syphilis, ranking of Nashville and Memphis among 64 cities with more than 200,000 population in United States, 1989–2001.

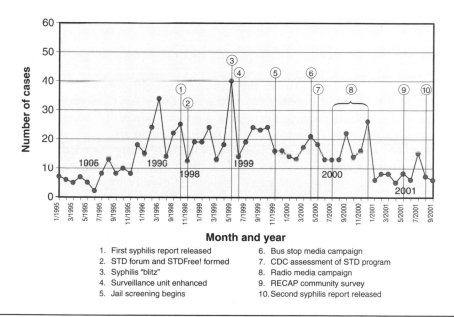

1. First syphilis report released
2. STD forum and STDFree! formed
3. Syphilis "blitz"
4. Surveillance unit enhanced
5. Jail screening begins
6. Bus stop media campaign
7. CDC assessment of STD program
8. Radio media campaign
9. RECAP community survey
10. Second syphilis report released

Figure 12.4   Nashville's current syphilis epidemic control efforts.

Communication. The emphasis on increasing awareness allowed everyone in the community to reach a level of understanding that affected them in some way, causing action and/or support, even in elected officials and those who likened this to the Tuskegee experience. The emotional barriers were removed because of people seeing the broad effect and consequence of not being involved. Up-front and patient communication allows issues and assumptions to surface that would get in the way later if left alone at the beginning.

Process improvement. The fact that the epidemic started two years before staff brought it to my attention strongly suggested that some systems needed to be looked at. Knowing that processes will change (and probably should) makes things easier.

Realistic and reasonable steps/actions. People want to and will get involved. True public engagement is healthy and energizing for staff, community, organizations, youth, and so on. When action is taken, measured, and celebrated, then capacity and capabilities flourish.

SUSTAINABILITY

Make the effort everyone's business. By involving many sectors of the community, eliminating syphilis became everyone's business.

Results. Results matter. Once the business showed results, the momentum escalated.

Process improvements. (See above.) In the book *Shaping Things* by Bruce Sterling, it is pointed out that if reflection does not occur after each cycle, then sustainability will not happen. "Checking" allows for decisions to be refreshed for the next cycle of events.

SUMMARY

Quality is an integrated part of the culture of an effective and high-performing organization. The metropolitan Nashville and Davidson County, Tennessee, community is fortunate to have such strong and resourceful leadership. Hindsight shows that many of the approaches implemented in this success story are discussed frequently in other chapters of this text. Celebrate the wisdom and experience in your local health department. Use the stories and recommendations in this text to tie your existing efforts to a structured quality improvement system that will provide even more performance excellence in the future.

Chapter 13

Data Management and Basic Statistics

John W. Moran and Grace L. Duffy

This chapter is about how to convert data into useful knowledge and information that will allow us to know when to take action, make improvements, or leave things alone. As managers we are constantly making decisions that impact our organization with little or no hard data. Sometimes we rely on experience, instinct, or just plain common sense. Imagine how much better our decisions could be if we had real-time accurate data to rely on when making a decision. Imagine having data that showed a trend line describing where the process under study had been performing in the past, where it is trending, if it is in control or out of control, and its historical variability. If you had this type of data, imagine how less stressful decision making would be when confronted with a problem or process requiring action. When we have accurate and timely data that we can convert into useful knowledge and information, we have vastly improved our business and operation intelligence.

This chapter will help make that type of data a reality when you apply the principles of a good data management strategy.

Data by itself has no value since it just shows information. Information requires interpretation and presentation for it to have value. Decision makers add value through interpretation, which transforms data into knowledge, and then communicate the results in a manner that makes the data visible, understandable, and actionable.

Parts of this chapter are based on a previously published book by ASQ Quality Press entitled *A Guide to Graphical Problem Solving*, written by J. Moran, R. Talbot, and R. Benson, published in 1990. We have expanded and made enhancements to that original work to make it relevant to public health.

A data management strategy is composed of four elements as shown in Figure 13.1.

1. *Collecting.* Developing a process to obtain the raw data

2. *Consolidating.* Translating through the use of data tables

3. *Interpreting.* Summarizing the data through the use of descriptive statistics

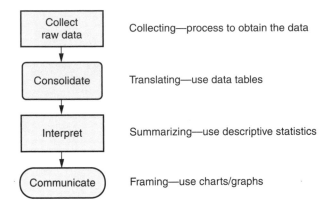

Figure 13.1   Elements of a data management strategy.

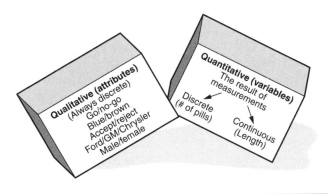

Figure 13.2   Kinds of data.

4. *Communicating.* Framing the data visually through the use of charts and graphs

The goal of the data management strategy is to visually display information to facilitate analysis and communication.

As illustrated in Figure 13.2, all the world's data may be classified or grouped into two very broad classifications: qualitative and quantitative.

Qualitative data are called attribute data and are always discrete (individually distinct) variables. Discrete variables are naturally discontinuous since they are classified into two or more chunks such as *pass* or *fail* or *poor, fair, good,* or *excellent* classifications. Some examples of qualitative data are as follows:

- Yes/no

- Infected/not infected

- Perfect/imperfect

- Pass/fail

- Positive/negative
- Good/bad
- Male/female
- Red/yellow/green/blue
- Dead/alive

While qualitative data are always discrete, quantitative data may be either discrete or continuous. This is because there are two different ways to measure quantitative data: by counting or measuring. Discrete variables can be counted or enumerated, such as the number of pills in a bottle. Continuous (uninterrupted) variables are measured, such as height, weight, blood pressure, birth weight, and number of on-time appointments kept.

We usually obtain the data through sampling in a planned and unbiased manner. It is beyond the scope of this chapter to discuss sampling techniques in detail. Sampling is done in a systematic statistical manner from a population as shown in Figure 13.3.[1]

As shown in Figure 13.3, we know the truth about a population *only* when we can count or measure *every* member in the population. This is rare! More often we take a small part of a population called a *sample*. We use the sample data to make inferences about the much larger population. In Figure 13.3 there are shown some symbols for population parameter and sample statistics; these will be explained later in the chapter.

Before collecting any data we must answer the following questions to ensure that we collect the right data for the right reasons:

- What is the purpose for collecting this data?

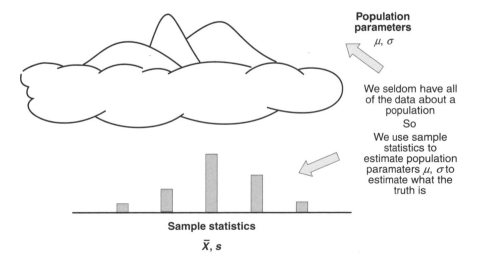

Population parameters

μ, σ

We seldom have all of the data about a population

So

We use sample statistics to estimate population parameters μ, σ to estimate what the truth is

Sample statistics

$\bar{X}, s$

Figure 13.3   Population versus samples.

- What type of data is going to be collected?
  - Qualitative?
  - Quantitative?
- Where will it be collected?
- Who will collect it?
- When will they collect it?
- What will we do with it after we collect it?
- How will we summarize and present the data?

Data collection is not an arbitrary action that is done in an unplanned and haphazard manner. If it is done this way it is a waste of time and energy and will not give us any useful information that we can use to take action on. Data collection needs to be done in a very rigorous and focused manner following a systematic process that is detailed in this chapter.

We want to make sure that our data collection process is simple and unbiased and those collecting the data understand what it will be used for in the future. It is imperative that those collecting the data understand the process functions that they will be observing to extract the sample data, all involved in the data collection are trained so they will collect unbiased data in the same manner, and the recording mechanism (check sheets) for the data samples are as simple as possible and not open to interpretation or manipulation.

Getting good data takes some planning, development of some rules of collection, and education of those involved. The first step is to make sure all doing the data collection walk the process under study to be thoroughly familiar with its operation. Define the data collection points in the process; make those data collection points in easily accessible areas of the process but not where they would intrude on a customer. Use simple data collection forms that do not leave any interpretation to the data collector. Make sure you clearly define the measurement unit on the data collection form and try to keep it consistent over all categories. This often requires a trial run of the data collection process to iron out any bugs in the data collection form. To make sure the data are unbiased, the times of collecting the data need to be established and a sampling plan selected and communicated to all involved in this effort. One good rule to follow is not having an "other" category since this often becomes the default in the collection process. You need to design a data collection form that has 99 percent of the collection categories defined so as to minimize the "other" category. If the "other" category must be used, have a space for the collector to write down why it was used and what was observed.

Getting poor data is a relatively simple process to do by not training anyone on what to do, having unclear directions, using terminology on the data collection form that is ambiguous, having inconsistent measurement units, and using data collectors who are unfamiliar with the process under study.

You can only trust the data when you trust where the data came from, and that trust is established through a sound data collection process that is executed seamlessly.

Once we have collected the raw data from sampling, the process of interpretation begins, and it is made easier by using some of the basic quality improvement tools such as:

- Flowcharts—understand the process from a macro view
- Cause-and-effect diagrams—understand causes not symptoms
- Pareto diagrams—determine the vital few
- Histograms—understand data distribution
- Check sheets—data collection form designed to make analysis simple
- Pie charts—understand how the data are broken up

A good data display helps the interpreter understand the data:

- What is it trying to tell us?
- What is it trying to say?
- Where is it pointing?
- What is it indicating?
- What action should we take?

The question that always comes up is— once the data are collected, what are the next steps in the process? Figure 13.4 is a data flowchart designed to help you think through all the steps involved in going from collection to display of the data.

Once the data are properly collected and classified we now have to decide how to communicate its results. There are numerous ways to do this summarization of the data and graphically communicate the results. The two most common methods are using a histogram and frequency polygons. There are many advantages to using these two methods:

- They are easy to make and use
- They present data in an easy-to-grasp form
- They provide simple statistical estimates of a distribution
- They help show the shape of the data distribution
- They aid in spotting particular data
- They display the relationship between variables

All of these factors work together to provide the effective and timely communication of relevant data. The data flowchart shown in Figure 13.4 illustrates the many ways of handling both qualitative and quantitative data. It shows the sequential development of many of the statistical measures and graphics that can be used.

An example of a frequency polygon is shown in Figure 13.5 for on-time and late WIC appointments.

The frequency distribution shown in Figure 13.5 is not a graph; it is the raw material from which a graph may be constructed. The histogram of the on-time/ late for WIC appointments frequency distribution is shown in Figure 13.6.

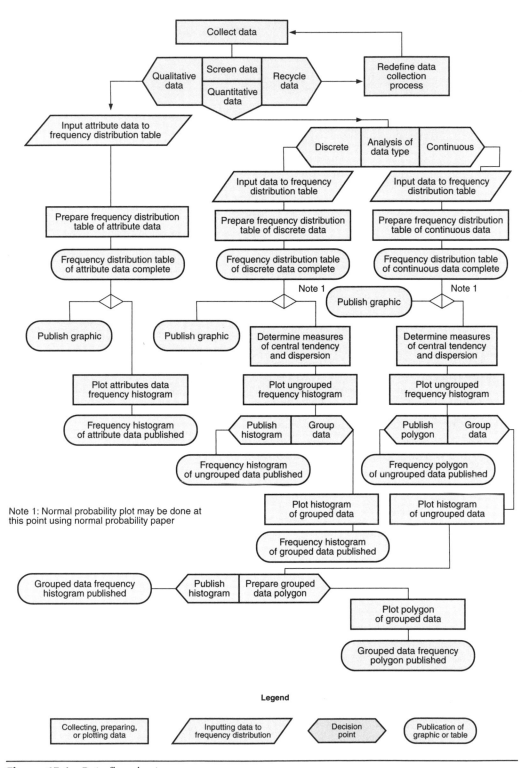

Figure 13.4 Data flowchart.

Attribute	Frequency
On time for WIC appointments	15
Late for WIC appointments	10

Figure 13.5   Frequency distribution table of on-time/late occurrences.

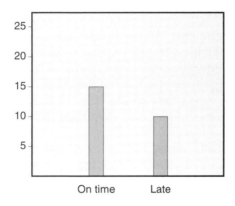

Figure 13.6   Histogram of on-time/late occurrences..

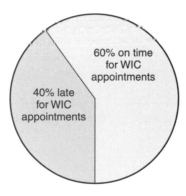

Figure 13.7   Pie chart of on-time/late occurrences.

Another way of depicting the on-time/late WIC appointment data is a pie chart as shown in Figure 13.7. A pie chart is a circle graph divided into pieces. A pie chart is used to display the sizes of parts that make up a set of collected data and is usually used when presenting data as percentages of the total for different data categories. A pie chart is easy to view and understand and shows a good qualitative view of the data.

When we have quantitative data the frequency distribution table can be expanded to help sort collected data into categories and prepare the data for statistical analysis.

It is beyond the scope of this chapter to present an in-depth presentation of statistical analysis, but the basics of analyzing population and sample data central tendency and variability will be presented through a case study.

Whenever we hear the word "statistics," the quote, "There are three kinds of lies: lies, damned lies, and statistics," comes to mind. This well-known saying is part of a phrase attributed to Benjamin Disraeli and popularized in the United States by Mark Twain. The semi-ironic statement refers to the persuasive power of numbers, and succinctly describes how even accurate statistics can be used to bolster inaccurate arguments. When we use statistics as part of our communication strategy we must ensure they are accurate. The population and sample basic statistics of central tendency and variability are calculated by the software we use, but we will display the formulas to give the readers an insight into the process used to calculate the values that are the basis of understanding why the various columns are set up in the frequency distribution tables displayed in the following case study.

A local public health department's septic permitting team decides to do a sample of septic tanks in a particular locality to determine whether the floating scum layer in the septic tank is within one inch of the top of the outlet baffle. They designed a statistically valid sampling plan that calls for 100 septic tanks to be measured. If it is within one inch of the top, the septic tank needs to be pumped. A sample of 100 septic tanks was measured and the data were recorded in the ungrouped frequency distribution table shown in Figure 13.8.

With these data it is possible for the septic permitting team to calculate three measures of central tendency: the mean, the median, and the mode. The measures of central tendency are descriptive statistical calculations that are done by most of the software you may utilize. We will give an overview of the calculations as a statistical refresher.

Measured in inches	Tally	Absolute frequency
.506	I	1
.505	II	2
.504	IIII	4
.503	IIIII IIIII	10
.502	IIIII IIIII IIIII	15
.501	IIIII IIIII IIIII III	18
.500	IIIII IIIII IIIII IIIII I	21
.499	IIIII IIIII IIII	14
.498	IIIII IIII	9
.497	IIII	4
.496	I	1
.495	I	1

Figure 13.8 Ungrouped frequency distribution table.

The *mean* is the arithmetic average of the 100 measurements taken by the septic permitting team and is calculated by adding all the measurements together and dividing by 100. The sample mean in this case is .5006 inches.

The *median* is simply the middle value in the sample. In this sample we have an even number of measures (100); therefore we average the middle two measurements as follows:

50th measurement	.500 inches
51st measurement	.501 inches

$$1.01 \text{ inches} \div 2 = .5005 \text{ inches}$$

Thus, the sample median, MED = .5005 inches.

If the sample had an odd number of data, we would have selected the middle value and no averaging would have been required.

The *mode*, the last measure of central tendency, is the easiest to obtain. It is simply the measurement that most frequently occurs. By inspecting the data in Figure 13.8, it is easy to see that the sample mode is .500 inches. This value has the greatest absolute frequency of 21 occurrences.

From these data it is clear that there is one mode. Sometimes, however, there can be more than one modal value, as shown in Figure 13.9. One of the benefits of plotting the data is that plots can clearly show whether a distribution is unimodal or multimodal.

The three measures of central tendency help us to understand how the data are distributed:

- Symmetrical—normal—bell shaped

- Skewed—left or right

- Rectangular

It is always best to plot the data and confirm the shape of the data. In our example the mean, median, and mode were in close agreement, and this indicates a symmetrical, unimodal distribution.

The septic permitting team could stop here, but they know that the three measures of central tendency (the mean, median, and mode) alone only tell part of the story! Of equal importance is the variability of the septic tank measurements around the mean, that is, the spread or dispersion of the data around the mean of .5006 inches.

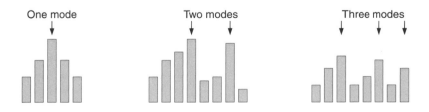

Figure 13.9   Unimodel, bimodal, and multimodal distributions.

"A central theme of the statistical approach to data analysis is this: variability always exists. No experiment can be repeated exactly. Variability can never be totally eliminated."[2] Variation is not all bad since it always displays a pattern or a distribution of itself, and these patterns or distributions can tell us a great deal about the process itself and the causes of problems found in the process. A histogram can be constructed from the data to help us identify and interpret these patterns of variability.

There are three measures of variability: the range, the variance, and the standard deviation. The *range* is a measure of dispersion, the *variance* indicates how much spread is in our sample data, or the *scatter,* and the *standard deviation* indicates the amount of dispersion of the data about its mean. There are important differences in the way we compute the variance and the standard deviation depending on whether we have a population or a sample. Most of the time we deal with a sample as the septic permitting team is doing. Figure 13.10 shows the formulas for calculating the measures of variability.

Note: In these formulas, *n* represents the number of items in the sample and *N* is the number of items in the population. The software the septic permitting team used calculated the three measures of variability and the results are as follows:

$$\text{Range} = 0.011 \text{ inches}$$

$$\text{Sample variance } S^2 = 0.00000417 \text{ inches}^2$$

$$\text{Standard deviation } S = 0.0020 \text{ inches}$$

Now all the key statistics—three measures of central tendency and three measures of variability—have been calculated. These may be used as a comparison against historical data on the septic tank measurements to determine whether:

- The center of the process has shifted

- The variability of the process has increased

- Combination of both of the above

Now the septic permitting team has an abundance of data and decides to use graphing techniques as a means of further analyzing and communicating its findings.

For a sample	For a population
Range = R	Range = R
R = Highest value – Lowest value	R = Highest value – Lowest value
Sample variance, S^2	Population variance, σ^2
$S^2 = \dfrac{\Sigma_{i=1}^{n}\left(X_i - \bar{X}\right)^2}{n-1}$	$\sigma^2 = \dfrac{\Sigma_{i=1}^{N}\left(X_i - \mu\right)^2}{N}$
Sample standard deviation, S	Popular standard deviation, σ
$S = \sqrt{\dfrac{\Sigma_{i=1}^{n}\left(X_i - \bar{X}\right)^2}{n-1}}$	$\sigma = \sqrt{\dfrac{\Sigma_{i=1}^{N}\left(X_i - \mu\right)^2}{N}}$

Figure 13.10   Formulas for calculating measures of variability.

The septic permitting team's first step in graphing is to use the data already collected and expand it into a format called an ungrouped frequency distribution table, as shown in Figure 13.11. This is the foundation for building the graphics. The tally column begins to show the shape of how the data are distributed, which will be verified when they are plotted.

Take the following cautionary measures when constructing frequency distribution tables and graphs:

- Do not throw any data away

- Know what type of data you are dealing with—qualitative or quantitative

- Know if the data are discrete or continuous

- Label everything appropriately

- Keep it clear and simple

- Use the data flowchart (Figure 13.4) as a guide while working through the process

With the frequency distribution table complete, the septic permitting team constructed a frequency polygon as shown in Figure 13.12.

The data plot shows that we have a normal-looking distribution that is unimodal, and it is easy to observe once the data are plotted from the ungrouped frequency distribution table.

The polygon is based on ungrouped data and there is a provision for each and every septic tank measurement. Sometimes it is helpful to group data into clusters or "cells." This clustering can simplify the calculation process and may also give a better understanding of the shape of the underlying distribution.

When ungrouped data are grouped, the class becomes a class interval that includes several different measurements. The class interval is called a "cell." The

Measured in inches	Tally	Absolute frequency	Absolute cumulative frequency	Relative frequency	Cumulative relative frequency
.506	I	1	100	0.01	1.00
.505	II	2	99	0.02	0.99
.504	IIII	4	97	0.04	0.97
.503	IIIII IIIII	10	93	0.10	0.93
.502	IIIII IIIII IIIII	15	83	0.15	0.83
.501	IIIII IIIII IIIII III	18	68	0.18	0.68
.500	IIIII IIIII IIIII IIIII I	21	50	0.21	0.50
.499	IIIII IIIII IIII	14	29	0.14	0.29
.498	IIIII IIII	9	15	0.09	0.15
.497	IIII	4	6	0.04	0.06
.496	I	1	2	0.01	0.02
.495	I	1	1	0.01	0.01

Figure 13.11   Ungrouped frequency distribution table.

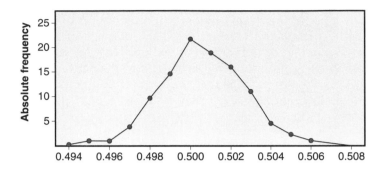

Figure 13.12   Frequency polygon.

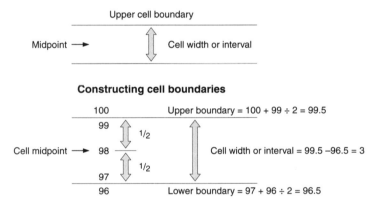

Figure 13.13   Procedure for construction of data cells.

cell has width and is defined by upper and lower boundaries. The procedure for the construction of cells is shown in Figure 13.13.

The frequency distribution table shown in Figure 13.14 shows the results of grouping the 100 measurements taken by the septic permitting team into five cells.

The polygon and histogram shown in Figure 13.15 are then constructed using the grouped data. Note that in plotting the grouped data polygon, only the midpoints and their grouped frequencies are used. In plotting the grouped data histogram, the cell boundaries are shown.

SUMMARY

As we have noted in the figures shown on how to convert data into information, it is important to remember that the results obtained from any histogram will depend on the data with which the histogram is constructed. If the data are inaccurate then any result obtained will also be inaccurate. Data collection is not an arbitrary action that is done in an unplanned and haphazard manner. If it is done this way it is a waste of time and energy and will not give us any useful

Cell boundary	Cell midpoint	Measured in inches	Tally	Grouped absolute frequency	Absolute cumulative frequency	Relative frequency	Cumulative relative frequency
.5075							
	.506	.507		3	100	0.01	1.00
		.506	I				
.5045		.505	II		99	0.02	0.99
		.504	IIII		97	0.04	0.97
	.503	.503	IIIII IIIII	29	93	0.10	0.93
.5015		.502	IIIII IIIII IIIII		83	0.15	0.83
		.501	IIIII IIIII IIIII III		68	0.18	0.68
	.500	.500	IIIII IIIII IIIII IIIII I	53	50	0.21	0.50
.4985		.499	IIIII IIIII IIII		29	0.14	0.29
		.498	IIIII IIII		15	0.09	0.15
	.497	.497	IIII	14	6	0.04	0.06
.4955		.496	I		2	0.01	0.02
		.495	I		1	0.01	0.01
	.494	.494		1			
.4925		.493					

Figure 13.14   Grouped frequency distribution table.

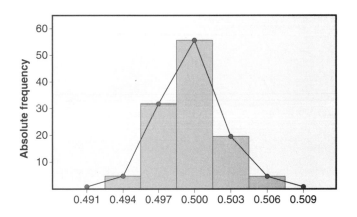

Figure 13.15   Frequency polygon and histogram–grouped data.

information that we can use to take action on. Data collection needs to be done in a very rigorous and focused manner following a systematic process that has been detailed in this chapter.

Getting good data takes some planning, development of some rules of collection, and education of those involved. You can only trust the data when you trust where the data came from, and that trust is established through a sound data collection process that is executed seamlessly.

Obtaining good data is one step in the quality improvement process. The statistics and graphs developed from data do not give solutions but give us directions of where to focus our future analytical effort. Measurement is the driver of improvement.

Chapter 14

Basic Tools of Quality Improvement

John W. Moran and Grace L. Duffy

There are many tools and techniques that can be used when trying to prioritize quality improvement projects, clarify a complex issue, solve a quality improvement problem, or improve a problem process. In order to help the reader, this chapter and the next one, Chapter 15, "Advanced Tools of Quality Improvement," have been developed to guide the reader through the maze of tools and techniques that are available.

Each tool will be presented in the following format in the four categories shown below. This will not be an exhaustive description of the tool but one that will allow the reader to have a quick reference source on a tool's use and application.

- *What it is.* A description of the basics of the tool

- *When to use it.* General guidance on the most common application of the tool

- *How to use it.* The basics of the process and procedure of applying the tool to a situation

- *Example.* An example of the use of the tool to clarify the three categories above.

This chapter concentrates on the basic tools of quality improvement, which are designed to assist a team when solving a defined problem or project. These tools will help the team get a better understanding of a problem or process they are investigating or analyzing.

Tools discussed in this chapter:

1. Bar chart

2. Brainstorming

3. Cause-and-effect diagram

4. Check sheet

5. Control chart

6. Five whys and five hows

7. Flowchart

8. Force field analysis

9. Histogram

10. Nominal group technique

11. Pareto chart

12. Pie chart

13. Run chart

14. Scatter diagram

15. SIPOC+CM

16. Solution-and-effect diagram

This is not an all-inclusive list of the basic tools of quality improvement but it is a listing of the most commonly used in process improvement and problem solving.

Figure 14.1 shows a simple flowchart of how to use the basic quality improvement tools in a problem-solving sequence to resolve an issue of importance to a team or individual. This is a general flow and does not meet all problem situations that could arise. When using basic tools of quality improvement a team or individual should think through an approach they would use and then adopt the best sequence of basic quality improvement tools to fit the particular situation they are trying to solve.

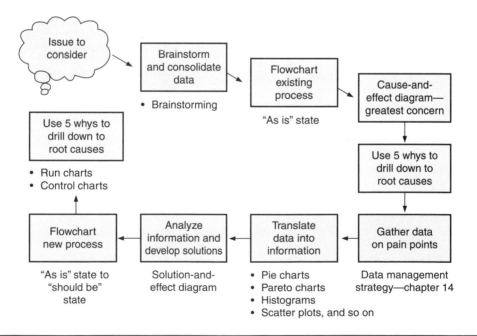

Figure 14.1 General approach on how to use the basic tools of quality improvement.

BAR CHART

What It Is

- A bar chart or bar graph is a chart with rectangular bars of lengths proportional to the value that they represent.

- It is a way to communicate information visually.

- Bars can be oriented horizontally or vertically.

- Bar graphs consist of two axes (x and y) and labeled horizontal or vertical bars that show different values for each bar. A numerical scale is indicated along the side of the bar chart.

When to Use It

- Bar charts, like pie charts, are useful for comparing classes or groups of data collected and when comparing two or more values.

- Double bar graphs can be used when there are two pieces of information on each item.

How to Use It

- A bar chart can be constructed by putting the collected data into groupings or classes. There is no set pattern to develop groups or classes since they are determined by the developer.

- Then determine the number of data points that reside within each group or class and construct the bar chart from the data collected.

- Develop a numerical scale to plot the groups or classes against. It is best to have the same scale for all of the groups or classes, but the scales can be different.

- If the groups or classes do not have the same scale, be sure to prominently indicate it so the reader is not tricked by the data displayed using different scales.

- Be sure that the interval between classes is consistent. Hour to hour, day to day, week to week, or month to month are consistent intervals.

- When viewing a bar chart focus on:
  - The tallest bar
  - The shortest bar
  - Growth or shrinking of the bars over time
  - One bar relative to another
  - Change in bars representing the same category in different classes

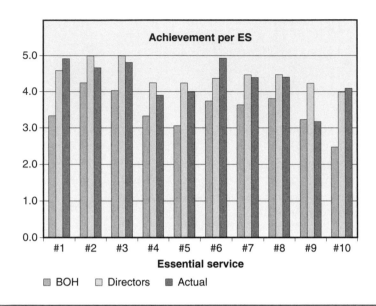

Figure 14.2 Bar chart.

Example

See Figure 14.2 for a bar chart example.

BRAINSTORMING

What It Is

- A group creative technique that was developed in the late 1930s by Alex Faickney Osborn (1888–1996) in a book called *Applied Imagination*. In this book he proposed that groups could double their creative output by using the method of brainstorming.

- Brainstorming is a method for a group to generate a large number of ideas around an issue of interest.

When to Use It

- When a method is needed to help break out of stale, established patterns of thinking that keep producing the same results

- When new opportunities need to be developed

- Where you want to improve the output that your group offers to customers

- When you want to involve everyone in the process since this process allows all participants to express their ideas without being judged

How to Use It

- Assemble the right group of people to discuss the issue under consideration. This is key to a successful brainstorming session.

- Energize the group and get everyone to contribute ideas.

- Clearly state and define the issue to be discussed to the group.

- Set a time limit (20 minutes) and a goal for number of ideas (50 to 100) to be generated for the brainstorming session.

- Keep the session focused on the issue at all times.

- Do not allow criticism or judgment of ideas during the brainstorming session.

- Begin by having participants shout out solutions to the problem while the facilitator writes them down.

- When ideas slow down go into a rotation mode—if a participant has no idea they must say pass when it is their turn in the rotation.

- Always welcome creativity.

- Encourage participants to build on other people's ideas

- Record all ideas on a flip chart and keep them visible.

Example

See Figure 14.3 for a brainstorming example.

Opportunities

- Education (presentation, speeches, speakers)
- Brochures: DIS role
- Referral sources
- Accessibility
- High-risk population—identify
- Collaborate with CBOs, private MDs, hospitals, and other departments within health department
- Increase awareness (presence in community)
- Do more screenings (outreach activity)
- Cross-training of staff
- Train/prepare for supervisor role
- Lead DIS

- Utilize DIS specialty/degree
- Bilingual DIS
- Use cell phone for language line
- Allow DIS to attend free training
- Supervisor appreciation breakfast
- Retreat—staff/fun
- Annual STD health fairs
- Kudos—monetary acknowledgments
- Provider visits
- Accommodate patients (field bloods)
- Hire staff—train and leave to go to CDC
- More media visibility

Figure 14.3   Results of brainstorming on opportunities available to the Orange County, Florida, Health Department STD team for increasing effectiveness, Summer 2006.

CAUSE-AND-EFFECT DIAGRAM

What It Is

- This tool was developed in 1943 by Kaoru Ishikawa at the University of Tokyo.

- Cause-and-effect diagramming graphically relates the symptom or problem under investigation to the factors or causes driving it.

- Resembles a fish skeleton and sometimes called a fishbone diagram or Ishikawa diagram.

- Systematic approach to analyze the problem and find the root cause is more efficient and effective.

When to Use It

- When a problem-solving team needs to consider the complexity of a problem and to take an objective look at all the contributing factors and not just the symptom that is most obvious.

- When the team needs to determine both the primary and the secondary causes of a problem.

- When a team needs to not use their usual approach of working on the obvious symptom when confronted with a problem.

How to Use It

- Write the issue as a problem statement on the right-hand side of a piece of flip chart paper and draw a box around it. Then draw an arrow from the left side of paper pointing toward the box.

- This issue is now the effect, which is a sign or indication of what is happening or being seen.

- Using brainstorming generate ideas as to what are the main causes of the effect—whatever makes something happen. Question what the problem is, who is impacted, and how and where it occurs to get the group started analyzing the issue. Label these as the main branch headers.

- Typical main headers are:

  - Four M's—Manpower, Materials, Methods, Machinery

  - People

  - Policies

  - Materials

  - Equipment

  - Lifestyle

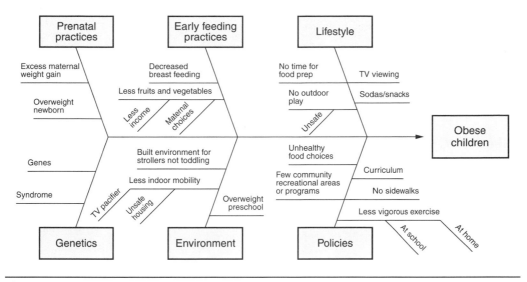

Figure 14.4 Cause-and-effect diagram.

- Environment

- And so on

- For each main cause category brainstorm ideas as to what are the related sub-causes that might affect the issue.

- Use the five whys technique when a cause is identified to drill down into the details. Keep repeating the "Why?" question until no other causes can be identified.

- List the sub-causes using arrows.

- When the cause-and-effect diagram is finished it is time to decide what few areas should be focused on to develop solutions to solve the effect.

Example

See Figure 14.4 for a cause-and-effect diagram example.

CHECK SHEET

What It Is

- Simple data recording form for collecting data in an easy, systematic, and organized manner

- Useful in collecting and classifying useful information to make informed decisions

- Tally of items or indicators of how often things occur

- Often used in conjunction with other QI tools to assist in problem analysis

- A simple data display method that helps the viewer understand the data:

  - What it is saying?

  - What it is trying to tell us?

  - Where it is pointing?

  - What it is indicating?

When to Use It

- When data need to be collected about a particular issue or problem in an easy and systematic way

- When a data recording form is needed that helps classify the data collected into groups or classes as it is being recorded

- When data needs to be converted from information to knowledge through interpretation by decision makers

How to Use It

- To develop a check sheet we need to first answer the following questions:

  - Why are we collecting the data?

  - What type of data is going to be collected?

  - Who is going to collect the data?

  - What is the timing of the data collection?

  - Where will it be collected?

  - Is there any other relevant information that should be collected at the same time?

  - What is the sample size?

- Then we need to decide what type of check sheet to use:

  - Defective item check sheet

  - Defective location check sheet

  - Defective cause check sheet

  - Checkup confirmation check sheet

  - Root cause analysis check sheet

Vendor: _____   Service provided: _____   Contract #: _____

Performance requirement	Measurement	Measurement unit	Vendor performance	Target

Figure 14.5   Vendor performance check sheet.

Example

See Figure 14.5 for a check sheet example.

CONTROL CHART

What It Is

- Developed May 16, 1924 by Walter Shewhart of Bell Labs to improve the reliability of their telephony transmission systems. He realized that continual process adjustment in reaction to nonconformance actually increased variation and degraded quality.

- A statistical study of how a process changes over time.

- Data plotted in time order sequence

- A way to monitor and control process variation and make the proper corrective actions to eliminate the sources of variation.

When to Use It

- When we need to determine whether we have common cause (predictable) or special cause (unanticipated) operating within a process. Dr. Deming stated that all the problems encountered in processes are caused by:
  - Common causes about 80 to 85 percent of the time
  - Special causes about 15 to 20 percent of the time
- When determining how stable a process is over time.
- When determining where and how to take corrective action in a process under study.

How to Use It

- Choose the appropriate control chart for your variable or attribute data.

- Collect process data

- Construct the control chart by calculating from the process data:

  - Centerline for the average—*X*-bar

  - Upper line for the upper control limit—UCL

  - Lower line for the lower control limit—LCL

- Compare the ongoing current process data to these three plotted lines and look for out-of-control signals:

  - If the data fluctuate within the limits, it is the result of common causes within the process and it is in control.

  - If one of the data points falls outside of the control limits it could be the result of special causes and can indicate that the process is out of control, and corrective action may be needed after a thorough investigation of the cause.

  - A run of eight points on one side of the centerline. This pattern indicates a shift in the process output and needs investigation.

  - Two of three consecutive points outside the two-sigma warning limits but still inside the control limits could indicate a process shift.

  - A trend of seven points in a row upward or downward. This may be a result of gradual deterioration in the process.

- This is not an all-inclusive list of out-of-control warning signals, but a few to show examples. Refer to a textbook on statistical process control for a full list of possible out-of-control signals.[1]

Example

See Figure 14.6 for a control chart example.

FIVE WHYS AND FIVE HOWS

What It Is

- The *five whys* and *five hows* are a detailed questioning process designed to drill down into the details of a problem or a solution and peel away the layers of symptoms.

- The technique was originally developed by Sakichi Toyoda and he states "that by repeating why five times, the nature of the problem as well as its solution becomes clear."

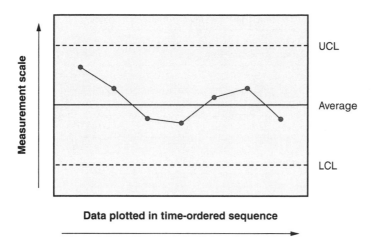

Figure 14.6   Typical control chart.

- The five whys are used for drilling down into a problem and the five hows are used to develop the details of a solution to a problem.

- Both of them are designed to bring clarity and refinement to a problem statement or a potential solution and get to the root cause or root solution.

- Edward Hodnet, a British poet, observed that "If you don't ask the right questions, you don't get the right answers. A question asked in the right way often points to its own answer. Asking questions is the ABC of diagnosis. Only the inquiring mind solves problems."

When to Use It

- When we want to push a team investigating a problem to delve into more detail. The five whys can be used with brainstorming or the cause-and-effect diagram to develop more details of the root causes of a problem.

- The five hows can be used with brainstorming and the solution-and-effect diagram to develop more details of a solution to a problem under consideration.

- Both methods are techniques to expand the horizon of a team searching for answers. These two techniques force a team to develop a better and more detailed understanding of a problem or solution.

How to Use It

- Draw a box at the top of a piece of flip chart paper and clearly write down the problem or solution to be explored.

Too much TV and video games	*Why?*
Few community-sponsored recreation programs	*Why?*
No family recreational activities	*Why?*
No safe play area	*Why?*
Lack of resources	*Why?*

Figure 14.7   Five whys of less vigorous exercise.

Less TV and video games	*How?*
More community-sponsored recreation programs	*How?*
More family recreational activities	*How?*
Safe play areas	*How?*
Additional resources	*How?*

Figure 14.8   Five hows of more vigorous exercise.

- Below the statement box draw five lines in descending order
- Ask the "Why" or "How" question five times and write the answers on the lines drawn from number one to five.
- It may take less or more than five times to reach the root cause or solution.

Example

See Figures 14.7 and 14.8 for five whys and five hows examples.

FLOWCHART

What It Is

- Flowcharting is the first step we take in understanding a process; it is usually in the form of an organized combination of common shapes, lines, and text.

- Flowcharts provide a visual picture of all the steps a process uses to complete its assigned task or output.

- Flowcharts show how interactions occur within and outside of a process and make the invisible and often forgotten tasks very visible.

- As W. Edwards Deming stated, "If you can't describe what you are doing as a process, you don't know what you're doing."

When to Use It

- When there is a need to establish the *"as is"* baseline or current state for analysis or to establish a baseline to measure improvements.

- When there is a need to identify wasteful activities or steps in a process.

- When there is a need to uncover possible sources of variation or where improvements could be made.

- When there is a need to show or train employees in an improved or new process.

How to Use It

- Start by clearly defining the process under study and its boundaries by listing the start and end points.

- Decide on the level of detail of the flowchart to be developed—macro or micro view.

- Use the common flowchart symbols to develop the chart by gathering information on how the process works. This can be done by experience, observation, conversation, interview, or research. The goal is to clearly define each step in the process.

- After you have completed the flowchart, walk through it in real time if possible to verify each step in the flowchart.

- Identify time lags and non-value-adding steps on the flowchart since they may be areas of potential improvement.

- There is no one right way to develop a flowchart, but the following guidelines provide a general structure:

  - Start with a simple one-line description or title of the process being flowcharted, for example, "How to . . . "

  - Using a top-down hierarchy, start with an oval symbol named *Start*.

  - Connect each successive action step in the logical sequence of events.

  - Reference detailed information through annotations or connectors.

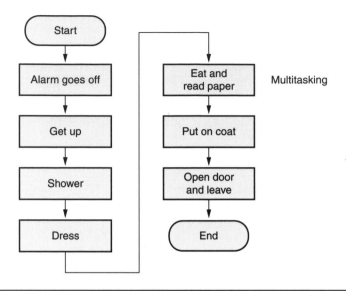

Figure 14.9   Morning activity flowchart.

      – Follow the process through to completion, denoted by an oval
      symbol named *End*.

Example

See Figure 14.9 for a flowchart example.

FORCE FIELD ANALYSIS

What It Is

- Force field analysis was developed by Kurt Lewin in 1969 when
  he stated, "An issue is held in balance by the interaction of two
  opposing sets of forces—those seeking to promote change (driving)
  and those attempting to maintain the status quo (restraining)."

- A process to look at the balance of power in a changing situation.
  Helps identify the important opponents and allies. Presents the
  positives and negatives of a situation so they are easily comparable.

When to Use It

- When there is a need to understand how to influence the opponents
  and allies

- When there is a need to prepare a plan for removing restrainers
  and increasing drivers of change

- When there is a need to consider all aspects of making a desired change

- When there is a need to encourage agreement about the relative priority of factors on each side of the force field with opponents and allies

- When there is a need for a team or group to understand the root causes of a problem and its solution

How to Use It

- Assemble the right team to participate in the force field analysis.

- Start by drawing a large letter T upside down on a flip chart.

- Write the issue under study at the top of the flip chart. This is the current state.

- Next describe to the participants where the current state would evolve to if no action was taken. This is the undesired state.

- Engage the participants in defining the desired state and write it as a goal on the far right side of the flip chart.

- Create a force field diagram by brainstorming driving and restraining forces on achieving the desired state. The driving forces are written on the right side of the upside down T and the restraining forces are on the left.

- Determine the strength of each force and indicate it on the force field diagram as high, medium, or low. We want to work on the high strengths first since they have the most impact on reaching our desired stated.

- Develop an action plan to move to the desired state, indicating how to increase the strength of driving forces and decrease the strength of restraining forces.

Example

See Figure 14.10 for a force field analysis example.

HISTOGRAM

What It Is

- A bar graph that shows the frequency of data collected

- A tool for clearly summarizing, displaying, analyzing, and interpreting collected data

- A tool to sort collected data into categories and the frequency or count of each category

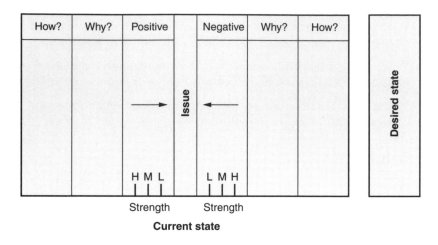

Figure 14.10 Force field analysis matrix.

- A graphical representation and summary that displays the amount of variation found in collected data

When to Use It

- When there is a need to understand the underlying shape/spread (normal, Poisson, binomial, chi square, and so on) or symmetry (symmetric or skewed) of a process under study

- When we are interested in the shape of the population from which the data are gathered

- When there is a need to know if a process is in control

- When there is a need to know if we should take any action based on some observed data from a process

How to Use It

- Develop a frequency table from the collected data arranged in single data points or in classes of equal size.

- Then construct the histogram:

  - Plot the histogram as an x and y axis plot—data points (ascending order) or groups are on the x-axis and the frequency (count) on the y-axis.

  - For each data point or class draw a bar to the height that corresponds to the frequency of the observed values. When we draw a bar for a class of values it is centered on the midpoint of the class of values it represents.

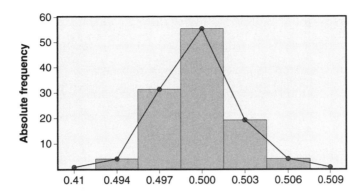

Figure 14.11   Frequency polygon and histogram–grouped data.

- If you plot individual data points, the height of the bar will indicate the number of times that value occurred.

- If you used grouped data then the width of each bar will represent a class of values and the height of the bar will indicate the number of times that value occurred.

- Once the histogram is completed, review the graph and look at the type of pattern it represents and make a determination of how the process is functioning. This chapter covered the types of statistical calculations that can be made from data to help in the review.

Example

See Figure 14.11 for a histogram example.

NOMINAL GROUP TECHNIQUE

What It Is

- A structured process that helps teams to prioritize a large list of items to a short list of action items by:

  - Helping to prioritize by consensus a list of potential ideas, causes, or solutions

  - Allowing every team member to rank choices through voting

  - Building team ownership of choices by consensus

  - Managing the quiet or expressive teammates

When to Use It

- When a new or established group needs to make a decision

- When the topic might be political, difficult, or sensitive
- When the team is in deep disagreement over what the root cause is
- When a decision is needed in a timely manner
- When a team is unable to reach consensus by other methods

How to Use It

- On a piece of flip chart paper, write out a clear definition of the problem or objective under consideration.
- Brainstorm and record ideas about the problem or objective under consideration.
- Review, discuss, and classify each of the recorded idea into groupings.
- Determine the voting scheme, such as:
  - 1—Worst method
  - 2—OK method
  - 3—Better method
  - 4—Best method
- Each team member gets four votes as shown above and assigns them to each group.
- Tally the votes, and if no clear winner emerges use the list from the previous vote and take another vote.
- When the final vote is completed, tally the votes and prioritize the items.

Example

See Figure 14.12 for a nominal group technique example.

PARETO CHART

What It Is

- Joseph Juran popularized the Pareto principle in 1950 after observing that a high proportion of quality issues resulted from only a few causes.[1] Vilfredo Pareto (1848–1923), an Italian economist, invented this method of information presentation toward the end of the 19th century, and it became known as the Pareto principle or 80/20 rule.
- The underlying rule of the Pareto principle is that 80 percent of the total problems observed are the result of 20 percent of the possible causes.

Issue: Expand community partners

Possible partners:
A. St. Luke's Congregation
B. United Way
C. Over 55 Community Association
D. County PTSA board
E. City government department

- The local public health leaders, with assistance from their community board, identified the most promising community partners for a new youth mentoring program.
- With only enough project capacity to collaborate with three of the five identified partners, the board used nominal group technique to choose the final partners.
- The three candidates with the highest total tally were selected as community partners for this youth engagement project.

Multivoting/NGT tally table						
Voter	Jack	Sally	Sheila	Bill	Grace	Total
A	3	2	5	2	4	16
B	1	3	2	3	2	11
C	2	1	3	1	1	8
D	5	5	1	5	3	19
E	4	4	4	4	5	21

Figure 14.12   Nominal group technique example.

- If you concentrate on the vital few over the trivial many you can eliminate the majority of your problems.
- The chart is similar to the histogram or bar chart, except that the bars are arranged in decreasing order from left to right along the *x*-axis.

When to Use It

- When there is a need to know what are the really important issues facing our team or organization
- When there is a need to know which 20 percent of causes are contributing to 80 percent of the problems
- When there is a need to know where to focus our efforts to achieve the greatest improvements
- When there is a need to know what priorities our team should focus on
- When there is a need to understand what the impact of our implemented solution has been
- When there is a need to analyze data about the frequency of problems or causes in a process
- When there is a need to understand what constitutes broad causes by looking at their specific components
- When there is a need for a communication tool to inform others about our findings

How to Use It

- Clearly define the problem to be investigated.

- Determine the categories that you are going to use to collect data about.

- Use check sheets to collect the data for the Pareto chart.

- Record total occurrences in each category for the interval measured, the grand total, and the percentages for each category.

- Rank order the categories from most to least by the percentages calculated.

- Draw the Pareto chart:
  - y or vertical axis should be labeled from zero to whatever the grand total is using convenient even multiples for a scale.
  - Begin at the left side of the x or horizontal axis with the largest category. Label the categories on the bottom of the axis.
  - Draw a bar to represent the amount of each category observed parallel to the y-axis.
  - Title the graph.
  - Draw a cumulative percentage line.

- Interpret the graph by looking for the two or three categories that tower above the others.

- Once you improve the first few critical items, redo the Pareto analysis, and discover what other factors have risen to the top now that the biggest ones have been improved.

Example

See Figure 14.13 for a Pareto chart example.

PIE CHART

What It Is

- A *pie chart* is a circle graph divided into pieces that show a good qualitative view of the data.

- Each piece displays the size of some related piece of collected data.

- Usually used when presenting data as percentages of the total for different data categories.

- Used to display from two up to six fractions of the whole of the collected data.

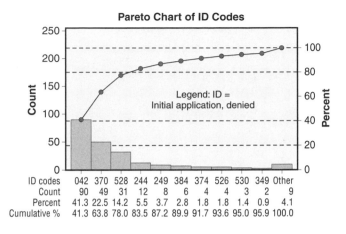

Figure 14.13   Pareto chart.

- An easy and simple graphical display of data to view and understand.
- Useful for a single series of data and when there are not too many slices of the pie.

When to Use It

- When there is a need for a relatively easy way to display and communicate qualitative data
- When there is a need to communicate the differences between values or alternatives
- When we need to display data points as a percentage of the whole
- Some cautions:
  - Not useful with quantitative data since it is difficult to interpret the angles of the wedges and the magnitude of the data
  - Can not show progress toward a goal
  - Difficult to compare multiple series of data

How to Use It

- Clearly define the issue or problem for which the data will be collected.
- Develop a check sheet that will describe each category of data to be collected.
- Develop a data collection strategy and collect the data.
- Tally the results for each category and calculate the grand total of all the data collected.

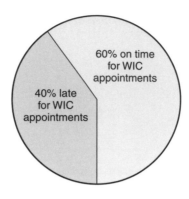

Figure 14.14 Pie chart.

- Convert each category to a percentage of the whole by dividing the data total for each category by the grand total and multiplying that result by 100.

- Draw the pie chart using the calculated percentages for each category to determine the size of each slice of the pie.

- Pie charts can be done by hand or using software such as Excel.

- Look at the largest slices to determine the most important categories.

Example

See Figure 14.14 for a pie chart example.

RUN CHART

What It Is

- Run charts originated from the control charts that were designed by Walter Shewhart in the 1920s at Bell Telephone Laboratories in New York.

- Run charts are line graphs of a variable under study over time with a median line displayed and showing time patterns.

- The median line divides the data into two equal halves—the median is the middle value in our data sample.

When to Use It

- When a plot of data over time will reveal information about a process under study.

- When we suspect that a process may be experiencing some shifts in its functioning. Run charts may show data patterns such as:

- Trends

- Mixtures

- Outliers

- Cycles

- Instability

- Sudden shifts

- When we want an easy-to-use method to show how a process is performing over time without calculating control limits.

- When there is a need for a simple way to confirm your knowledge of the process.

How to Use It

- Clearly define a process to study that is of interest to a team or a management group.

- Design a data management strategy to collect sample data. A minimum of 25 samples must be collected.

- Once the data is collected, determine the median as shown in Chapter 13.

- Draw a run chart by plotting the time order sequence on the x-axis and the corresponding data points on the y-axis.

- Draw the median line on the graph.

- Review the run chart and determine what the data plot is trying to convey. Understand the reason for any unusual patterns, shifts, or cycles.

Example

See Figure 14.15 for a run chart example.

SCATTER DIAGRAM

What It Is

- A nonmathematical graphical method to determine if a possible visual relationship exists between two variables under study.

- It is an x and y plot of measured values with one variable on the x-axis and the change in the other variable on the y-axis. The purpose of the plot is to show what happens to one variable (dependent) when the other variable (independent) is changed.

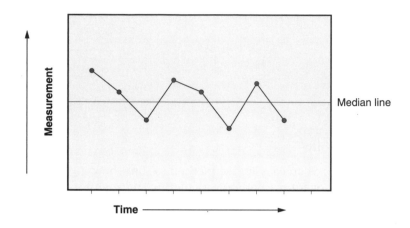

Figure 14.15   Run chart.

- Statistical correlation analysis is used to interpret scatter diagrams. Figure 14.16 shows a positive correlation, an increase in variable x is related to an increase in variable y; if the correlation were negative, an increase in x would be related to a decrease in y. If the correlation is close to zero, the variables have no linear relationship.

When to Use It

- When a cause-and-effect diagram points out a possible relationship between two variables, the scatter diagram can visually show if a relationship exists.

- When there is a need for a quick and easy way to graphically identify the possible relationship between two variables.

- When there is a need for a nonmathematical method to easily show, interpret, and communicate to others about the possible relationship of two variables.

How to Use It

- Identify the two variables to be investigated to see if there is a relationship.

- Identify one variable as the independent and one variable as the dependent variable from experience or knowledge of the process.

- Develop a data collection strategy and collect the data in pairs (x,y) using a check sheet.

- Draw the x and y axes of the graph and label them.

- Construct the two axes the same length with values increasing from left to right and bottom to top of the graph.

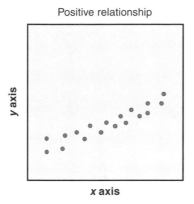

Figure 14.16   Scatter diagram.

- Plot the paired (x,y) data on the graph.
- Determine if there is any relationship between the two variables under study:
  - Positive relationship—as the independent variable (x) increases, the dependent variable (y) increases, and the reverse is also true.
  - Negative relationship—as the independent variable (x) increases, the dependent variable (y) decreases, and the reverse is also true.
  - No relationship—change in the independent variable (x) has no effect on the dependent variable (y).
- Caution:
  - Scatter diagrams are easy to visualize and interpret but also easy to misinterpret.
  - A relationship may appear to exist in the diagram but it may not be a true cause-and-effect relationship between the two variables. Always further investigate observed relationships with a more rigorous mathematical approach such as regression analysis.

Example

See Figure 14.16 for a scatter diagram example.

SIPOC+CM DIAGRAM

What It Is

- SIPOC is a data collection form that is used before we start to construct a flowchart since it helps us to gather relevant information about the process.

- Assists in gathering information about suppliers, inputs, processes, outputs, and customers of the process.

- SIPOC is high-level view of the "as is" state of a process under investigation.

- The +C stands for *constraints* facing the system and the +M for the *measures* to be used.

When to Use It

- When first starting to investigate a process and a team needs to understand the basics that make up the process.

- When a team needs a way to get the collective knowledge of the team members about a process recorded in an easy-to-view format.

- When we need to make a concise communication to others about a process and the parameters that it encompasses.

How to Use It

- On a piece of flip chart paper draw the SIPOC+CM diagram with seven blocks indicating the components of SIPOC+CM.

- Clearly identify the process under study and define the process boundaries (start and end points) so that everyone involved understands the limits of the analysis.

- On the SIPOC+CM form identify the data available for each of the following major categories:

  - Suppliers—who or what (internal or external) provides the raw materials, information, or technology to the process.

  - Inputs—the material or information specifications that are needed by the process.

  - Process—a high-level flowchart of the key five to seven core activities that comprise the process. This is a "35,000-foot" view of the process. The detailed steps will be developed in the flowchart.

  - Outputs—what the process produces as products, services, or technology.

  - Customers—who are the main users of the process's output?

  - +C—constraints facing the system or process.

  - +M—measures being used or to be used.

- Review the form for completeness with relevant stakeholders, sponsors, and other interested parties.

Begins with:
Identifying required service standards of performance.

Constraints:
Limited funds for benchmarking other public health organizations.
Human resources is short two staff and overworked already.

Ends with:
Trained and effective employees committed to using the standards in all areas.

Measures:
LPH standards of performance completed.
Percent of standards signed by employees.
Percent of job descriptions updated.
Training materials for standards completed on time.
Percent employees completing training.

Process/activities:
Benchmark other PHDs for standards of service performance.
Gather and review all current job descriptions for existing standards and expectations.
Research current journals for trends on behaviorally-based characteristics.
Work with HR and senior management to establish LPH standards.
Update all job descriptions and performance planning models to new standards.
Develop training materials to roll out new standards for current employees and new hires.
Announce rollout timelines and measurements.
Work with supervisors and employees to put standards into each performance plan.
Gather feedback, adjust, report, and maintain.

Inputs:
LPH system values and vision.
Current job descriptions and job performance expectations.
Benchmarking from other PHDs and service organizations.
Training on interviewing and employee selection criteria.
General idea of client, inspector, nurse, and other staff expectations.

Outputs:
Approved standards of service performance excellence for PHD.
Training modules developed for all levels of management and employees.
Announcement campaign to provide awareness and support of standards.
Rollout of training to all staff.
Training to supervisors on how to use the standards in performance planning.

Supplier(s):
PHD senior management, human resources, benchmarking organizations, consultant on hiring and interviewing, clients, health officer, nurse, supervisors, and employees.

Customers:
Employees, human resources, supervisors, PHD clients, senior management partners, nurses, community.

Figure 14.17   High-level SIPOC+CM form.

Example

See Figure 14.17 for a High-level SIPOC+CM example.

SOLUTION-AND-EFFECT DIAGRAM

What It Is

- This tool is the reverse of the cause-and-effect diagram since we are now focusing on solution rather than cause.

- This tool identifies changes and recommendations made to solve a problem.

- The "effect" is made into a positive statement, such as from "What are the causes of childhood obesity" to "How to prevent childhood obesity."

- Resembles a fish skeleton and sometimes called a fishbone diagram.

- Systematic approach to analyzing the possible solutions to find the root solution.

- May be more efficient and effective than cause-and-effect when multiple solutions are available.

When to Use It

- When a problem-solving team needs to consider the complexity of a proposal and to take an objective look at all the contributing factors and not just the solutions that are most obvious.

- When the team needs to determine both the primary and the secondary solutions to a problem and delve into the details in a more in-depth approach.

- When a team needs to not use their usual approach of taking the path of least resistance when confronted with a problem to solve.

How to Use It

- Write the issue as a solution statement on the left-hand side of a piece of flip chart paper, opposite the cause-and-effect diagram, and draw a box around it. Then draw an arrow from the right side of the paper pointing toward the box.

- Write the issue as a positive statement on the left-hand side of the page and draw a box around it. Then draw an arrow from the left side of the paper pointing toward the box.

- This positive issue of working toward a solution is now the effect.

- This issue is now the effect, which is a sign or indication of what could happen and be implemented as a solution.

- Use brainstorming to generate ideas as to what are the main components of the effect—whatever makes something happen. Question what the solution is, who is impacted, and how and where it can occur to get the group started analyzing the solution. Label these as the main branch solution headers. Typical solution headers are similar to the cause-and-effect headers:

  – Four M's—Manpower, Materials, Methods, Machinery

- People

- Policies

- Materials

- Equipment

- Lifestyle

- Environment

- And so on

- For each main solution category brainstorm ideas as to what are the related sub-solutions that might affect our issue.

- Use the five hows technique when a solution is identified to drill down into the details. Keep repeating the "How?" question until no other sub-solutions can be identified.

- List the sub-solutions using arrows on the diagram.

- When the solution-and-effect diagram is finished it is time to decide what few areas should be focused on to develop solutions to solve the effect.

Example

See Figures 14.18 and 14.19 for solution-and-effect diagram examples.

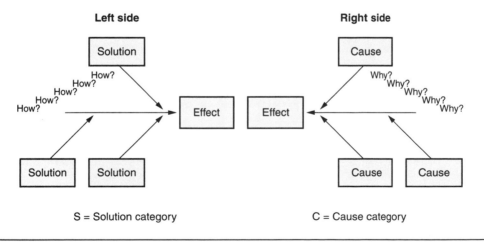

Figure 14.18 Solution-and-effect diagram.

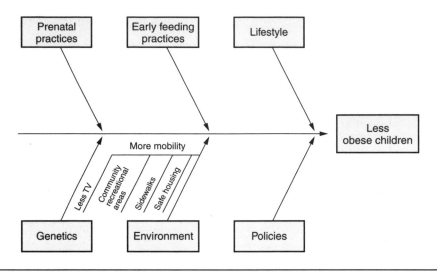

Figure 14.19 Solution-and-effect diagram for childhood obesity example.

Chapter 15

Advanced Tools of Quality Improvement

John W. Moran and Grace L. Duffy

T he advanced tools of quality improvement help us to clarify organization-wide issues into clearly defined issue statements that describe the root cause of the issue. The issue statement clarifies the current state and describes the future state we desire to move toward. The advanced tools of quality improvement are vehicles to help us sort through the many interrelated possibilities we have at the strategic level and help narrow them down into the vital few issues to focus our resources upon to make the biggest positive impact on the organization. These vital few issues are usually hidden and not apparent when we first start to explore a strategic issue, but the tools in this section provide the means to focus a team on the few priorities that will move the organization to its desired future state as quickly as possible.

The advanced tools of quality take a system approach of continuous refinement of the issue as we move from one tool to the next in a defined sequence of application. This is a process of constant refinement to help us clearly understand the issue being investigated and its interrelated components. When used in a sequence of application as shown in Figure 15.1, they form a dynamic process that helps us to continually refine our issue/problem statement, which narrows the scope and the approaches to solve the problem.

Figure 15.1 shows a basic flowchart of how to use the advanced tools of quality improvement in a problem-solving sequence to resolve an issue of importance to a team or individual. This is a general flow and does not meet all issue/problem situations that could arise. When using the advanced tools of quality improvement a team or individual should think through an approach they would use and then adopt the best sequence of advanced tools of quality improvement to fit the particular situation they are trying to solve.

In order to help the reader this chapter has been developed similarly to Chapter 14 to guide the reader through the maze of advanced tools and techniques that are available.

Each tool will be presented in the following format in the four categories shown below. This will not be an exhaustive description of the tool but one that will allow the reader to have a quick reference source on a tool's use and application.

- *What it is.* A description of the basics of the tool

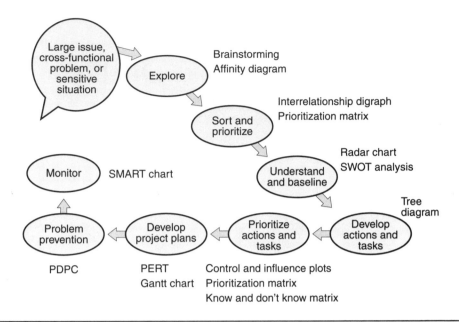

Figure 15.1 General approach on how to use the advanced tools of quality improvement.

- *When to use it.* General guidance on the most common application of the tool

- *How to use it.* The basics of the process and procedure of applying the tool to a situation

- *Example.* An example of the use of the tool to clarify the three categories above

As stated by Lao Tse, Chinese philosopher, "For every complex question there is a simple answer and it is usually wrong." The advanced tools of quality deal with complex issues in a manner that forces those analyzing the issue to focus on hidden interrelationships that are not obvious without detailed analysis. This detailed analysis forces those analyzing an issue away from the simple answer.

As shown in Figure 15.2, the advanced tools use a funnel approach to clarify issues.

Tools discussed in this chapter:

1. Affinity diagram

2. Control and influence diagram

3. Gantt chart

4. Interrelationship digraph

5. Matrix diagram

6. Process decision program chart

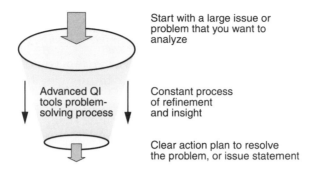

Start with a large issue or problem that you want to analyze

Advanced QI tools problem-solving process

Constant process of refinement and insight

Clear action plan to resolve the problem, or issue statement

Figure 15.2   Funnel approach to clarifying issues.

7. Prioritization matrix

8. Radar chart

9. SMART matrix

10. SWOT analysis

11. Tree diagram

Before we present the advanced tools of quality improvement the authors will present a technique they have found useful when beginning a process requiring these advanced tools: developing focusing and issue statements.

This process develops a clear issue or problem statement that can be communicated to a team assigned to make change. This clear issue or problem statement forms the basis for the use of the tools to investigate the issue or problem.

When developing focusing and issue statements stay at a strategic level in the explanation and try not to get too operational; let the team develop the details.

Also, when developing the focusing and issue statements do not suggest or imply any solutions.

Focusing statement—current state. Describe some background on the issue/problem that has been selected for those who will be working on it.

- What is the current state?

- Why is this important?

- What is it costing us—time/dollars/staff, and so on?

- What is the impact on our customers/clients?

- What is the impact on our division/agency/department?

Example:

Too few state and local public health agencies are measuring their success based on improvements in community health outcomes. Through development of agencywide performance management systems and the routine employment of quality improvement (QI) techniques, public health agencies can improve their performance, become more accountable to the public and policy makers, and achieve better community health outcomes. At the present time, performance management and QI are not well-integrated into most public health agencies.

Issue statement—moving to the future state. Give the team working on the issue some of your thinking, in broad terms, on what the future state should look like.
    Describe:

- What are the important aspects of the future state?

- What is driving us to this future state?

- What might be the consequences of not moving to the future state?

- What might change?

- What is the proposed timeline?

Example:

> *To improve the current public health situation and begin moving public health to the cutting edge of quality and innovation, how will XYZ accomplish this within the next three years?*

In other exercises, as we narrow down to solutions to reach the future state, we will use the description as a decision criteria so it needs to be very clearly defined.

Components of the issue statement. Describe the components of the issue statement in discrete high-level elements. A form can be used for this as shown in Figure 15.3. In this section we want to answer the questions:

- Do we as a group have complete control over the element?

- Can we implement a solution to this element when we develop it?

- Do we have to involve and influence others to get the element resolved?

- Is this element outside our control and influence ability?

For each element check the column(s) that apply.
    From here select the area(s) of focus, develop a ranking of the elements to focus on, and write the problem statement for the quality improvement project.

Elements	Control	Implement	Involve and influence	Outside our control and influence

Figure 15.3 Control and influence matrix.

Problem statement. At this level we begin to look at things more operationally rather than strategically. We still want to keep the problem statement broad and not suggest a solution.

Example:

How will we focus our department's resources on the shifting socioeconomic situation of the clients now requiring services from us?

How will we serve people now needing health services?

How will we implement a property maintenance program to preserve our community's character?

The clearer we can be when we charter a team to make improvements, the better the chances they will be able to make that change. Clear intentions/directions save the team time and energy trying to figure out exactly what their sponsor wanted them to do.

Figure 15.4 shows a graphic depiction of this process.

AFFINITY DIAGRAM

What It Is

- It was created in the 1960s by Japanese anthropologist Jiro Kawakita.

- Tool for gathering, grouping, organizing, and understanding large amounts of information.

- Helps to identify and draw out common themes from a large amount of information and reveal any hidden linkages.

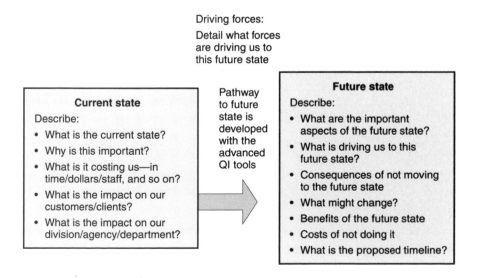

Figure 15.4   Moving from current to future state.

- Partners well with brainstorming to organize a large number of ideas/issues.

When to Use It

- As the next step in organizing the output of a brainstorming event into relevant themes or categories for analysis

- To actively involve stakeholders in the specifics of a situation in which you require their understanding, experience, knowledge, and support

- To further analyze data, ideas, or observations for eventual hypothesis testing, prioritization, and decision making

How to Use It

- Develop and post a broad clear purpose, problem, concern, or issue statement to focus the group at the macro level.

- Materials needed:

  - Sticky notes or 3 × 5 cards

  - Marking pens

  - Large work surface such as a wall, table, or floor

- Start with individual silent brainstorming and have the participants record each of their ideas with a marking pen on a separate sticky note or card. Each statement needs to be a complete and positive statement—no one-word statements.

- Each participant reads and randomly posts their ideas on the wall or work surface one at a time.

  - Other participants can ask for clarification when an idea is read, but there is no debate, just clarification.

  - Do not place the notes in any order since you do not want to determine categories or headings in advance. Use the whole posting area to randomly post ideas.

- Once all the ideas are posted the participants do a silent consensus process:

  - The entire team gathers around the posted notes

  - No talking during this step

  - Look for ideas that seem to be related in some way

  - Move the sticky notes and place them side by side

  - Repeat until all notes are grouped

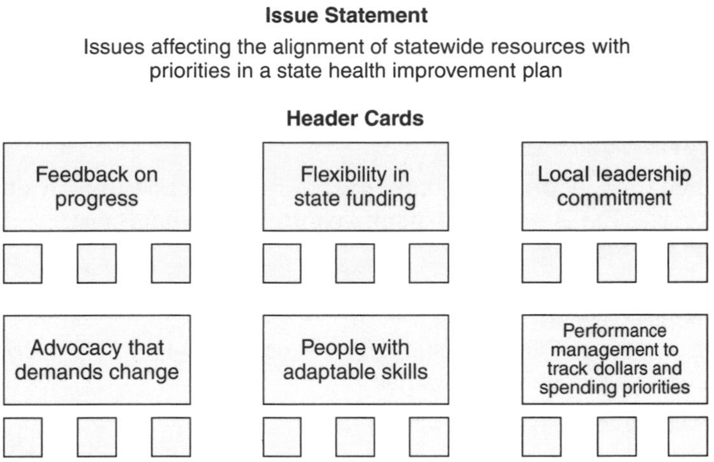

Issue Statement

Issues affecting the alignment of statewide resources with
priorities in a state health improvement plan

Header Cards

Feedback on progress	Flexibility in state funding	Local leadership commitment
☐ ☐ ☐	☐ ☐ ☐	☐ ☐ ☐
Advocacy that demands change	People with adaptable skills	Performance management to track dollars and spending priorities
☐ ☐ ☐	☐ ☐ ☐	☐ ☐ ☐

Figure 15.5   Affinity diagram example.

  – Okay to have "loners" that don't seem to fit a group (outliers)

  – It's all right to move a note someone else has already moved

  – If a note seems to belong in two groups, make a second note

• After the ideas are grouped, the participants discuss what the grouping patterns show or have uncovered.

• Select a heading for each grouping of ideas.

• Place the heading at the top of the group and highlight it in a bright color.

• Take the time to do this step well since it is the foundation for the other tools in the process.

Example

See Figure 15.5 for an affinity diagram example.

CONTROL AND INFLUENCE DIAGRAM

What It Is

• This is a conceptual tool to help give guidance on what to focus on when trying to pick an area to improve.

• This tool focuses a team on the areas where they have both control and knowledge. It is important for a team to focus its resources on areas where they can make an impact quickly.

- In public health we may work more in the influence part of the diagram or quadrant shown in Figure 15.6.

When to Use It

- When we need to understand the boundaries of a problem situation, such as what is under the team's control and what is not

- When we first start a team and want to understand the knowledge and experience of the team members

- When we want to understand in what areas a team may need assistance or outside expertise

- When we first start a team and want to understand or anticipate what might be potential roadblocks

- When we want to know what areas we should stay away from

How to Use It

- Draw a four-quadrant square as shown in Figure 15.6 and label the top two columns as Control and No control. Then label the left side rows as Knowledge and No knowledge.

- Fill in each quadrant with the team and indicate in what areas the team members have:

  - Control and knowledge—these areas we can focus on

  - Control and no knowledge—these are areas we can focus on with expert assistance

  - No control but have knowledge—these are areas in which we can do some influencing

  - No control and no knowledge—these are areas we should stay away from since they will just waste the team's resources.

- Once all the quadrants are filled in, go through a prioritization process (nominal group technique, interrelationship digraph, prioritization matrix, and so on) for all the quadrants except the No control and No knowledge one.

- Once the prioritization process is complete the team will be able to visualize what areas to focus on that will have the most impact on the problem under study.

Example

See Figure 15.6 for a control and influence diagram example.

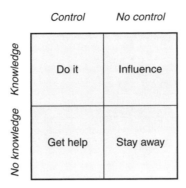

Figure 15.6   Control and influence diagram.

GANTT CHART

What It Is

- The first Gantt chart was developed by Karol Adamiecki, who called it a *harmonogram,* and because he did not publish his chart until 1931, this famous chart bears Henry Gantt's name (1861–1919) since he designed his chart in 1910 at the Franklin Arsenal.

- It is a matrix diagram that shows work that has been planned and accomplished in the same space—it shows plans and progress.

- It is a tool that emphasizes work movement through time

When to Use It

- When we need a simple method to convey how progress is being made toward a goal.

- When we need a method that can show when a series of sequential actions/tasks must be completed.

- When we need to show who is responsible for each assigned action.

- When we need to identify and eliminate obstacles that might impede progress toward a goal.

How to Use It

- Draw an L-shaped matrix and divide its top horizontal axis into three columns and the vertical axis into many rows (see Figure 15.7).

- Label the first column "Tasks," which will be listed below it in sequence.

Task: Saginaw County HD	29-Feb	7-Mar	14-Mar	21-Mar	28-Mar	1-Apr	10-Apr	15-Apr	21-Apr	1-May	8-May	13-May	19-May	28-May	6-Jun	13-Jun	Responsibility
Finalize self-assessment analysis	X																
Align with SCPHD MOD Squad	X																
Identify priority project candidate	X																
Plan PHF consultant visit		X															
Set agenda and travel schedule		X															
Saginaw/PHF PI meeting			X														
Plan pilot PI project and milestones			X	X													
Validate PHF hours remaining of 33			X		X		X			X		X	X	X			
Teleconference consultant update																	
Decide team meeting schedule					X	1:30	2:30	1:30	10:00	10:30	10:00	10:00	10:00	10:00			
Hold formal team meetings					X												
Complete team charter					X												
Flowchart desired staff training proc																	
Analyze causes of staff exp issues																	
Select solutions as appropriate																	
Design pilot PI activities																	
Establish measures and outcomes																	
Kickoff staff expertise PI pilot test																	
Gather measures and analyze																	
Analyze and modify process as needed																	
Senior management interim reports																	
Rollout of updated processes																	
Monitor behavioral changes																	
Measure process for improvement																	
Create report of improved outcomes																	
Final senior mgmt report & storyboard																	
Final NACCHO/PHF report for 5/31/08															X		

Legend: Complete ▢   Watch ▢   Late or at risk ▢

Figure 15.7   Simple Gantt chart created in Microsoft Excel.

- The second column will be subdivided into as many columns of week ending dates as necessary to finish the project's tasks. In many cases this will be an estimate, and more dates can be added if necessary as the project progresses.

- The third column is labeled "Responsibility" and will indicate for each action/task who the responsible party is.

- The vertical axis lists all the sequential actions/tasks to be performed for a project:

  - Each row contains a single task identification

  - Each action/task completion end date is indicated under the week ending date column

- The team monitors the actions/tasks to determine which are on schedule, which are slipping but recoverable, and those that are in trouble and will not make their completion date.

- Those tasks that are slipping or in trouble are analyzed for root cause, and corrective actions are developed and implemented to get them back on schedule.

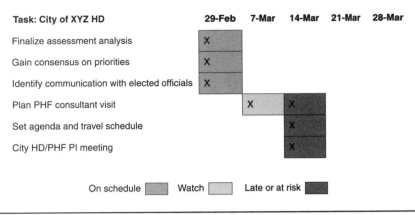

Figure 15.8   Traffic light Gantt chart.

- Another variation of the Gantt chart is the *traffic light Gantt chart* (see Figure 15.8). This chart uses the colors of a traffic light to indicate progress on a Gantt chart:

  - Green—on schedule

  - Yellow—caution—some slippage in completion date but recoverable

  - Red—behind schedule and needs intervention and analysis to determine why it is behind schedule and what can be done to get it back on track

- For a more complex project a *program evaluation review technique* (PERT) can be utilized, but this is a time- and resource-intensive process requiring software to keep the chart up to date. A discussion of PERT is beyond the scope of this book.

Example

See Figures 15.7 and 15.8 for Gantt chart examples.

INTERRELATIONSHIP DIGRAPH

What It Is

- A visual technique to help a team understand how the various elements of a defined issue are related.

- A follow-on to the affinity diagram process that uses the header cards to:

  - Prioritize and find the real critical issues—not reactions to symptoms—of a complex issue or problem

  - Discover the hidden linkages between the header cards

  – Identify the driving elements and those that are bottlenecks

When to Use It

- When there is disagreement between team members on what is the real root cause or driver of a problem situation

- When a team needs to prioritize the header cards from an affinity diagramming session

- When we want to show a simple tabular summary of the prioritization of the affinity diagram header cards

How to Use It

- Use the header cards from the affinity diagram and spread them out on a large work surface covered with flip chart paper.

- Start with one of the header cards and compare it to all the other header cards. Continue this process until all the header cards have been compared to all the others.

- When comparing header cards use an "influence" arrow to connect related header cards.

- The arrows should be drawn from the header card that influences to the one influenced. A question to ask when comparing header cards is:

  – Does this card cause any others to happen or is it a result from another card(s)? If the answer is *"yes,"* draw an arrow connecting them. If the answer is *"no,"* do not draw an arrow connecting them and move on to the next paired comparison.

  – Then determine the strength of the relationship by assigning a "1" for a weak relationship, a "5" for a medium relationship, and a "10" for a strong relationship.

- Use only one-way arrows. The arrow should point toward the effect and away from the cause:

  – Outgoing arrow = basic cause—if solved, spillover reaction on a large number of other issues

  – Incoming arrow = secondary issue or bottleneck

- Once all the comparisons are completed, count the number of *in arrows, out arrows,* and the total strength assigned for each header card.

- The header card with the most outgoing arrows and highest strength will be a driver of root causes. The one with the most incoming arrows and highest strength will be a bottleneck, outcome, or result.

- The tabular results of the arrows and strength can be captured on the interrelationship digraph (Figure 15.9) or in a matrix (Figure 15.10).

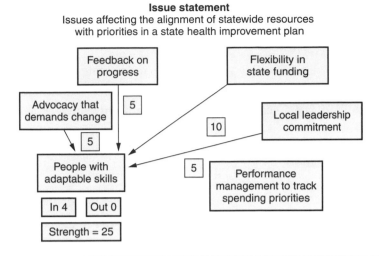

Figure 15.9 Interrelationship digraph (ID)—bottleneck/outcome/result.

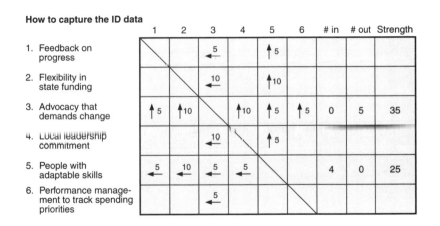

Figure 15.10 Interrelationship digraph matrix.

Example

See Figures 15.9 and 15.10 for interrelationship digraph examples.

MATRIX DIAGRAM

What It Is

- A method to show relationships/strength between items
- Can show the relationship between two, three, or four groups of information/issues/tasks

- A method to display information about the relationship between items of two, three, or four groups of information/issues/tasks

- A way to help prioritize tasks or issues to facilitate decision making

- A method to help identify the connecting points between items

When to Use It

- When we need to show a lot of data in a simple array

- When we need a method to show relationships between items

- When we need to determine relationships between elements

- When we need a method to help prioritize tasks or issues

- When we need a method to find the common thread or identify the connecting points between large groups of ideas

How to Use It

- First decide on which type of matrix is needed for the task at hand:

  - L-shaped—shows relationships between any two different groups of information—compare A to B.

  - T-shaped—two L-shaped diagrams connected together showing the relationships of two different factors to a common third one—compare A to B and A to C but not B to C.

  - X-shaped—extends the T-shaped matrix into an X-shaped matrix—compare four groups A, B, C, D. You can compare A to B to C to D to A but you can not compare A to C or B to D.

  - Y-shaped—identifies interactions between three different factors—A, B, C. You can compare A to B, B to C, and A to C in a circular fashion.

  - C-shaped—identifies the interaction between three different factors—A, B, C. It allows for a comparison all three factors simultaneously—comparison is a dot in the matrix. This is a three-dimensional matrix and difficult to use or construct without software.

- Draw the appropriate matrix on a piece of flip chart paper and fill in the comparison factors information.

- Have the team members fill in the relationships between the comparison factors on the matrix.

- Once the comparison information and relationships have been tabulated, list the prioritized items.

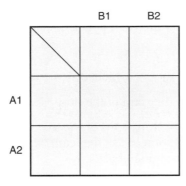

Figure 15.11   L- shaped matrix.

- Focus the team on the top three items and decide which ones need further analysis.

Example

See Figure 15.11 for a matrix diagram example.

PROCESS DECISION PROGRAM CHART (PDPC)

What It Is

- A process that helps an implementation team to systematically identify what might go wrong in a plan under development.

- A method by which you can anticipate problems in advance so you can either revise the plan to avoid the problems or be ready with the best response when a problem occurs.

- The process decision program chart is another version of the tree diagram with a couple of extra steps to identify risks and countermeasures for the action or tasks.

When to Use It

- When the risk of failure for a project is high or there is a very tight implementation timeline

- When implementing a large and complex plan

- When the plan must be completed on schedule

- When the price of failure is high

- When a team needs to think through what could go wrong with an implementation plan before they make a presentation to decision makers

- When countermeasures need to be developed to prevent or offset potential problems

How to Use It

- Start with the tree diagram of the proposed plan.

- For each task on the third level of the tree, brainstorm what could go wrong. The question to ask the team is, "If we wanted this to fail, how could we accomplish that?"

- Review all the potential problems and eliminate any that are improbable or whose consequences would be insignificant.

- For the remaining potential problems, brainstorm possible countermeasures.

- Decide how practical each countermeasure is by using criteria such as:

  - Cost

  - Time required

  - Ease of implementation

  - Effectiveness

  - And so on

- For each countermeasure developed, ask the following questions to ensure that the team has considered all possibilities:

  - What assumptions are we making that could turn out to be wrong?

  - What has been our experience in similar situations in the past?

  - Does this depend on actions, conditions, or events outside our control?

  - Are these potential problems controllable or uncontrollable?

Example

See Figure 15.12 for a PDPC example.

PRIORITIZATION MATRIX

What It Is

- A qualitatively rigorous decision-making tool

- Utilizes an L-shaped matrix to capture the data

- Uses a pair-wise comparison process of items under consideration

- Utilizes set decision criteria to guide the pair-wise comparisons

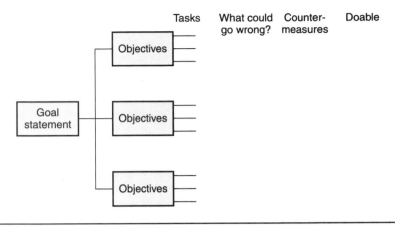

Figure 15.12   Process decision program chart.

- Utilizes a weighting criteria to score the pair-wise comparisons

When to Use It

- When we need consistency in a decision-making process

- When we want to select firm decision criteria to guide our decision-making process before starting team consensus

- When we do not want an arbitrary prioritization process

- When we want to have a numerical scale to represent each judgment on the pair-wise comparisons

- When we want a quick and efficient method to prioritize a list of potential alternatives or actions

- When we want a simple way to present a group's collective prioritization on a complex issue

How to Use It

- Utilize the header cards from the affinity diagram or brainstorm a list of issues/actions to be prioritized.

- Develop the decision criteria to be utilized when making the pair-wise comparisons before starting the process. Some criteria could be:

  - Improved quality

  - Lower costs

  - Improved delivery

  - Improved outcomes

  - Better service

- Draw an L-shaped matrix on a piece of flip chart paper and be sure to have enough rows for all the items under consideration on the vertical axis, and on the horizontal axis have one more column than rows so you can total the scores for each item.

- Label the rows with the items under consideration; the column labels should correspond to the row numbers.

- Blank out the intersections of the same item in a row and column. This will result in a diagonal block through the L-shaped matrix.

- Take the cards two at a time and ask the following question:

  - Does having X contribute more than Y in achieving the goal, based on our decision criteria?

  - Let the experts decide the answer to the question—expertise will rotate in the group on different pair-wise comparisons.

- Once there is agreement on the answer to the question you must decide on how much using the following rating scale:

  - 1—equally important

  - 5—significantly more important

  - 10—exceedingly more important

  - 1/5—significantly less important

  - 1/10—exceedingly less important

- Assign the agreed-upon value to the issue/action contributing more than the other compared action in the matrix. The one not contributing more gets the reciprocal score. If both are equally important they both get a score of 1.

- It is best to do the pair-wise comparisons quickly—your first inclination is usually correct.

- When all the pair-wise comparisons are completed, total the scores and prioritize the issues/actions from the most important (highest score) to least important (lowest score).

- Remember, you must stick to the decision criteria throughout the process and can not change them. If you change the decision criteria it will probably change the prioritization.

- This process can be used in conjunction with the tree diagram as shown in Figure 15.17.

Example

See Figure 15.13 for a prioritization matrix example.

	1	2	3	4	5	6	7	8	9	10	
1		1/5	10	1/5	1/10	10	5	1/5	5	1/5	30.9
2	5		10	1	5	10	5	5	10	1	52
3	1/10	1/10		5	1	1/5	1/10	1/10	5	1/5	11.8
4	5	1	1/5		1/5	5	1/5	1/5	5	1/5	17
5	10	1/5	1	5		1/5	1/5	1/5	5	1/10	21.8
6	1/10	1/10	5	1/5	5		1/5	1/10	5	1/10	15.8
7	1/5	1/5	10	5	5	5		1	5	1/5	31.6
8	5	1/5	10	5	5	10	1		5	1	42.2
9	1/5	1/10	1/5	1/5	1/5	1/5	1/5	1/5		1/10	1.6
10	5	1	5	5	10	10	5	1	10		52

Figure 15.13 Prioritization matrix.

RADAR CHART

What It Is

- A graphical technique that can depict strengths and weaknesses together
- Gives a clear, concise picture of current and future states
- Consensual picture of a team's agreement on the state of a series of attributes or categories

When to Use It

- When you need to develop a baseline of a series of attributes
- When you need a way to help a team reach a visual consensus quickly
- When a team needs a method to capture the range of feelings or perceptions
- When we need a simple way to reach consensus on areas for improvement
- When we need a way to identify areas of excellence in a series of categories or attributes

- When we need to visually show improvement goals and performance gaps together

How to Use It

- Draw a circle on a piece of flip chart paper and divide it into as many spokes as there are categories or attributes to chart.

- It is best not to have more than eight categories or attributes since more make it difficult to visualize and the graphic looks crowded.

- The measurement scale needs to be determined; the farther from the center of the radar chart, the better the score.

  - The measurement scale can be quantitative (0–5) or qualitative (Strongly agree [SA], Agree [A], Disagree [D], Strongly disagree [SD])

- Empower a team around a topic and let them make an individual assessment of each category or attribute using measurement criteria.

- Then develop a consensus score for each measurement criterion.

- Plot the consensus score for each measurement criterion. Also show the range of scores on each measurement criterion—see where the consensus score came out.

- Connect the scores and a pattern will develop.

- Identify the low-scoring items (improvement opportunities).

- Identify high-scoring items (pockets of excellence—areas to learn from).

- Once we have determined the areas to focus on or improve we can use the other tools of quality improvement to analyze the opportunities.

- The radar chart can be used to show the future state we want to achieve for each category along with the consensus score. This will show the improvement gap to be closed.

- Revisit this chart on a regular basis and plot improvement gains— observe whether the gap is closing between the current and future states.

Example

See Figure 15.14 for a radar chart example.

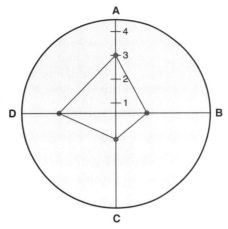

A public health agency decided to rate themselves on how well they were doing on performance management. They rated themselves from a 1—very poor to a 4—very good on the following four criteria:

A. Performance standards

B. Performance measures

C. Reporting of progress

D. Quality improvement

Figure 15.14   Radar chart example.

SMART MATRIX

What It Is

- A communication and planning tool to identify the specifics of actions or tasks.

- SMART stands for *specific, measurable, attainable, resources,* and *time.*

- It is an L-shaped matrix designed to capture the key points of a team's project objectives.

- A process to review how actions are being implemented around various attributes.

When to Use It

- When a team needs to analyze an implementation plan's tasks to ensure they are on track

- When we need to understand the amount of resources needed to implement a plan

- When we need to understand how the various tasks are sequenced and related

How to Use It

- On a piece of flip chart paper draw an L-shaped matrix with five columns labeled Specific, Measurable, Attainable, Resources, and Time.

- Write the implementation plan title in the upper left of the chart.

- Detail the specific tasks to be performed. Make the task statement detailed and well defined. The example in Figure 15.15 shows a combination of task and objective statements providing measures, outcomes, and time frames.

- For each detailed specific task:

  - Define a measure or indicator that can be tracked.

  - Determine how will it be attained in actionable terms that are realistic and feasible.

  - Indicate the amount and type of resources required to complete each task identified.

  - Identify the timeline for completion.

- Once the matrix is completed, review the results with the implementation team to ensure that everything has been accounted for and recorded.

- Review the matrix to make sure the timeline is realistic and everything is not due to be completed on the same day.

- Review the matrix and get a feel for the total amount of resources that are required and determine if they are available or if adjustments need to be made.

Figure 15.15 shows a table summarizing the detailed conversation generated by using the SMART matrix. Notes within the matrix indicate areas of resource constraints that require attention from project sponsors and department leadership.

Example

See Figure 15.15 for a SMART matrix example.

SWOT ANALYSIS

What It Is

- SWOT stands for *strengths, weaknesses, opportunities,* and *threats.*

- A process to complete a systematic assessment of an organization's internal and external operating environment.

- A methodology to identify the major attributes that affect the organization's ability to achieve its vision and to improve and protect its competitive position.

- A process to align future initiatives with outcomes of SWOT analysis as tied to company vision and goals.

Task/objective	S	M	A	R	T
Reduce overtime for clerical staff by 15% by the end of 3Q09	X	X	X	Training Process mapping Office schedule Electronic filing	12 mos
Recruit five nursing assistants for the vaccination program by July 15, 2009	X	X	Discuss at 12/15/09 senior management meeting	Hire tickets Salary budget Available talent pool	8 mos
Enroll the new quality improvement coordinator into team training for 4Q08	X	X	X	Training budget Appropriate class Travel funds Time away from current duties	2 mos
Visit three substance program community partners each month between 12/08 and 7/09	X	X	X	Director and health officer schedule Travel budget Agency car	5 hrs/mo
Obtain two additional grants totaling $85K for toxic waste cleanup by 2Q09	X	X	Few funding sources for toxic waste cleanup	Grant writer Chemical analysis equipment Chemist	3 mos
	Specific	Measureable	Attainable	Resources	Time

Figure 15.15 SMART matrix.

When to Use It

- When an organization needs to assess and understand how its current resources and capabilities position it in the competitive environment in which it operates

- When we need input as to the operating and market environment before a strategic planning process begins

- When we need answers to the following questions:

  - How can we maximize each *strength* we possess as an organization?

  - How can we minimize each *weakness* we have as an organization?

  - How can we exploit each *opportunity* we uncover as an organization?

  - How can we defend the organization against each *threat* we face in our environment?

How to Use It

- On a piece of flip chart paper draw an L-shaped matrix with four columns labeled as Strengths, Weaknesses, Opportunities, and Threats.

- Next define the time horizon of the analysis: one, three, five years out?

- On the top of the flip chart sheet define the current state and a desired future state in detail as a clear, concise, and attainable objective to be achieved.

- Brainstorm and fill in the four columns with the team and then eliminate those that do not seem reasonable, and identify those that need to be verified and those for which we already have data. Make sure the entries on the SWOT chart are specific, not vague. Some examples:

  - Strengths: brand name, reputation, cost advantage, location

  - Weaknesses: high costs, lack of access to key resources, limited funding

  - Opportunities: new markets, unfulfilled customer needs, joint ventures

  - Threats: new competitors, less funding

- Keep the process simple and do not overanalyze until items have been verified.

- Force the team members doing the SWOT analysis to be realistic about current strengths, weaknesses, opportunities, and threats facing the organization.

- Distinguish between the current and future state.

- Remember, a SWOT analysis is subjective and needs to be confirmed with data.

Example

See Figure 15.16 for a SWOT analysis example.

Future state: _____

Clearly define objective: _____

Strengths	Weaknesses	Opportunities	Threats
• Brand name • Reputation • Cost advantage • Location	• High costs • Lack of access to key resources • Limited funding	• New markets • Unfulfilled customer needs • Joint ventures	• New competitors • Other service providers

Current state description: _____

Figure 15.16   SWOT analysis.

TREE DIAGRAM

What It Is

- A method to take a broad objective and break it down into its subcomponents in a step-by-step approach.

- A tree diagram starts with one item that branches into two or more items in a logical manner.

- A tree diagram helps you move your thinking step by step from generalities to specifics.

When to Use It

- When a tool is needed to focus a team on a logical thinking process, from a major goal to detailed tasks

- After an affinity diagram or interrelationship digraph and key issues are selected and need to be detailed

- When we need to break down broad categories into finer and finer levels of detail and go from the general to specific—objectives to tasks to measures, and so on

- When a plan must be generated/mapped out, broad objectives must be broken down into specific implementation detail, root causes need to be identified, or assignable tasks must be created

- When contingency planning with anticipated obstacles is required

- When a simple communication tool is needed to explain details to others

How to Use It

- Develop a goal statement and write it at the far left of a piece of flip chart paper and put a box around it.

- Then utilize the ideas developed in the affinity diagram brainstorming session and arrange the ideas from broad to specific for each header card in a tree diagram format. Ask a question that will lead you to the next level of detail.

- If the affinity diagram process was not used, ask the following questions about the goal statement:

  - "How can this be accomplished?"

  - "What causes this?"

  - "Why does this happen?"

  - "What tasks must be done to accomplish this?"

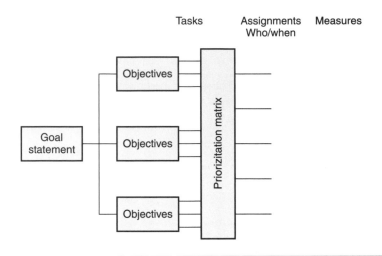

Figure 15.17   Tree diagram.

> – Brainstorm all possible answers.

- Write each idea to the right of the first statement. Show links between the tiers with arrows.

- Once the tree diagram is completed, do a check and make sure all the items at each level are necessary for the one on the level above. Check your logic and flow. Ask the following check question at each level of the tree diagram:

  - If all the items at this level were present or accomplished, would they be sufficient for the one on the level above?

  - Once the tree diagram is checked it can be used to prioritize tasks, develop contingency plans, or assign responsibilities. A prioritization matrix can be used to identify the most important tasks before assigning staff, deadlines, and measures.

Example

See Figure 15.17 for a tree diagram example.

Chapter 16

Applying Lean Six Sigma in Public Health

Grace L. Duffy, Erica Farmer, and John W. Moran

WHAT IS LEAN SIX SIGMA?

Lean Six Sigma is a methodology that integrates concepts and tools from lean operations and Six Sigma methodologies. The concept of *lean* evolved from a series of quality and performance improvement models dating back to the work of W. Edwards Deming and Joseph A. Juran in the 1950s. Organizations must eliminate waste and reduce time to market for services and products to remain competitive. Unless all available resources are directly engaged in the fulfillment of a customer need, something is being wasted. There will always be a competitor who can do the same function for less, or faster, or better given the same resources.

As defined by the Turning Point Performance Management Collaborative,[1] *performance management* in public health is the practice of actively using performance data to improve the public's health. This practice involves the strategic use of performance measures and standards to establish performance targets and goals, to prioritize and allocate resources, to inform managers about needed adjustments or changes in policy or program directions to meet goals, to frame reports on the success in meeting performance goals, and to improve the quality of public health practice. Six Sigma offers a robust family of measurement and performance tools designed to meet a broad range of customer requirements. Lean enterprise uses an overlapping set of tools to identify and eliminate waste from all activities performed by the organization.

Lean addresses reduction of waste and cycle time, while Six Sigma focuses on customer acceptance. A useful way to distinguish between the two sides of Lean Six Sigma is to think of the profit equation most familiar to the business community:

$$\text{Revenues} - \text{Expenses} = \text{Profit}$$

In the public health community, this equation might be better represented as:

$$\text{Funding} - \text{Expenses} = \text{Available capital}$$

The expense side of the profit equation is addressed by lean enterprise tools. Reducing waste and non-value-added expenses leaves more for meeting the highest priority needs of the public health community. The funding side of the profit

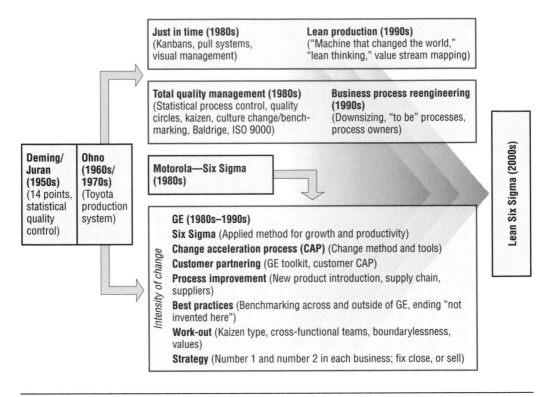

Figure 16.1   Evolution of Lean Six Sigma methodology, which builds on the practical lessons
learned from previous eras of operational improvement.

Source: IBM Global Business Services analysis.

equation is more frequently addressed by Six Sigma approaches of being customer-
focused and expanding the reputation and respect of the public health organization within the greater community of stakeholders, contributors, and potential
clients.

Figure 16.1 illustrates a series of business, quality, and performance models
used by global industry leading up to the current Lean Six Sigma methodology.
The Japanese developed significant expertise in reducing variation after World
War II. This talent provided Japan with a highly competitive platform for meeting customer requirements, reducing cycle time, and managing for continuous
improvement. United States industry became aware of Japanese competitiveness in the 1970s when Toyota began publishing the results of their improvement
efforts. U.S. businesses and universities spent much of the 1980s benchmarking
with Japanese companies to bring these innovative techniques to America.[2]

To better understand Lean Six Sigma, a review of lean enterprise and Six
Sigma tools and concepts is our starting point.

LEAN ENTERPRISE OR LEAN OPERATIONS

Lean concepts are applicable beyond the traditional manufacturing shop floor.
Companies have realized great benefit by implementing lean techniques in the

office functions of manufacturing firms as well as in purely service firms such as banks, hospitals, restaurants, public health organizations, and others. Lean manufacturing in this context is known as *lean enterprise*. *Lean operations* is another term also used to identify tools and activities of lean beyond traditional manufacturing. Public health departments (PHDs) are becoming aware of the benefits of a lean approach through collaborative projects with corporate and government community partners and through peer communications at conferences and meetings around the United States.

A definition of lean used by the Manufacturing Extension Partnership (of NIST/MEP, a part of the U.S. Department of Commerce) is "a systematic approach in identifying and eliminating waste (non-value-added activities) through continuous improvement by flowing the product at the pull of the customer in pursuit of perfection." Lean focuses on value-added expenditure of resources from the customer's viewpoint. Another way of putting it would be to give the customers:

- What they want

- When they want it

- Where they want it

- In the quantities and varieties they want

A planned, systematic implementation of lean leads to improved quality, better cash flow, increased reputation and demand, greater productivity and throughput, improved morale, and higher profits.

The basic premise of lean operations is reducing expense through streamlining of work processes. Tools and concepts from lean commonly used in the Public Health and/or service industries include:

1. Eight types of waste

2. Value stream mapping

3. Spaghetti diagram

4. 5S

The Eight Types of Waste

The eight types of waste is a quick method to engage teams in a Lean Six Sigma project. A simple technique is to create a 6 × 6 laminated card containing a list with definitions of the eight types of waste (see Table 16.1). This reference card becomes a visual aid as team members engage in brainstorming with the team and a communication engagement tool that team members can share with their coworkers while engaging in their daily work activities.

Value Stream Mapping

Value stream mapping is a means of representing flow of the product or service through the process. A few of the important components of this flow include value-added activities, non-value-added activities, non-value-added but necessary activities, work in process (WIP), inventory (queues), processing time, and lead time.

Table 16.1 Lean enterprise eight types of waste.

Waste	Description	Public health example
Overproduction	Products being produced in excess quantity and products being made before the customer needs them	Duplicate septic system applications opened as a result of missing information
Waiting	Periods of inactivity in a downstream process that occur because an upstream activity does not produce or deliver on time	Paperwork waiting for management signature or review
Unnecessary motion	Extra steps taken by employees or movement of equipment to accommodate inefficient process layouts	Immunology testing equipment stored in cabinets far from DIS work area.
Transportation or handling	Unnecessary movement of materials or double handling	Department vehicles stored in one facility, requiring constant movement of vehicles to and from high-traffic locations
Overprocessing	Spending more time than necessary to produce the product or service	Combining client survey instruments into one form rather than developing specific instruments for each program
Unnecessary inventory	Any excess inventory that is not directly required for the current customer's order	Overestimating emergency evacuation support materials, requiring additional locked storage cages, inventory counting and reconciliation
Defects	Errors produced during a service transaction or while developing a product	Ineffective scripts for initial intake applications. Unclear directions for filling out required forms.
Intellect	Inefficient use of resources based on job level, skill, knowledge, and experience	Hiring Master's level case managers to support call center response lines
Duplication	Having to reenter data or repeat details on forms	Poorly designed community assessment and needs checklists
Unclear communications	Time spent clarifying information between customer and service provider, management and employees	Inattention to multilingual client population. Insufficient supervisory training.
Lost opportunity	Failure to retain a customer or gain a new customer, failure to establish a rapport, ignoring customers, unfriendliness and rudeness	Poor relations with community partners. Lack of effective communication skills for frontline office personnel.

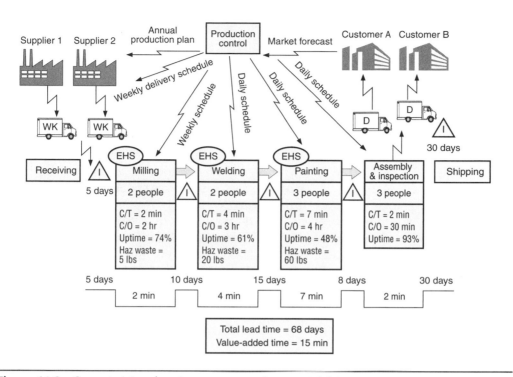

Figure 16.2   Current state value stream map—environmental data.

Source: U. S. Environmental Protection Agency, *Lean and Environment Toolkit* (2008). Accessed September 14, 2008 at http://www.epa.gov/lean/toolkit/fig3.htm.

Figure 16.2 is a value stream map created by a team assessing the environmental impact of a processing plant within their community. The goal is to work with the community partner not only to improve the quality of the wastewater returned to the water source, but to reduce their non-value-added activities elsewhere in the plant.

Hazardous waste is measured at each processing area in the plant. The primary purpose of the map is to focus on and reduce the amount of hazardous waste created, as well as improve the plant's disposal processes. In addition, the time between functions is measured in an attempt to use internal resources more effectively. By rebalancing workload in an efficient way, the plant management can provide more community residents with productive employment.

Non-value-added activities discovered included required management signatures when a project lead could be empowered to approve supplier orders and verify receipt of shipments. Work in process savings came from rebalancing activities between clerical and technical support staff. Clerical workers requested increased responsibilities and were rewarded for expanding their job skills. Technical staff was freed from repetitive administrative actions to focus on the backlog of chemical testing and reporting. Empowering the clerical staff by moving more tasks to a lower salary category enabled management to bring another technical professional into the organization, further reducing the backlog and adding additional skills to the team.

Spaghetti Diagram

A spaghetti diagram is a visual representation using a continuous flow line to trace the path of an item or activity through a process. The continuous flow line enables process teams to identify redundancies in the work flow and the opportunity to expedite process flow.

The diagram in Figure 16.3 reflects a study done by a health department administrative office. The intent of the study was to identify ways to shorten the walking time from one activity to another for frequently performed tasks. Another benefit of the visual drawing is to highlight major intersection points within the room. Areas where many walk paths overlap are causes of delay. Waiting is one of the eight wastes of lean, as is unnecessary motion.

A secondary benefit of creating the spaghetti diagram was the collaboration of the staff most impacted by the current workplace design. A brainstorming session was facilitated by the health department quality improvement coordinator to identify areas of congestion and wasted movement among the office personnel. Focusing on a common goal brought the team closer together while highlighting the purpose for placement of some work areas.

5S

5S is a visual method of setting the workplace in order. It is a system of workplace organization and standardization. The five steps that go into this technique all start with the letter "s" in Japanese (*seiri, seiton, seison, seiketsu,* and *shitsuke*). These

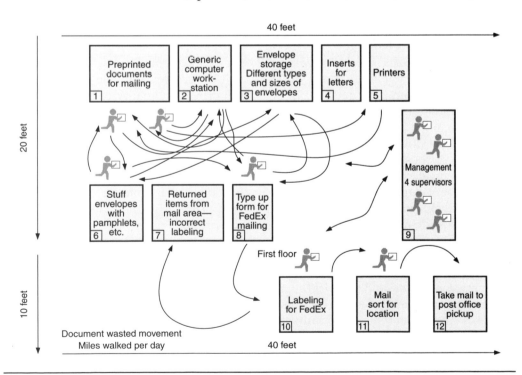

Figure 16.3   Spaghetti diagram showing health department administrative office flow.

five terms are loosely translated as *sort, set in order, shine, standardize,* and *sustain* in English. Table 16.2 shows the definitions of the five standardization and organizing tasks most employed in a lean enterprise action within a company.

5S can be instituted in any location. An environmental health department used 5S to:

1. *Sort* in-process applications for septic system permits

2. *Set in order* all applications by placing them in "green folders" for visual recognition

3. *Shine* the desks and work areas by locating all "lost" in-process applications, which were causing the average turnaround time for processing to be extended

4. *Standardize* the septic system permit application process by flowcharting and documenting the steps for consistency and ease of training new employees

5. *Sustain* the process by including measures and review points for the office senior coordinator and first line supervisor

The tools described in Table 16.3, page 231, are part of a larger set originally designed to support traditional manufacturing organizations. These tools proved so useful that industries of all sorts, from healthcare to services to not-for-profit to small business, are experiencing excellent results.

Figure 16.4 is a classic diagram called the "House of Lean," showing the basic tools of lean. These tools have been transferred wholesale into the Lean Six Sigma discipline. A short explanation of each of the tools in the House of Lean follows.

Table 16.2   Categories and descriptions of 5S.

5S	Description	Public health
Sort	Distinguish needed items from unneeded items and eliminate the latter	Identify and resolve all septic system permits on hold for additional information
Set in order (simplify)	Keep needed items and set them in order so they are easily accessible	Put all active applications in green folders for easier recognition
Shine (sweep)	Keep the work area swept and clean	Maintain cleanliness of front reception and waiting areas
Standardize	Standardize clean-up, that is, the first three steps *sort, set in order,* and *shine*	Include workforce in the documentation of process flows for all department activities. Train staff on correct procedures for all processes.
Sustain (self-discipline)	Make it a routine to maintain established procedures	Institute measures at critical monitoring points for all processes. Schedule ongoing management reviews.

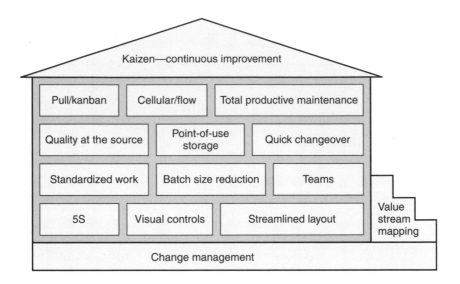

Figure 16.4   The House of Lean.

The building blocks include:

1. *5S.* A system for workplace organization and standardization. The five steps in this technique all start with the letter "s" in Japanese (*seiri, seiton, seison, seiketsu,* and *shitsuke*). These five terms are loosely translated as *sort, set in order, shine, standardize,* and *sustain* in English. See Table 16.1 for examples of their use in a public health improvement project.

2. *Visual controls.* The placement in plain view of all tooling, parts, production activities, and indicators so everyone involved can understand the status of the system at a glance. Labeling of storage cabinets, closets, and other workstation resources is an example of this tool, along with diagrams of frequently performed activities for either clients or staff.

3. *Streamlined layout.* Workplace designed according to optimum operational sequence. The value stream mapping example in Figure 16.2 illustrates a use of this tool.

4. *Standardized work.* Consistent performance of a task, according to prescribed methods, without waste, and focused on human movement (ergonomics). A spaghetti diagram prompted a local public health department to standardize their office flow, as exhibited in Figure 16.3.

5. *Batch size reduction.* The best batch size is one-piece flow, or "make one and move one!" If one-piece flow is not appropriate, reduce the batch to the smallest size possible. This tool was used by the environmental health services department by entering applications into the database

immediately on client payment at the front desk rather than waiting for a cluster of applications to be received before assigning numbers.

6. *Teams.* In the lean environment, the emphasis is on working in teams, whether they are 1) process improvement teams or 2) daily work teams. Lean Six Sigma incorporates the use of teams whenever possible to provide multiple perspectives for decision making and problem solving.

7. *Quality at the source.* Inspection and process control by frontline employees so they are certain the product or service that is passed on to the next process is of acceptable quality. This approach is very useful in a local public health department. Since staffing is usually tight, having skills readily available in more than one person in the office saves time and provides backup within the office.

8. *Point-of-use storage.* Raw material, parts, information, tools, work standards, procedures, and so on, are stored where needed. The spaghetti diagram example in Figure 16.3 is an excellent example of how one health department studied their common work area to maximize availability of supplies and work stations for effectiveness of staff within the office.

9. *Quick changeover.* The ability to change staff or equipment rapidly (usually in minutes) so multiple products in smaller batches can be run on the same equipment. This tool is translated from a production to a service environment by providing cross-training of health department staff to allow quick movement from one project or client requirement to another within a small office.

10. *Pull/kanban.* A system of cascading production and delivery instructions from downstream to upstream activities in which the upstream supplier does not produce until the downstream customer signals a need. Originally, it was just a manual card system, but has evolved to more sophisticated signaling methods for some organizations.[3] The value stream mapping example in Figure 16.2 uses kanban to pull supplies from the chemical treatment vendors only when their inventory reaches the lowest level possible to assure that the next task can begin without waiting on additional materials.

11. *Cellular/flow.* Physically linking and arranging manual and machine process steps into the most efficient combination to maximize value-added content while minimizing waste; the aim is single-piece flow. This tool is reflected in the project that used the spaghetti diagram in Figure 16.3. The septic system permitting improvement team empowered a cross-functional group of clerical staff, inspectors, and management to create a seamless sequence of steps from client application, through processing, to permitting and final review.

12. *Total productive maintenance.* A lean equipment maintenance strategy for maximizing overall equipment effectiveness. Although the title of this tool seems complex, it is really quite simple. Every office has equipment

requiring scheduled maintenance, calibration, new release updates, and so on. A preprinted checklist or electronic reminder system for when administrative, technical, or other programmatic updates are required minimizes downtime or lack of availability of equipment when needed.

Change management is the foundation of the House of Lean because all improvement comes from change. Value stream mapping is seen as the stairway to lean because of the effectiveness of that tool in identifying opportunities for using the other tools to improve the organization as an interrelated system.

SIX SIGMA DEFINED

Six Sigma is a methodology that primarily focuses on identifying and reducing variation in a process. The primary metric of Six Sigma is the sigma level or defects per million opportunities (DPMO). In Six Sigma, the higher the sigma level, the better the process output, which translates into fewer errors, lower operating costs, lower risks, improved performance, and better use of resources.

Six Sigma is a continuous process improvement methodology that facilitates near perfection in the processes of your organization. It considers not only the average performance but also the variability of what your business presents to the customer. This variation is often the cause of what is considered the "hidden factory," or the penalty for not getting it right the first time. In terms of public health activities, it consists of rework costs to reprocess forms before delivery to the client, scrap costs, recovery from a bad client experience, concessions for late service or paperwork deliveries, and write-offs to assuage offended clients or stakeholders, just to name a few.

Considering that Six Sigma methods revolve around the impact of defects in a process, one may consider how a defect should be defined in public health practice, particularly on the local level. In general, a defect may be described as anything that results in customer dissatisfaction.

If deployed properly, Six Sigma will create a structure to ensure that you have the right resources working on activities that will meet or exceed your clients' or stakeholders' needs, reduce direct expense costs in your organization, and provide a framework for measuring and monitoring those efforts. This is also the answer to the question, "what should Six Sigma do for me?" If done correctly Six Sigma will:

1. Create an infrastructure for managing improvement efforts and focus your resources on those efforts

2. Ensure that those improvement efforts are aligned with your client and stakeholder needs

3. Develop a measurement system to monitor the impact of your improvement efforts

Due to the importance of these outcomes, department leadership must be involved heavily in validating the benefit to the client and the health department, ensuring the strategic linkage to the department's vision, and visibly demonstrating that you are committed to the project. Without this, your change agents will not gain the traction that you expect and your Six Sigma program will not be successful.

THE DMAIC METHODOLOGY

Improvement teams use the DMAIC methodology to root out and eliminate the causes of defects through the following planning and implementation phases:

D: Define a problem or improvement opportunity.

M: Measure process performance.

A: Analyze the process to determine the root causes of poor performance; determine whether the process can be improved or should be redesigned.

I: Improve the process by attacking root causes.

C: Control the improved process to hold the gains.

Figure 16.5 gives an overview of the activities performed during each of the DMAIC steps in the Six Sigma continuous improvement cycle. Each of the DMAIC steps is defined below:

1. *Define.* Just as the name implies, this is where the defect, and moreover, the scope of the effort, is determined. Most often, you should expect project champions to partner with a Master Black Belt (MBB) to develop the parameters the Black Belt will operate within. They should work closely to define the defect, determine the client and organizational impact, assign target dates, assign resources, and set goals for the project, all of which is documented in a project charter (See Chapter 23), which becomes the "contract" with the Black Belt. Moreover, they must ensure that this contract aligns with the department strategy to avoid any disconnects between the goals of the project and the organization as a whole. Once this is complete, a Black Belt can begin using the tools, such as a process map and a cause-and-effect diagram, to uncover the specifics of an issue and get to the root cause of the defects. Process maps and cause-and-effect diagrams are described in Chapter 14, "Basic Tools of Quality Improvement." Table 16.4, page 232, describes the main responsibilities of Master Black Belts, Black Belts, and other team positions in a Six Sigma and Lean Six Sigma organization.

2. *Measure.* In this phase, the Six Sigma resource determines the baseline performance of the process, validates that the measurement system in place is accurate, verifies the cost of poor quality (COPQ)—the cost of not doing it right the first time—and makes an assessment of capability. This is the performance level of the process against customer requirements or expectations.

In other words, how *capable* is my process in meeting my customers' needs? Statistically speaking, *sigma* is a term indicating to what extent a process varies from perfection. The quantity of units processed divided into the number of defects actually occurring, multiplied by one million results in *defects per million*. Adding a 1.5 sigma shift in the mean results in the following defects per million:

1 sigma = 690,000 defects per million

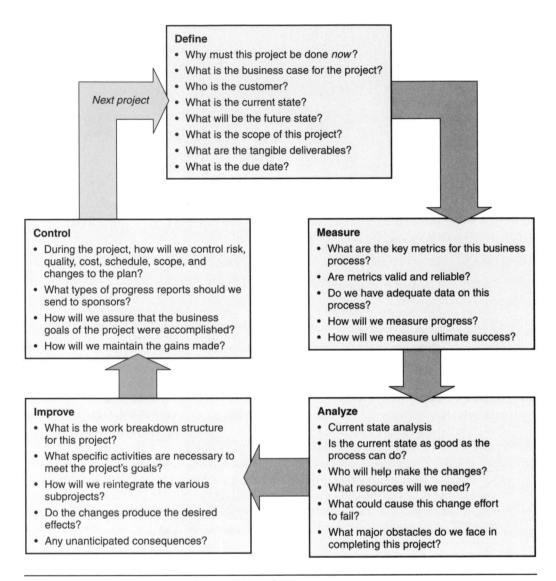

Figure 16.5   The Six Sigma project DMAIC cycle.

2 sigma = 308,000 defects per million

3 sigma = 66,800 defects per million

4 sigma = 6,210 defects per million

5 sigma = 230 defects per million

6 sigma = 3.4 defects per million

While much of the literature refers to defects relative to manufacture, Six Sigma may be used to measure material, forms, a time frame, distance, computer program coding, and so on. For example: if the cost of poor quality, at a four sigma level, represented 15 percent to 20 percent of sales revenue, an organization should be concerned.

Six Sigma, as a philosophy, translates to the organizational belief that it is possible to produce totally defect-free products or services—albeit more a dream than a reality for most organizations. With most organizations operating at about three sigma or below, getting to perfection leaves much work to be done.[4]

Identifying whether your process is capable of meeting customer requirements is the first checkpoint, or tollgate, where the determination to continue the effort is made. Some of the tools you should expect to employ are customer surveys, complaint data analysis, Pareto and run or control charts.

Figure 16.6 is an example from a consolidated call center supporting a large county health department (HD). The HD leadership met with a broad base of community stakeholders, clients, and service partners to learn of their priority needs for using the call center. In this case, prompt response time was a major external customer requirement, as identified in the statement, "I consistently wait too long to speak with a call center representative."

Likewise, a significant internal customer comment is, "Why are the monthly administration costs suddenly higher than the last three months?" These two statements, when associated with the major functions of the HD, prompted leadership to identify four measurement categories: *response time, service, utilization rate,* and *cost per call.*

3. *Analyze.* This is the phase where the technical expert, the Black Belt, scrubs the data collected to uncover the root cause(s) of the defect. Once they have isolated the potential factors, they use statistical, or hypothesis, testing to prove conclusively that the factor is indeed causing or contributing to the problem. Expect to see graphical analysis completed before any statistical testing is undertaken, and question any analysis that does not have the statistical analysis backing it up. Chapter 13, "Data Management and Basic Statistics," along with several other chapters in this text, provides additional guidance for effective statistical analysis in the public health arena.

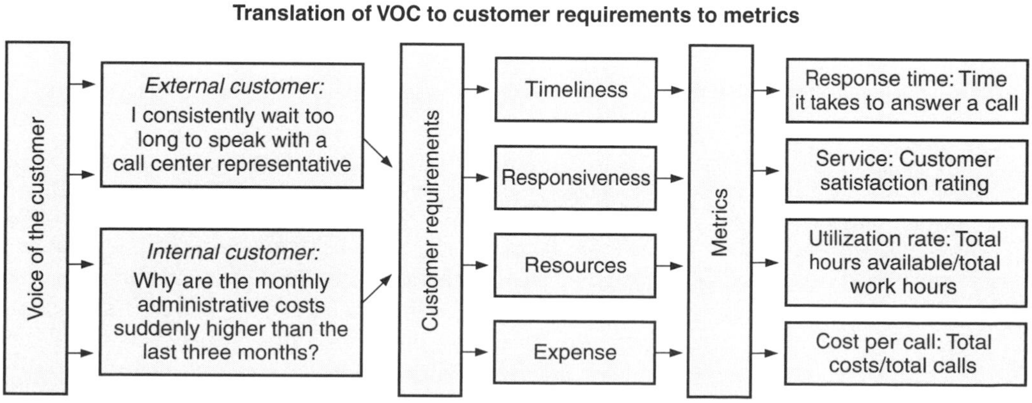

Translation of VOC to customer requirements to metrics

Figure 16.6   Performance metrics developed from customer requirements.

4. *Improve.* Now that the Black Belt knows what is causing the problem, he or she can predict what the performance of the process would be if they fixed the identified issues. This is achieved through a number of different approaches for identifying possible solutions. The Turning Point performance management system described in Chapter 2 is one such approach. Setting performance expectations is crucial as it facilitates the evaluation of the multiple solution sets, which should be documented in a decision matrix, allowing side-by-side comparisons of the proposed solutions and the expected performance. This is the final opportunity for you to halt the project prior to further investment and irreversible—at least without great cost—changes to the process.

5. *Control.* After implementation in the improve phase, the final phase is ensuring that the solution truly improved the process and that it is integrated into the health department daily operation. Some tools you can expect to see employed are control charts, dashboards or balanced scorecards, and updated process effectiveness. You must demand statistical proof that post-implementation performance is better than it was and that it is in statistical process control as described in Chapter 13. This ensures that if the process ever breaks again, the process owner knows when and how to react to the situation. Another element that is important for you to be involved in is the propagation of the standardization of the solution across other areas of the department. In other words, if a solution is found in one location and your organization has three others, then you need to ensure that the others gain the benefit of the project as well.

Six Sigma provides the framework to ask the right questions, depending on the process and desired outcome. Understanding the power of how a defect affects a process, operation, or practice is critical to the success of any Six Sigma initiative. In public health practice, defects can refer to birth, genetics, or topological conditions. But the scope of the defects would have to be expanded in public health practice to meet operational standards. Public health practice, (particularly public health program development, analysis, and oversight functions) may be enhanced with Six Sigma submethodologies such as define, measure, analyze, improve, control (DMAIC). Public health practice processes that may benefit from Six Sigma include:

- General administration (reducing the "lifecycle" of repetitive processes)

- Understanding risk and burden in local public health practice standards

- Development of strategies to master core public health competencies

Each of these processes has the potential of being broken down further by utilizing DMAIC methodology. Six Sigma methods share similarities with other evidence (quantitative)–based projects, specifically, the measure and analysis functionality of DMAIC methodology. This systemized approach complements and also challenges current paradigms that relate to the development of public health practice operations and procedures. DMAIC may also be crucial when local health departments perform statewide rollouts that may synchronize with Department of Health and Human Services (DHHS) initiatives.

Six Sigma is a very data-driven methodology. Implementing Six Sigma will cause significant demands for data collection and reporting. Expanding data and information use and the associated technology growth may create friction between your existing technology plans and the new needs being created to support projects (low-level data needs), control plans (low- and mid-level measures), and scorecards (high-level measures). Plan a way to prioritize these data needs. There should be a balance between the more strategic or structural needs for the high-level scorecards supporting the management system and the low- to mid-level needs of the DMAIC methodology.

COMBINING LEAN AND SIX SIGMA METHODS AND BENEFITS

As shared in the introductory paragraphs of this chapter, the concepts and tools of lean and Six Sigma complement each other strongly in the operational environment. Lean enterprise applications address the short-term requirements of reducing waste, effectively balancing resources, and improving productivity within the operating unit.

Six Sigma provides strong overlapping tools and methodologies, including new technologies, while bringing in additional approaches for client-focused orientation, and opportunities to increase the organization's reputation within both the local and wider community.

Figure 16.7 compares high-level activity steps for lean and two of the Six Sigma approaches most often discussed in business literature.[5] The lean flow begins with analyzing existing systems, whether performing as designed or needing

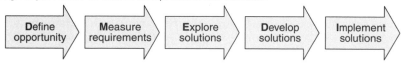

Lean Six Sigma incorporates and deploys the key methods, tools, and techniques of its predecessors.

Lean focuses on waste elimination in existing processes.

| Analyze opportunity | Plan improvement | Focus improvement | Deliver performance | Improve performance |

Six Sigma focuses on continuous process improvement (DMAIC) to reduce variation in existing processes.

| Define opportunity | Measure performance | Analyze opportunity | Improve performance | Control performance |

Six Sigma also focuses on new process design/complete redesign (DMEDI) for wholesale redesign of processes as well as new products and services.

| Define opportunity | Measure requirements | Explore solutions | Develop solutions | Implement solutions |

Figure 16.7   Process flow comparisons of predecessor methodologies.

improvement. Subsequent steps guide the improvement team to identifying priority areas for reducing waste, eliminating defects, and improving performance.

The second flow in Figure 16.7 shows the DMAIC continuous improvement flow espoused by Six Sigma and described previously within this chapter. Third, another Six Sigma activity flow (DMEDI) has been identified to support new process design or complete redesign of an existing process. This flow incorporates steps to define the redesign opportunity, establishes measures as drivers for expected outcomes, explores solutions to the new design initiative, then develops and implements solutions based on return on investment and resource maximization decisions.

The Body of Knowledge identified for the combined Lean Six Sigma methodologies includes major areas of emphasis common to the separate disciplines of lean enterprise and Six Sigma:

- Systemwide integration

- Leadership involvement and visibility

- Business process focus

- Voice of the customer driven

- Change management oriented

- Project management dependent

While project success is imperative, Lean Six Sigma also recognizes the intense interdependence of one activity within the system with a multitude of other requirements. No one process works in a vacuum. What happens in one area of the department impacts and is impacted by other functions.

Table 16.3 lists a number of commonly used tools matched to the phases of either the DMAIC continuous improvement flow of Six Sigma or the phases of the lean enterprise methodology. The reader will notice an overlap in tool usage between the two methodologies. This is an additional benefit of combining the two approaches for total system improvement. In either approach, preplanning through effective project management is imperative to secure commitment of senior leadership for long-term realization of organizational and community goals.

Defining and communicating Lean Six Sigma roles and responsibilities is likewise critical to project success. Having the right members on the Lean Six Sigma team goes a long way toward assuring the success of final project outcomes.

Table 16.4 lists the major roles required for a Lean Six Sigma project and suggests job titles within a public health organization where the necessary skills might exist. Earlier chapters in this text cover significant success factors in the use of teams and teamwork in meeting the goals of the organization. That information will not be reproduced in this chapter. It is important, however, that the responsibilities of each of the major Lean Six Sigma roles be identified. Teams are used successfully without application of the Lean Six Sigma methodology. The reverse is not true. Lean Six Sigma is not successful without the effective implementation of a team environment.

Table 16.3   Lean Six Sigma tools.

DMAIC phases	Six Sigma tools	Lean phases	Lean tools
Pre-project	Project scoping Project prioritization Project plan	Pre-project	Project scoping Project prioritization Project plan
Define	Project charter Team charter Stakeholder analysis SIPOC, cross-functional map Voice of the customer Tollgate review	Analyze	One-piece flow Value stream mapping Spaghetti diagram Teams Run charts Benchmarking
Measure	Data collection plan Identify key metrics Gap analysis Process sigma calculation Capability study Control charts Tollgate review	Plan improvement	Error-proofing Visual controls Total productive maintenance Streamlined layout
Analyze	Pareto chart Ishikawa Diagram Five whys Run charts Relations graph Correlation Regression analysis Hypothesis testing Tollgate review	Focus improvement	Visual display 5S Value stream mapping Root cause analysis Five whys

Improve	Brainstorming
	Mistake-proofing
	Design of experiments
	Pugh matrix
	House of quality
	Failure mode and effects
	   analysis
	Tollgate review
		Deliver performance	Kaizen
			Kanban
			Changeover reduction
			Point-of-use storage
			Standardized work
			Failure mode and effects
			   analysis

Control	Control charts Process sigma Dashboards Balanced scorecards Storyboarding Tollgate review	Improve performance	Visual controls 5S Continuous flow and cell design Quality at the source Balanced scorecards

Table 16.4   Lean Six Sigma roles and responsibilities.

Traditional title	Public health title	Responsibility
Project Champion	Same	• Dedicated to see it implemented • Absolute belief it is the right thing to do • Perseverance and stamina
Project sponsor	Same	• Believes in the concept/idea • Sound business acumen • Willing to take risk and responsibility for outcomes • Authority to approve needed resources • Upper management will listen to her or him
Process owner	Functional manager or unit supervisor (Varies by local public health department)	• Is a team member • Takes ownership of the project when it is complete • Is responsible for maintaining the project's gains • Removes barriers for Black Belts
Master Black Belt	Senior data analyst, Quality subject matter expert, Department quality manager	• Expert on Six Sigma tools and concepts • Trains Black Belts and ensures proper application of methodology and tools • Coaches/mentors Black and Green Belts • Works high-level projects and those that impact multiple divisions or business units • Assists Champions and process owners with project selection, management, and Six Sigma administration
Black Belt	Quality tools specialist, Experienced project leader, Data analyst	• Leads, executes, and completes DMAIC projects • Teaches team members the Six Sigma methodology and tools • Assists in identifying project opportunities and refining project details and scope • Reports progress to the project Champions and process owners • Transfers knowledge to other Black Belts and the organization • Mentors Green Belts
Green Belt	Team leader, Project lead	• Committed to the team's mission and objectives • Capable of developing process maps, applying basic quality tools, creating charts, and engaging in basic statistical analysis • Experienced in planning, organizing, staffing, controlling, and directing • Capable of creating and maintaining channels that enable members to do their work • Capable of gaining the respect of team members; a role model • Is firm, fair, and factual in dealing with a team of diverse individuals

Continued

Table 16.4   Lean Six Sigma roles and responsibilities *(Continued).*

Traditional title	Public health title	Responsibility
		• Facilitates discussion without dominating • Actively listens • Empowers team members to the extent possible within the organization's culture • Supports all team members equally • Respects each team member's individuality
Yellow Belt	Team member	• Willing to commit to the purpose of the team • Understands lean and Six Sigma tools and concepts • Able to express ideas, opinions, suggestions in a nonthreatening manner • Capable of listening attentively to other team members • Receptive to new ideas and suggestions • Able to engage in analysis of Lean Six Sigma tools and concepts • Even-tempered, able to handle stress and cope with problems openly • Competent in one or more fields of expertise needed by the team • Favorable performance record • Willing to function as a team member and forfeit "star" status

SUMMARY

The one remaining issue you will need to follow up on is how to manage the change you are introducing into the system. The following are examples of change-related issues we have seen or heard in less than thorough deployments:

• Lack of resource support for the project team

• Lack of support for gathering data for a project

• Failure or resistance to implement a recommended solution

Any systemwide methodology for organizational improvement requires continual surveillance by senior leadership. The role of project champion, process owner, Master Black Belt, or other senior leadership position, is at the core of successful improvement activities.

Lean Six Sigma depends on both quantitative and qualitative data on which to make decisions affecting the issue under study. Much has been written in this text on the necessity for fact-based decision making. Opinions are not sufficient to justify major process or organizational change.

Unless data validate the observations or opinions of those proposing change, other stakeholders will undoubtedly resist the change. Data alone will also not motivate others to accept change. Involvement in the identification of opportunities for change and in the development of acceptable solutions is the basis of the Lean Six Sigma methodology. Strong teamwork, project management, consistent leadership, and ongoing data-based decision making are all characteristics of a successful Lean Six Sigma initiative.

Public health has long understood the requirement for strong data analysis and project management. The examples shown in this chapter further support the applicability of Lean Six Sigma as a core approach for quality improvement within our public health discipline.

Chapter 17

Community-Focused Performance Management

Paul D. Epstein, Jennifer R. J. Frost, Lyle D. Wray,
and Alina Simone

A s the definition of public health has expanded to become more deeply community focused, the performance management approach to public health must similarly expand to include significant roles for community members. The emergence of the consensus "10 essential services of public health" over the last 15 years has provided an important start in that direction, giving some structure to how public health can work as a community system that engages people and community partnerships while also tracking and using data to improve health outcomes and reduce disparities. At about the same time, research into broader local government and nonprofit practices produced a model of performance management providing effective tools for engaging the community in results-focused ways to improve the quality of life. The *effective community governance* (ECG) model that emerged matches up well with the essential services of public health. The model and related ECG practices can provide practical guidance to local health agencies for effectively involving the community while managing for results within the budgeting and performance planning systems of their government.

EFFECTIVE COMMUNITY GOVERNANCE AND THE ESSENTIAL SERVICES OF PUBLIC HEALTH

ECG provides an integrated framework that supports the development of effective health policy and performance management of that policy by systematically incorporating key themes of engagement of people, performance feedback, collaboration, and accountability. It establishes *engaging the community, measuring results, and getting things done* as three "core community skills" that help people and organizations make decisions about what actions to take in a community, and help them measure the community's performance in achieving results. Community engagement invests legitimacy in those decisions and performance measures. To be effective, a community—or community-serving organization—will align two or all three of these skills to perform the "advanced governance practices" of the governance model, as shown in Figure 17.1.

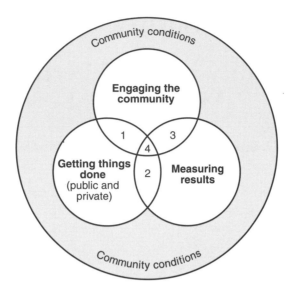

The four "advanced governance practices" are represented by the overlapping areas in the figure, which represent alignment of "core community skills" as follows:

1. Community problem solving: Aligns "Engaging the community" and "Getting things done."
2. Organizations managing for results: Aligns "Measuring results" and "Getting things done."
3. People reaching for results: Aligns "Engaging the community" and "Measuring results."
4. Communities governing for results: Aligns all three core skills.

Figure 17.1   Effective community governance model.

ECG, developed from research on community engagement and performance management practices of local government and nonprofit organizations across the United States, is described in depth in the book *Results That Matter* by Paul Epstein, Paul Coates, and Lyle Wray, with David Swain (Jossey-Bass 2006) and at www.effectivegovernance.net on the Web. In the ECG model:

- *Engaging the community* means not only engaging community organizations, but also engaging the people of the community— who live there, work or play there, go to school there, or have other interests.[1] So, it relates directly to essential services "3. Inform, educate, and empower people . . . " and "4. Mobilize community partnerships . . . " As noted below, in ECG engagement is a robust idea with many roles for people to play in improving community health.

- *Measuring results* refers to measuring community conditions as well as service performance, which relate directly to essential services "1. Monitor health status . . . " and "9. Evaluate effectiveness, accessibility, and quality of personal and population-based health services." As noted below, ECG encourages use of performance feedback for effective performance management, and those local health organizations that practice essential service "10. Research for new insights and innovative solutions . . . " can contribute those insights as part of the feedback loops used to improve performance.

- *Getting things done* refers to the many decisions, plans, and actions taken by public and private parties that affect community conditions. The "actions" relate to essential services involving implementation, as in essential services "7. Link people to needed personal health services . . . ," "2. Diagnose and investigate health problems and health hazards . . . ," and "6. Enforce laws and regulations. . . . " Just as important is the planning and decision making aspect of "Getting things done," which relates directly to essential service "5. Develop policies and plans that support individual and community health efforts."

EFFECTIVE COMMUNITY GOVERNANCE AS A COMMUNITY-FOCUSED APPROACH TO PERFORMANCE MANAGEMENT

Two "advanced governance practices" of the ECG model directly involve performance management:

- *Organizations managing for results,* in which organizations use measured results of community conditions and service performance to improve how they "get things done," not just once, but through regular, systematic feedback cycles described under "Use of Performance Feedback" below. If a health organization only uses its expert interpretations of data for decisions, this will be a strictly organization-focused approach. If the organization also consults people to understand health issues from the community's perspective, then they can make this a community-focused performance management approach.

- *Communities governing for results* align all three core community skills. As in "managing for results," organizations and communities achieving this advanced practice use measured results in regular feedback cycles to improve results. But their community engagement goes beyond obtaining input from people to better understand health issues to systemically engaging them at some level in planning, decision making, and implementing policies and services as described below under "Robust Engagement of Community Residents in Multiple Roles."

A local health organization that attempts either of these advanced governance practices can achieve community-focused performance management. As shown in Figure 17.2, the difference is that "managing for results with community

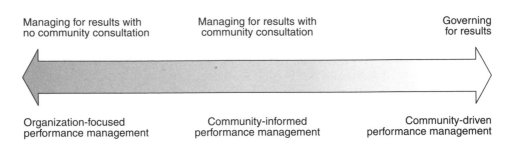

Figure 17.2   Continuum of community engagement in performance management.

consultation" is, in effect, "community-informed performance management" while "governing for results" comes closer to "community-driven performance management."

But how does this play out in practice? How does a local health organization really achieve community-focused performance management, at any level? That is best explained by examining the four "community improvement themes" of effective community governance that emerged from research of practices used in communities that exhibited the four advanced governance practices of ECG:[2]

- Robust engagement of community residents in multiple roles

- Use of performance feedback in organizational or community decisions

- Use of strong collaborations

- Linking desired results to resources and accountable people or organizations

The first two themes, which form the essence of community-focused performance management, are described in detail here. The last two themes are discussed briefly below and in somewhat more detail in the next chapter, "Community Balanced Scorecards for Strategic Public Health Improvement," which ends by discussing approaches for using those themes in strategic performance management.

ROBUST ENGAGEMENT OF COMMUNITY RESIDENTS IN MULTIPLE ROLES

In public health, community residents are not only the objects of a field of study, they are, or should be, agenda setters and allies in making community change happen and in making personal change happen for themselves and their families. These multiple facets of public health call for engagement of residents in a variety of roles. Robust or "authentic" engagement, in which community residents have real opportunities for influence, will produce more sustainable results than pro forma "paint by the numbers" public participation. Residents have local knowledge of their neighborhoods or rural districts, their family experiences, and their demographic groups that is often vital to properly define and solve local health problems. And they also have tremendous potential energy they can contribute to improving community health. To fully tap their knowledge and energy, local health organizations need to engage residents in multiple roles and work to support residents to strengthen them in those roles. In the following paragraphs, the major community resident roles of issue framer, collaborator, advocate, evaluator, and stakeholder are described. These descriptions are followed by Table 17.1, page 242, which provides a "quick guide" on ways to support residents in each of these roles.

Residents As Issue Framers

In public health, as in other community improvement endeavors, engaging residents in shaping a vision for the future is a critical step in developing an improvement strategy people will support. Around the country, residents have come together to articulate their quality-of-life goals and develop strategies to make these goals a reality. Improved health outcomes almost always figure prominently on the list of key elements in a community's shared vision.

The issue-framing process involves fundamental questions such as: "Who says this is a priority issue?" "Who gets to decide?" and "How is this issue linked to more fundamental issues underlying surface symptoms?" Often the definition of the problem—and who gets to characterize it—is a challenge in itself. Public health experts may review teen and young adult mortality statistics and say, "We have a youth violence challenge," while community residents might say, "We have a youth unemployment and police abuse problem." A fundamental process question is, "Once we have all the stakeholders involved, how can we arrive at a viable process that yields a workable definition of the problem, points in a clear direction, and supports an effective set of strategies and tactics to meet the challenge in a reasonable period of time?" Different communities have developed their own answers, but the most promising approaches combine the information health experts bring, such as findings from evidence-based practice and epidemiological studies, and the values, concerns, and local knowledge residents have, for setting a vision. To do this, health professionals can not simply provide lots of information to residents, even if the information is carefully explained in layman's terms. They need to give residents opportunities to deliberate, to question, and listen to one another and to the experts, so they can be authentic participants in making hard choices about priority goals, and develop a vision they feel is worth striving for.

These deliberative dialogs provide a consensus view on the path to a desirable future for the community, the main goals needed to bring this vision about, and the appropriate means—both professional and community-based—required to realize the shared vision. The MAPP program of the National Association of County and City Health Officials and the Centers for Disease Control and Prevention (see http://www.naccho.org/topics/infrastructure/mapp/index.cfm) is one promising and field-tested example of such an approach. MAPP engages residents as issue framers to participate both in visioning and in rigorous assessments of four different health-related aspects of community life.

Once a shared vision is developed and priority issues and goals identified, community residents can still be important issue framers at the next level of detail, helping define problems and craft solutions. For example, if a goal is to change the physical environment to encourage walking and exercise, residents may define the problem, in part, as auto-dominated streets and seek a "complete streets" solution. The complete streets movement seeks to tame the automobile and encourage walking and bicycling through sound transportation design, signage, and law enforcement. Applying a complete streets strategy involves community conversations on traffic calming and other pedestrian protection measures, and adjusting road-building standards to affect more than auto roadways.

The issue-framer role is by far the most pivotal role that a resident can play. By providing opportunities for residents to play such a role, the vision and actions for improving community health will be grounded in community realities and supported from the bottom up by the community itself.

Residents As Collaborators

If residents have been engaged as issue framers, they are more likely to feel they can make a difference in improving community health and take part in collaborating to improve health. Residents who collaborate with local leaders to reach shared public health goals can be donors, volunteers, teachers, mentors, and organizers. For example, public health agencies can partner with community groups to recruit community residents as collaborators in culturally appropriate distribution of health information, bringing information on nutrition, safe sex practices, and early-detection tests for preventable diseases to their friends, neighbors, and families. Residents can also identify and leverage "hidden assets" in the community that staff of public or nonprofit organizations are not aware of, such as retired people with special skills who can be tapped to supplement public services, or local businesses willing to donate supplies or equipment. For public health, all residents are perhaps, themselves, the most important community assets for achieving better health outcomes by collaborating to adopt healthier behaviors and encouraging their families to do the same. Given the influence of personal behaviors on health outcomes, this form of collaboration is an especially critical role of community residents.

Residents As Advocates

In communities across the country, residents advocate for public decisions and actions to protect or advance their own interests, their families' interests, or the interests of a group they belong to or support. Advocacy can be as narrowly focused as attempting to get a stop sign or traffic signal at an intersection to safeguard young children, or as broadly focused as seeking to change overall community health policy. If a public health agency helps residents advocate for their own interests and those of their families, the agency may reap future dividends. Some of those residents, or their community organizations, may be willing to visibly support the agency when the agency needs to show community support for policies it is advocating. Numerous civic organizations assist residents in their advocacy, either close to home or nationally. One exemplary program, Partners in Policymaking, for over 20 years has assisted parents and other family members of individuals with developmental disabilities to play an effective role in state and local policy making by providing training, support, and data. This award-winning program involves a range of advocacy teaching tools including online e-courses (http://www.partnersinpolicymaking.com/).

Residents As Evaluators

Community residents can be engaged in assessing whether the goals set out in a community process are indeed being achieved. Are playgrounds actually child friendly? Are streets actually safe and inviting for pedestrians and bicyclists? Are healthier food choices available within walking distance of their homes? Residents in communities from Connecticut to California have been organized and trained to take systematic surveys of the physical conditions in their neighborhoods and parks and record defined problems on electronic PDAs for transmission to relevant agencies. Other resident evaluators have helped generate questions for surveys of community residents and service users. New "Web 2.0" tools that enable users to easily generate content offer the prospect of new ways for residents to act as evaluators. Public health professionals may require evidence from "controlled" evaluations for many health-related decisions, but they should not ignore what they can learn from "uncontrolled" information residents contribute by using Google "map hacks," blogs, or popular interactive sites such as Flickr and YouTube. These can potentially provide leads on public health problems, issues, or opportunities they otherwise would not know about.

Residents As Stakeholders

This is the most widely cited role for residents and other community members, such as people who work, go to school, or own property in a community. The people who live in the community are stakeholders interested in their own health and that of their families, and they are also stakeholders as "customers" of public health services. Many local, state, and provincial governments, as well as nonprofit civic organizations, treat resident stakeholders as "owners" deserving of reports on community conditions and service performance, including data on public health services and outcomes. While this kind of information sharing is a step forward in transparency, community residents are much more than just customers of the healthcare system, "owners" of the results, and interested parties in their own health. They can and should play other major roles, besides stakeholders, such as those described above, in achieving personal and community health outcomes.

Table 17.1 provides guidance to local leaders on how they can expand opportunities for residents to play multiple roles in the community.

Table 17.1   Quick guide to supporting residents in major roles of community engagement.

Major roles	How you can support or strengthen the role
Residents as issue framers	Foster deliberative processes in which people listen to each other and make hard choices.
	Ensure that residents are engaged early to set agendas, define problems, and identify solutions.
	Encourage community-centered, boundary-crossing problem solving.
Residents as collaborators	Help residents voice opposition to get attention needed to be recognized as potential collaborators in achieving solutions.
	Help residents recognize different stakeholder interests and to think beyond opposition to forge effective compromise solutions.
	Organize opportunities for residents to contribute to their community as volunteers or "coproducers" in implementing solutions, including acting as "coproducers of their own better health."
	Help residents identify and leverage community assets (including themselves) to get big things done despite limited resources.
	Identify "spark plugs" to energize community coproduction projects, and support them in organizing the community.
Residents as advocates	Help residents get technical and political help and find the "leverage" they need.
	Help residents "learn the way things work" in the community, and help them learn from each other to be effective advocates.
Residents as evaluators	Help residents make their assessments rigorous, credible, and useful.
	Provide residents with periodic reports of performance data on issues and services of concern to them.
Residents as stakeholders	Help residents organize and associate with each other close to home.
	Ensure that residents have an opportunity to influence things they care about as stakeholders.

Source: P. Epstein, P. Coates, and L. Wray, *Results That Matter* (San Francisco: Jossey-Bass, 2006). Adapted from Table 2.1, p. 21.

USE OF PERFORMANCE FEEDBACK IN ORGANIZATIONAL OR COMMUNITY DECISIONS

Organizations serving communities with effective governance do not just collect data on service performance and community results, they *use* that information to make better organizational or community decisions to get better results in the future. Organizations that are the most effective users of performance information do not just use it on an ad hoc basis. Instead, they have performance management *systems* that feed back performance data through regular *cycles*. This feedback enables them to learn from past performance to improve future performance and community results. The plan–do–check–act model described earlier in this book is a tried-and-true "single-loop feedback cycle" used to improve process quality and service performance in many public and private settings, including public health. Some government and nonprofit organizations have expanded on single-cycle performance management. Their performance management systems have several feedback cycles for different kinds of strategic, policy, and operational decision processes, with different time horizons, to keep their decisions on all levels focused on producing the best results to meet the needs of their community or constituents.

The use of multiple performance feedback cycles is a best practice of effective community governance (ECG). Public health departments can tailor this best practice to fit their local decision environment, including a multiyear community health strategic planning process, their own or their government's annual budget process, and quarterly or more frequent operational performance reviews to keep daily service delivery and special initiatives on track. As noted later, the emerging accreditation system and other public health assessment processes can enhance public health performance feedback cycles for more accelerated performance gains. Also, community residents can be part of the process to turn these "managing for results" systems into "governing for results" systems in which residents' concerns and priorities influence the focus of services improved, problems solved, and community results achieved at several levels.

The Triple-Loop Learning Model

This model is a useful example to consider because it can work for virtually any community-serving organization. As shown in Figure 17.3, the inner cycle represents improving delivery of existing programs and services, which is the most frequent feedback cycle. At the Hartford Public Library, which uses this model, in the inner cycle managers review monthly operational performance data with staff of specific programs, services, and branches at least quarterly to interpret what the data mean, what services need improvement, and how they can be improved. For police departments and entire state and local governments that have adopted "stat" systems of frequent performance monitoring, the inner cycle can represent weekly or monthly performance accountability meetings and actions to correct performance problems identified. For public health, the inner cycle can be equivalent to reviewing process quality data and service performance as part of a plan–do–check–act cycle of performance feedback and improvement.

In the middle cycle, significant changes can be made to basic program designs and service plans (including dropping or replacing some programs) based on managers' assessment of measured results. Some grant-funded programs, for example, may go through such reviews semiannually or annually as part of required grant review and renewal processes. Some programs may only go through this level of review for redesign, or elimination if they exhibit persistent performance problems. As noted in Figure 17.3, the outer "strategic" cycle influences the middle cycle to ensure that program designs and service plans stay relevant to current strategies and resources. So on occasion even a high-performing program can be

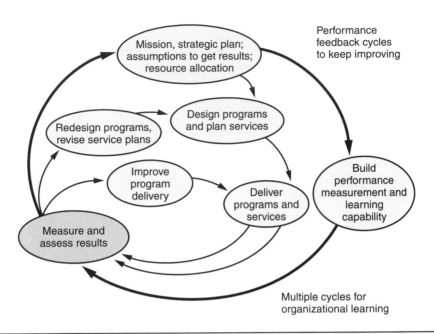

Figure 17.3   Triple-loop learning.

considered for significant change to become consistent with a new strategic direction or financial reality of the organization.

The outer loop of the triple-loop learning figure really represents several feedback cycles in one. Most major resource allocation decisions are made in the annual budget process. Major strategic changes are usually considered less frequently, and could come from a review of the main assumptions underlying the organization's strategy. Finally, the outer loop also involves improving how performance is measured and how the organization and its staff use performance information. It could involve revising measures to be more relevant or reliable, or learning new ways to use performance data to improve performance. In essence, this part of the outer loop keeps the organization's performance measures and the use of the data fresh and relevant to changing realities in the community. On occasion, these changes are also driven by newly available professional research. For example, the library has frequently used research on how young children become ready to read to evaluate how they design and measure early childhood and family literacy programs. Similarly, a health department can use evidenced-based research on community health issues as one of its sources for learning better ways to measure performance and use performance information.

Enhancing Triple-Loop Learning with Public Health Assessment and Accreditation Information

The emerging public health accreditation system and other assessment processes, such as the National Public Health Performance Standards Program (NPHPSP),

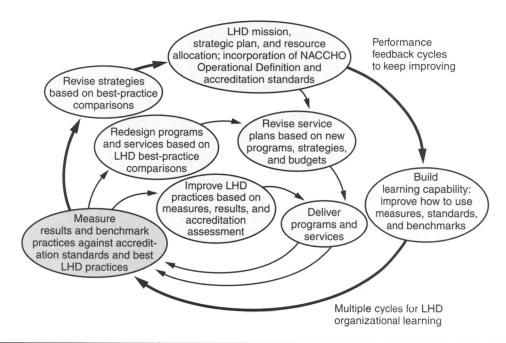

Figure 17.4   Triple-loop learning using accreditation and local performance measurement.

enable public health agencies to add a valuable new source of information to a triple-loop learning system of performance management. Figure 17.4 cites the pilot accreditation approach of the National Association of County and City Health Officials (NACCHO), which uses 225 "operational definition indicators," each representing a best practice for achieving standards related to the 10 essential services of public health. But enhanced triple-loop learning could work the same with the NPHPSP or other best practice–based assessments, as follows: in addition to measuring and reviewing its own performance, a local health department (LHD) can use comparisons against best practices inherent in these assessments as added performance management information. As shown in Figure 17.4, that can affect decisions on how to improve performance in the inner loop, how to design or redesign programs and services in the middle loop, and how to improve strategies in the outer loop.

These assessment processes involve many judgment calls concerning whether a health agency or system is meeting each specific standard. So, by itself, an assessment is inadequate for performance management. But, when combined with local measured results of a department's programs and services and local community health outcome measures, accreditation or other assessments can provide valuable additional information for determining how to improve performance. That can increase the learning and improvement power of the department's performance management system. Of course, NACCHO's operational definition indicators and the NPHPSP assessment instruments are not the only sources of best practices a health department may use. NACCHO and other organizations have databases of best practices that health departments can tap to find more approaches for improving their local practices, supplementing what they learn from their own accreditation assessment.

Tailoring Multiple Performance Feedback Cycles to a Government's Planning, Budgeting, and Reporting Systems

Public health agencies usually exist within much larger organizations, such as a state or local government. So they must follow the budgeting process of the larger entity. They also may have to follow other planning systems, for example, for multiyear strategic plans and annual service plans or "business plans" with annual service performance targeting and costing. The larger entity may also have internal or external performance reporting systems that the health department must follow. And some governments attempt to tie staff performance evaluations to service or program performance plans.

Health departments can tailor their own cycles of performance management to fit the budgeting, planning, and reporting processes of their larger entity and thus gain the benefits of multi-loop learning without creating duplicate systems. They can adjust the time horizons of their public health performance feedback cycles to match the schedules of the larger systems they work within. Some governments have already combined several key planning, decision, and reporting processes into an integrated multi-loop performance management system, as in Figure 17.5, which depicts Prince William County, Virginia's results-based system. Prince William County has four major performance feedback cycles: 1) adjustments during the year to improve service performance, 2) annual

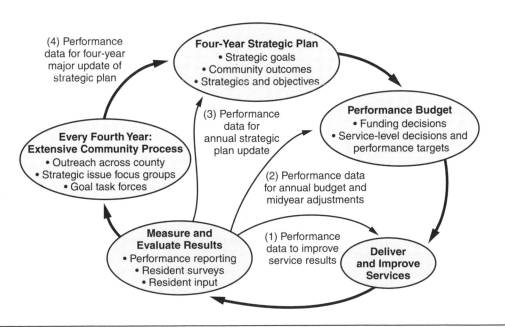

Figure 17.5 Governing for results cycles in Prince William County, Virginia.

performance budgeting and semiannual budget adjustments, 3) annual strategic plan updates, and 4) a major strategic planning process every four years. A local health department could easily match its own multi-loop learning cycle to fit this kind of local government cycle. More likely, their larger entity will have one or two of the cycles that Prince William County has, which the health department can match with its own performance management system. That will leave the department flexibility in the time horizons and approaches for other performance feedback cycles it wants to use for its own system of multi-loop learning.

Adding Community Engagement to Performance Management for a "Governing for Results" System

Figure 17.5 does not refer to *"managing* for results" in Prince William County but to the county's *"governing* for results cycles" because Prince William County has integrated community engagement into its performance management system. Prince William provides a well-developed example of community-focused performance management, described earlier in this chapter, consistent with the most complete "advanced governance practice" of the ECG model, which systemically combines *engaging the community, measuring results,* and *getting things done.* Figure 17.6 notes the ECG engagement roles played by community residents throughout the various cycles. Residents have their most important influence every four years when they are heavily engaged in a major update of the county's strategic plan, which

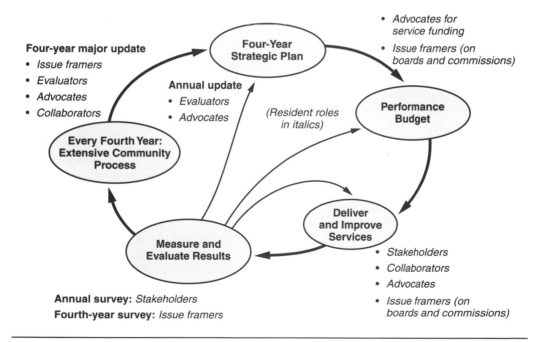

Figure 17.6   Major resident roles in Prince William County's governing for results cycles.

is the main driver of the rest of the system. However, as shown here, residents are never out of the process, and they have important roles to play in every performance cycle.

A local health department's larger government entity may not engage community residents to the degree that Prince William County does. But that should not stop the health department from pursuing its own community engagement approach to achieve the degree of community-focused performance management that department leaders feel is needed for effective public health policy and practices. Whether guided by its larger entity or following its own interpretation of good public health practices, a health department can give community residents many opportunities to play important roles in public health performance management.

For more on Prince William County, and other local government and nonprofit organizations that use multi-loop performance feedback cycles, see the book *Results That Matter* by P. Epstein, P. Coates, and L. Wray, with D. Swain (Jossey-Bass, 2006, chapters 3, 7, and 8) and the "Model in Action" section of the ECG Web site http://www.resultsthatmatter.net/site/model/index.php.

USE OF STRONG COLLABORATIONS

Collaborations between different health organizations and disciplines are important in any community and can be a challenge to manage even within the boundaries of the health sector. However, as many of the social and environmental determinants of health lie outside the formal health sector, collaborations with non-health organizations are also crucial for long-term community health improvement. ECG encourages partnerships that cross institutional and sectoral boundaries to achieve common goals such as improved health outcomes. Strong collaborations concurrently build community capacity while addressing difficult issues that no one organization, and often no one sector, can adequately address on its own. Of the essential services of public health, service "4. Mobilize community partnerships to identify and solve health problems," most directly deals with collaboration. But at some level, collaboration is needed to achieve success within each of the 10 essential services, from a local health department depending on private healthcare professionals to provide essential data, to collaboration between community organizations to engage and empower underserved populations, to collaborative research activities. ECG also encourages collaboration with the people of the community as well as with diverse community organizations. A health department that does both facilitates improved, culturally competent public health services and policies, builds community capacity, and strengthens all essential services of public health. Achieving results through collaborations involves special challenges as multiple accountability and decision-making structures come into play. But successful approaches to collaborative management have been emerging, as discussed near the end of the next chapter. In public health, including strong community collaborations in performance management is not an option. It is a requirement.

LINKING DESIRED RESULTS TO RESOURCES AND ACCOUNTABLE PEOPLE OR ORGANIZATIONS

Ultimately, the success of even the strongest collaborative public health approach depends on the extent to which accountability and commitment are shared by every partner involved. While it is important that each organization take responsibility and be accountable for results, the presence of a large number of players involved provides a special challenge in achieving this in a collaborative manner. Differing objectives and capacities of partnering organizations highlight the need for agreement on a common strategy for obtaining a desired outcome and clearly defined roles and responsibilities. Effective collaborations, therefore, rest on the ability of partnering organizations to build mutual trust and establish shared responsibility for commitments and results. In light of the challenges, new tools are evolving for devising collaborative community strategies and implementing them in a way that enables multiple organizations to fully understand and take responsibility for agreed-upon obligations. The "community balanced scorecard," described in the next chapter, is a tool for planning and managing a collaborative strategy to address community issues, such as public health, that no one organization or sector can address on its own. The end of the next chapter presents a related tool, the "community results compact," which can complement a balanced scorecard but does not require a scorecard for success. Community results compacts, as described in the next chapter, can also be useful for multiple organizations to collaborate successfully on performance management approaches described in this chapter. Whatever tools are used, public health performance management requires more than community-based policies and plans to succeed. It requires community organizations and leaders to back the plans with resources, to target their performance on contributing to mutually-desired outcomes, and to be accountable for meeting their resource commitments and performance goals.

Chapter 18

Community Balanced Scorecards for Strategic Public Health Improvement

Paul D. Epstein, Alina Simone, and Lyle D. Wray

T he *balanced scorecard* has been variously referred to as a tool for performance measurement, performance management, evaluation, strategy management, and strategic planning. It can be all those things. But the real power of a balanced scorecard is in the *strategic alignment* it achieves for an organization or community. That is as true for public health quality improvement as it is for any other endeavor. The brief history below provides an overview of how balanced scorecards have evolved to provide strategy alignment in for profit businesses, governments, and nonprofit organizations. The challenge for public health systems, which require cooperation between many organizations and stakeholders to succeed, is to achieve strategic alignment of a communitywide system, not just one organization. The rest of this chapter describes ways to do that.

EVOLUTION OF BALANCED SCORECARDS

Since being introduced in the early 1990s, the balanced scorecard has steadily become the strategic management system of choice within the private sector. As it has grown to be adopted by most of the Fortune 1000 companies, the benefits of the scorecard have also attracted an increasing number of adherents in governments, universities, hospitals, and nonprofit organizations. The balanced scorecard is a powerful tool, but it can not be applied in the same way to mission-driven public and nonprofit organizations as it is to private businesses with their focus on profit and delivering financial value for shareholders. In particular, public health management teams require an approach to the balanced scorecard that recognizes their need to engage residents and other stakeholders and to collaborate across organizations and across sectors. We call such an approach a *community balanced scorecard* (CBSC).

Before examining community scorecards, it is useful to review the traditional organizational balanced scorecard system. The organizational balanced scorecard, as created by Robert Kaplan and David Norton for businesses in the early 1990s, asks organizations to develop strategic objectives and performance measures from four different perspectives. These perspectives stack up on one another in cause-and-effect fashion whereby the achievement of goals at each level depends on the achievement of goals from each preceding level. The perspectives Kaplan and Norton introduced to businesses in the 1990s are still those most commonly in use:

Financial

↑

Customer

↑

Internal Processes

↑

Learning and growth (or organizational capacity)

As shown here, for businesses the "top" perspective, where organizations declare the final outcomes they seek to achieve, is "Financial." Public and nonprofit organizations have experimented with a variety of different perspectives, sometimes using more than four. But they most typically have used a variation of the business perspectives and moved a version of the financial perspective down one or more levels to align all strategic objectives toward the final goal of serving their constituency, as in the following example:

Customers, stakeholders, or constituents

↑

Financial stewardship (or resource management)

↑

Internal processes

↑

Learning and growth (or organizational capacity)

The perspectives form the framework for the tool at the heart of the scorecard, the *strategy map,* in which an organization distills its most important strategic objectives and maps a chain of assumed cause-and-effect relationships between the objectives and up through the perspectives. Then they are ready to drill down further: to create performance measures and initiatives for each objective, to "cascade" the scorecard down from the executive level through each department, and to anchor budgeting and employee evaluation systems to the strategy map. What emerges is a comprehensive strategic management system, complete with performance indicators, that compellingly aligns the priorities of the organization so each department and even each employee is aware of their role in helping the organization achieve its strategic goals. Thus, the strategy map is a crucial communications tool used for aligning strategy within the organization and also useful to present to potential investors, donors, volunteers, journalists, and others *external* to the organization, as a powerful means of conveying purpose. (Sample public health strategy maps are shown later in this chapter.)

The process of creating a strategy map is just as important as the strategic objectives that populate its perspectives and the cause-and-effect arrows that connect them. Management teams piloting the balanced scorecard development process are encouraged to include employees from different departments and different levels of the organization to amplify the impact of examining the organization from multiple perspectives.

COMMUNITY BALANCED SCORECARDS FOR PUBLIC HEALTH STRATEGIC ALIGNMENT

For the most part, balanced scorecards are used by organizations seeking to improve themselves and increase the value they deliver to their shareholders or stakeholders. However, in addressing public health issues leaders must look beyond the walls of their own organizations. Their work necessitates a collaborative effort that incorporates researchers, health providers, policy makers, social service providers, educators, businesses, and residents of their communities, all as active players in improving health outcomes. Consistent with the idea of "multiple citizen roles" in the previous chapter, when residents and other stakeholders are actively engaged in improving health, they are no longer simply "customers" or "constituents" of services, suggesting scorecard perspectives different from the typical ones, as in the examples later in this chapter. Also, with the need for collaboration between multiple players and organizations, it is not enough for a public health organization to achieve strategic alignment internally; what is needed is communitywide strategic alignment. Hence, a community balanced scorecard, which requires a collaborative approach. But the approach need not be overly elaborate or complex, as the individual collaborating organizations need not have organizational balanced scorecards of their own for a community balanced scorecard to succeed.

In short, the community balanced scorecard is designed for important issues that can not be resolved by one organization or sector alone. Introducing a community element to the traditional balanced scorecard yields four major benefits that are particularly applicable to public health:

- Pulls the community together around common outcomes desired by residents and other stakeholders

- Brings together decision makers and leverages assets from all sectors for shared results

- Aligns key community collaborators behind a common strategy for faster, measurable results

- Creates mutual accountability for results

ALIGNMENT WITH A COMMUNITY VISION FOR PUBLIC HEALTH

When adopted by governments and nonprofits, organizational balanced scorecards are built on the existing foundation of the organization's mission and vision. Similarly, a community balanced scorecard should align with the "community vision." There is a rich history of different "visioning" approaches in community-building efforts in the United States over the last 30 years. For public health, the MAPP process ("Mobilizing for Action through Planning and Partnerships") of the National Association of County and City Health Officials (NACCHO) and the

Centers for Disease Control and Prevention provides a useful template for how a community health coalition can develop a "public visioning" or "community diagnosis" process to produce a widely shared vision for improving health outcomes (see http://www.naccho.org/topics/infrastructure/mapp/index.cfm). The shared vision is important for aligning the efforts of the various collaborators needed for substantial community health improvements. A shared vision is a first step in achieving agreement on mutually desired public health outcomes for the community. Then the collaborators and stakeholders can develop a community balanced scorecard for achieving those outcomes. In doing so, they will have a powerful strategy that aligns resources, initiatives, performance measures, and targets with the community's vision for better public health.

CASCADING COMMUNITY BALANCED SCORECARDS BY "THEME"

Large organizations using balanced scorecards traditionally achieve strategic alignment by "cascading" the scorecard down from the executive level through their organizational units. Some organizations also create cascaded scorecards for *themes* based on strategic issues that cut across the organization. This can help break down organizational "silos" as staff from different units work together on "theme teams" to create thematic scorecards. For community balanced scorecards, organizational cascading may not be important, but thematic cascading is especially valuable. The themes can each reflect a different strategic dimension of issues addressed, and the theme teams would include members of the different organizations in the community whose participation is vital to successfully address the issue. For example, public health strategic themes can be geographic if there are underserved districts in a region. Or they may be demographic to focus on target populations. Or themes may focus on serious chronic health conditions affecting the community, or on strategic causes of mortality. Some cascaded scorecards may combine several types of themes. For example, a theme could focus on a hard-to-serve population, such as the homeless, and, based on conditions in a particular community, the theme could be made more specific to focus on homeless addiction, mortality, mental health, or veterans' issues.

USING THE 10 ESSENTIAL SERVICES OF PUBLIC HEALTH TO MAP A COMMUNITY HEALTH STRATEGY

The work done over the years to establish the 10 essential services of public health provides a solid foundation for using community balanced scorecards in public health. The essential services, or their equivalent in NACCHO's Operational Definition of a local health department, can readily be linked in cause-and-effect logic chains that focus on improving health outcomes in a community, as in the strategy map shown in Figure 18.1.

In this strategy map, which can be the basis for a CBSC, the ten essential services (with shortened and rephrased wording to fit in the graphic) are the strategic objectives in the bottom three perspectives. The top perspective, "Community health status," has a strategic objective that represents the ultimate long-term goals

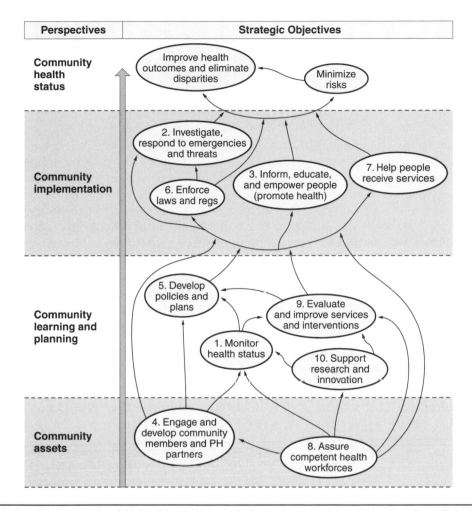

Figure 18.1   Potential public health community balanced scorecard strategy map based on the 10 essential services and operational standards of public health.

of a public health system: "Improve health outcomes and eliminate disparities." It also has the objective "Minimize risks" as a strategic way to improve outcomes.

The arrows between strategic objectives demonstrate the specific logic of the strategy from bottom (causes, or "drivers") to top (desired results).

Another way to grasp the logic of the strategy is to take a summary look backward across perspectives from the ultimate goal to the foundation of the system, as follows:

Community health status includes health outcomes, *which are improved by:*

> *Community implementation* including investigations, enforcement, health promotion, and health services, *which are made more effective by:*

> *Community learning and planning* including policies and plans, evaluation, health status monitoring, and research, *which are made more effective by:*
>
>> *Community assets* including engaged community members and public health partners, and competent health workforces.

Note in the strategy map that the "Community assets" of competent workforces and an engaged community and public health partners directly support *both* "Community learning and planning" *and* all the objectives in the "Community implementation" perspective. So, developing and engaging these assets forms the rock-bottom foundation needed for a successful community health strategy.

The strategy map in Figure 18.1 is not intended to describe the appropriate public health strategy for every community. Any community's strategy should be based on the shared vision of the partners in the local public health system, and the community's particular health needs, related social and environmental risks, and capacity, as may be determined by a community health assessment. Instead, this map can be used as a "reference strategy map" for a local public health system, to help system partners find their community's strategy faster by looking for their own local strategic variations from the reference map rather than starting from a blank page. The thematic CBSC examples that follow suggest possible variations to fit particular strategic public health themes in a given community.

THEMATIC SCORECARDS FOR LONG-TERM AND ACUTE COMMUNITY HEALTH STRATEGIES

Many government and nonprofit health and human service programs have been established to address acute problems that developed, became serious, and need attention. Often these are "downstream" problems that became serious because "upstream" social or physical issues in a community, region, state, or the nation were not adequately addressed earlier. The public health field recognizes the need for *upstream action* by stressing health promotion and disease prevention efforts (for example, exercise, good nutrition, smoking cessation) that can reduce the need for *downstream treatment* of serious, often chronic health conditions (for example, diabetes, obesity, respiratory diseases). Expanding the picture, public health agencies can try to influence broad *upstream policies* (for example, no-smoking laws, planning and zoning codes requiring sidewalks, parks, and mixed uses to encourage walking and exercise, subsidized markets with affordable, healthy food in poor neighborhoods).

In reality, public health agencies need to address acute downstream health problems at the same time as they try to address upstream prevention and community social and environmental issues. A community balanced scorecard helps health agencies strategically address both, making it a powerful tool for community public health.

Thematic CBSCs focused on specific public health issues in a community can be used for strategies that address both fundamental upstream conditions and acute downstream problems needing immediate attention. It is also likely that some efforts will address "midstream conditions" after a problem has occurred but before it becomes acute, as in the examples below. The theme of "Health of the local homeless population" in a city, county, or region is a good example as it has clear upstream, midstream, and downstream elements.

A Sample CBSC Strategy Addressing Upstream, Midstream, and Downstream Issues

The strategy map in Figure 18.2 could describe a potential community strategy for a local public health system to broadly address the homeless health issue. This map is based on the essential services of public health (as numbered) with some objectives changed to reflect this theme. For example, instead of one objective for essential service 5 (Develop polices and plans), this map has two:

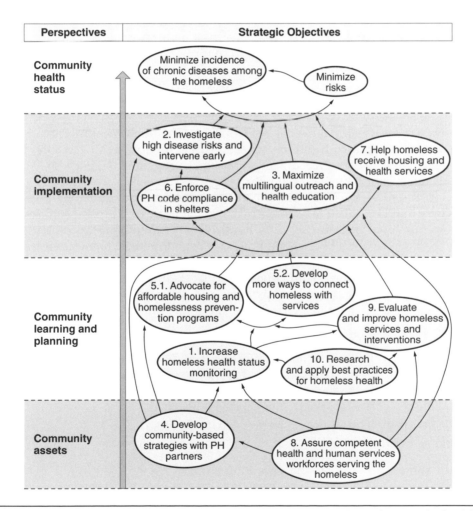

Figure 18.2 Potential community balanced scorecard strategy map for addressing the health of the local homeless population.

- 5.1—Advocate for affordable housing and homelessness prevention programs, *which addresses the upstream issue of preventing homelessness; this is important as just being homeless is a large health risk.*

- 5.2—Develop more ways to connect homeless with services, *which addresses the downstream need of ensuring that homeless get needed health services.*

Also, the objective for essential service 7 (Help people receive services) is:

- 7—Help homeless receive housing and health services, *which addresses the "midstream" issue of housing people who are already homeless and the downstream issue of health services for homeless people.* "Housing services" can include simply getting people living on the streets into shelters, as people with no shelter at all have the highest health risks of all homeless. "Housing services" can also include helping homeless move into permanent housing.

Essentially, this strategy says, "While we attempt to treat the immediate problem, we'll also make longer-term efforts to reduce the size of the problem."

What If a Community Issue with Public Health Implications Is Assigned to a Non-Health Agency?

A strategy such as the above assumes that the local public health system involves more than traditional health organizations. The public health "system" for this strategy may also include organizations that provide emergency shelter, fund or develop affordable housing, help people get housing subsidies, and provide social, financial, or legal services to intervene before families or individuals become homeless. So, it may be likely that a non-health organization (for example, a department of homeless services, housing, or community development) will be the lead agency for a broad community strategy to reduce homelessness. If so, a local health department or board of health should be a policy advocate to be sure the strategy addresses health issues, and that the lead agency, collaborators, and policy makers understand the upstream and downstream public health aspects of homelessness. That can increase the community's urgency to fund housing and homelessness prevention to reduce the size of the public health problem while also ensuring that adequate health services are provided for people while they are homeless. A CBSC can be just as effective if its development is stimulated by an advocate as if it is stimulated by a lead agency so long as the major partners understand the strategy and agree to implement their parts of it.

A CBSC Strategy That Takes a More Acute Focus on an Immediate Problem

If the same community found a growing number of homeless turning up in emergency rooms with very serious infectious diseases, such as tuberculosis or HIV/AIDS, they could develop a still more targeted strategy, such as that presented

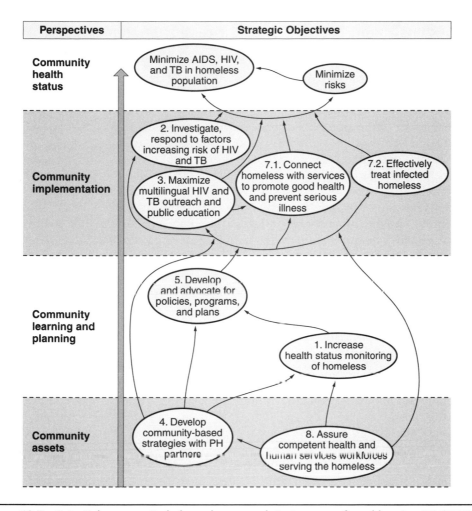

Figure 18.3   Potential community balanced scorecard strategy map for addressing HIV/AIDS and TB in the local homeless population.

in the strategy map in Figure 18.3. This strategy is more focused on solving the immediate acute problem, but it also has both "midstream" and "downstream" elements, as in the two objectives for essential service 7 (Help people receive services):

- 7.1—Connect homeless with services to promote good health and prevent serious illness. *In the broader strategy above, this might be a "downstream" objective. In this strategy, it is a "midstream" objective focused on preventing the more acute problem of homeless becoming infected with HIV/AIDS or TB.*

- 7.2—Effectively treat infected homeless, *a downstream objective of helping people survive and improve though they already have HIV/AIDS or TB.*

Relationships among "Parent" and "Cascaded" Strategies in a Community

All three strategy maps could conceivably be used by the same local public health system as part of a well-aligned strategy to improve community public health outcomes. The first, most general map could represent the overall community strategy for improving public health. Community leaders could determine which public health issues are important enough to develop thematic strategy maps for. If "Health of the homeless population" is one of those issues, then the second map, which represents a broad strategy to address the entire problem, is a "cascaded thematic map" that relates back to the first map. A community may stop at that level, focus on implementing that strategy for homeless health, and also develop thematic strategy maps for other important public health issues. Or, if the community has an acute problem of many homeless developing HIV/AIDS and TB, they may take cascading a step further, and develop the third strategy especially for dealing with this acute problem.

Note that the third map does not include objectives for all ten essential services of public health. This can be valid because, for example, public health leaders determined that they want to act quickly on the problem, so have left out objectives for "evaluation" and "research" (essential services 9 and 10) and will act based on what they know and what they learn from better health status monitoring. They may also see the acute-level strategy as primarily one of identifying high-risk and infected homeless and getting them treated quickly and sustainably, so they did not include an enforcement objective (essential service 6). If the public health system is pursuing research, evaluation, and enforcement at the broader level of the overall homeless health strategy, that can be sufficient to inform the acute-level strategy.

Overall, these examples show that a cascaded strategy map need not match other cascaded maps or a "parent" strategy map objective for objective so long as a clear relationship between the strategies comes through when examining the maps. They should all be clearly focused on achieving the same broader vision of improving public health, and they should have some consistency in their logic of getting to that vision, even if the particulars vary from theme to theme. The 10 essential services of public health give public health agencies and community health systems an easy way to ensure that their various cascaded thematic strategies align with each other and with the overall community strategy for improving public health. As in the examples above, though many strategic objectives are worded differently and the number of objectives differ on each map, each objective except the two "ultimate outcome" objectives in the top perspective clearly relate back to one of the essential services. If the same community used all three strategy maps, it would be clear how they all relate to a single overall community public health improvement strategy.

Completing the Community Balanced Scorecard: Adding Initiatives and Indicators

To turn a strategy map into a complete community balanced scorecard, specific performance indicators and initiatives are added to the strategic objectives. The initiatives are services, projects, or actions aimed at achieving the objective. The performance indicators define how to measure whether the objective is accomplished. Key performance indicators can also be targeted over time to indicate expectations for improvement. The scorecard table (Table 18.1) shows possible initiatives and indicators for the strategy map in Figure 18.3 focused on HIV/AIDS

Table 18.1   Scorecard table: community balanced scorecard for addressing HIV/AIDS and TB in a city's homeless population.

Perspective	Objective	Initiative	Indicator
Community health status	Minimize AIDS, HIV, and TB incidence in homeless population		Number and percent of homeless: • With AIDS • With HIV but not AIDS • With TB
	Minimize risks		Number and percent of homeless: • With untreated mental illness or drug abuse • Living on streets
Community implementation	(2) Investigate and respond to factors increasing risk of HIV and TB	Search for and respond to concentrations of homeless with drug-resistant infections	• Number of drug-resistant concentrations found • Average time to mitigate
	(3) Maximize multilingual HIV and TB outreach and public education	• Deploy multilingual outreach staff to engage high-risk homeless and encourage participation in shelters and medical services • Create multilingual HIV and TB info coasters, napkins, and paper cups for use at shelters, and encourage shelter staff to reinforce message	• Number of homeless who move from streets to shelter • Percent of homeless who know behaviors and conditions that increase risk of contracting HIV and TB

Continued

Table 18.1   *Continued.*

Perspective	Objective	Initiative	Indicator
Community implementation *(continued)*	(7.1) Connect homeless with services to promote good health and prevent serious illness	• Connect homeless with a regular source of health services to achieve, maintain good health • Monitor courses of mental health and drug treatment to keep homeless clients from dropping out	• Percent of homeless with regular source of healthcare • Percent of homeless clients who maintain mental or drug treatment as long as needed
	(7.2) Effectively treat infected homeless	Provide monitored treatment for TB and HIV to infected homeless	• Number of TB and HIV infected homeless on monitored treatment • Percent on monitored TB treatment who complete treatment successfully
Community learning and planning	(1) Increase health status monitoring of homeless	• Expand HIV and TB testing of shelter populations • Create a mobile HIV and TB testing clinic for the hidden homeless	Number of homeless who undergo HIV and TB testing
	(5) Develop and advocate for policies, programs, and plans	Advocate for an increase in budget for monitored treatment	Number of staff dedicated to monitored treatment
Community assets	(4) Develop community-based strategies with public health partners	Create an HIV and TB prevention, detection, and treatment work group of public health professionals, homeless people, homeless service providers, researchers, and advocates	Number of organizations that commit to implementing the work group's plans

Continued

Table 18.1   *Continued.*

Perspective	Objective	Initiative	Indicator
Community assets *(continued)*	(8) Assure competent health and human services workforces serving the homeless	• Train homeless service providers to recognize factors that increase risk of HIV and TB • Train outreach workers to recognize symptoms and dangerous conditions	Percent of provider and outreach staff who know behaviors, symptoms, and conditions that increase risk of HIV and TB

and TB in the homeless population. Cause-and-effect logic should still be inherent in the indicators and initiatives. As an example, consider a common thread running through initiatives for three objectives (5, 7.1, and 7.2): an emphasis on "monitoring treatment" of this hard-to-reach, hard-to-serve population. This is not only important for treating infections that develop drug-resistant strains, such as TB (objective 7.2). It is also important as a way to keep mentally ill or drug abusing homeless sticking with their treatment so they are less likely to lapse back into high-risk behaviors that make them prone to serious infection (objective 7.1). To make this possible, objective 5, which includes policy advocacy, has "Advocate for an increase in budget for monitored treatment" as an initiative. If this is successful, as measured by an increase in the indicator "Number of staff dedicated to monitored treatment," then the initiatives involving monitoring treatment for objectives 7.1 and 7.2 are more likely to be successful. At the top of the scorecard table there are indicators but no initiatives for the two objectives in the top perspective, "Community health status." This also reflects cause-and-effect logic in that all the initiatives below are expected to add up to improving the indicators for the top two objectives. In some strategies, the "top objectives" may have their own initiatives, but it is possible, as in this strategy, to view the top objectives as outcomes that are completely the result of the success of the objectives below, so they would have indicators but not initiatives.

Building Scorecards Incrementally, Implementing Change Along the Way

Once the partners in a community health system have mapped a common strategy, they may not have data collection techniques for desired indicators, know which indicators are best, or have the funding to fully design and implement each initiative. But that should not stop the partners from beginning to implement their strategy to the community's benefit. Getting started based on "what you know" and "what's practical now" can build momentum for strategic improvement while community partners learn to improve performance indicators and initiatives. It is not necessary to start implementing all objectives at once to make an impact. Where they can, community partners should make strategic choices of implementing some objectives likely to show early results to build support for the strategy, and other objectives that lay crucial long-term groundwork for desired outcomes. Once a community strategy is developed and has the support of key partners, it is important to start putting it into action. Don't ignore the need to "populate" all the objectives with strategic initiatives and useful, valid indicators. But that can be done in parallel with early action. For the good of the community, community balanced scorecard developers should move to action at an early stage, and perfect their scorecards as they go.

USING LEADING AND LAGGING INDICATORS IN AN EVIDENCED-BASED APPROACH TO MANAGING PUBLIC HEALTH STRATEGY

A critical methodological question left to address, after community health partners have populated their strategy map with objectives, initiatives, and indicators, is: "How can we use a community balanced scorecard to manage the strategy for achieving the community's public health goals?" Partly this is a community process issue of managing collaborations, as described in the last two sections of this chapter. Partly this is a technical issue of using data from performance indicators to determine how well the strategy is working and making changes to better achieve public health goals. In fact, balanced scorecards provide an evidence-based approach to managing strategy consistent with the public health ideal of evidenced-based solutions. Specifically, scorecard data can be used as evidence to test the core assumptions in the strategy map that comprise the route to improved community health. The key to this approach is to incorporate a good mix of leading and lagging indicators pegged to the strategic objectives. Kaplan and Norton also refer to these as "performance drivers" and "outcome indicators."

Leading indicators are those measures that will yield results in the near or mid term. Commonly, these include inputs and outputs, such as:

- *The number of staff dedicated to monitored treatment of homeless people with tuberculosis*

- *The number of TB-infected homeless on monitored treatment*

For some strategies, measures of capacity can also be leading indicators, such as *the number of organizations that commit to implementing the work group's plans.*

Lagging indicators, such as the *total number of homeless with TB* in the community, measure the results of long-term processes.

Short-term or medium-term outcomes, such as the *percent of monitored homeless who complete their full course of TB treatment successfully* (that is, until they are healthy and safely noninfectious), may occur after achieving an output, such as getting people into monitored treatment, *but they are still "leading indicators" of the ultimate desired outcome,* a total reduction of homeless people with TB.

If the hypotheses embedded in the strategy map about how outcomes can be achieved are correct, then improving the results of leading indicators should "drive" successful results of lagging indicators. For example:

- A communitywide strategic objective may target a lagging indicator of a *50 percent reduction in the number homeless people with TB* by 2015.

- The scorecard table suggests many leading indicators that can be targeted to contribute to that goal. Targets for two leading indicators could be, for example:

  - *80 percent of monitored homeless complete their full course of TB treatment successfully by 2010*

  - *800 homeless people are in monitored treatment by 2009*

Tracking of leading indicators can trigger red flags that enable management teams to make midcourse corrections. If leading indicator targets are not being met, then management will know years before getting results on lagging outcomes that they need to make changes in how they implement their strategy. If leading indicator targets are met but they are failing to drive lagging indicators, it may mean there is a disconnect somewhere in the logic chain, so key assumptions and even strategic goals need to be revisited. At the implementation level, close analysis of leading indicators can lead to a reassessment of program design to increase effectiveness, or a reallocation of budget funding or staff, thereby channeling resources toward the activities that will drive better long-term results.

BUILDING COMMUNITY ENGAGEMENT STRATEGY INTO THE PUBLIC HEALTH STRATEGY

Community engagement is required to fulfill the essential services of public health. But it does not mean creating a bloated bureaucratic structure or putting every management decision up for a vote before scores of resident or stakeholder committees. Smart community engagement is strategic. It is about identifying community health priorities, engaging and listening to residents who can explain the cultural and socioeconomic ground-level realities that will determine how programs play out, and most importantly, it is about harnessing the energy of people who are ready to work toward improving community health.

In a community balanced scorecard, a targeted community engagement strategy is built into the overall community health improvement strategy. Community residents are not just customers of services or stakeholders with special interests. The preceding chapter emphasized that residents can play many roles in improving their communities, and described several important resident roles. The key to harnessing residents' energy and knowledge of their neighborhoods or cultural groups is to support them in playing multiple roles constructively. The "Quick guide to supporting residents in major roles" (Table 17.1, page 242) in the previous chapter provides practical guidance in how to do just that.

In public health, supporting residents can vary from providing health information to neighborhood organizations, to training residents to gather and analyze such data themselves, or beyond, to soliciting their policy recommendations based on resident-led research. One example of such constructive engagement is *community-based participatory research* (CBPR), an approach designed to "involve community members as partners rather than as mere research subjects, use the community's knowledge to help develop interventions, inform community members about how research is done and what its results are, and . . . provide immediate benefits to the community."[1] CBPR has recently been applied in Harlem, in New York City, as a means of understanding how residents perceive local health problems and their causes, and to determine the best use of information technology in addressing these problems. The resulting data, culled from structured discussions with community residents, has implications for the application of technology designed to help Harlem residents prevent, manage, and ameliorate serious health problems.

As residents and other stakeholders can play multiple constructive roles, community engagement can be built into multiple perspectives and strategic objectives of a community balanced scorecard. Ultimately, public health agencies depend on residents becoming personally engaged in healthy behaviors, thus making them a part of even the top perspective in the sample strategy maps in this chapter as they personally reduce health risks. The rewards of incorporating citizens in strategic management of community health mirror the benefits of the balanced scorecard itself: addressing a goal from multiple perspectives to yield solutions that are ultimately more substantial, far-reaching, and likely to last.

HOW COMMUNITY COLLABORATION CHANGES BALANCED SCORECARD DYNAMICS

The balanced scorecard was first implemented within the familiar top-down power structures of the business world, with a fixed set of perspectives that emphasized the bottom line: financial success. When the BSC was introduced in government and nonprofit settings, the original perspectives were adapted, becoming more fluid in order to align the objectives of organizations driven by different goals, those of improving the lives of their constituents and their communities. With the introduction of the community balanced scorecard, the traditional dynamics are expanded again, this time to encompass a partnership-based approach where leadership and accountability are shared in order to address far-ranging problems beyond what any one organization or sector could cope with.

The benefits of the community balanced scorecard are best achieved with a clear and transparent approach to managing CBSC development and implementation. This can include a communication plan that outlines how accountability for results is distributed and shared, and a system for feeding back information on progress made toward accomplishing initiatives and performance targets. The approaches in the previous chapter under "Use of Performance Feedback . . . " can be expanded to communities for managing CBSCs for community learning and improvement. A strong consensus among leaders of organizations collaborating on the CBSC regarding strategic goals and methodology is also essential. Partners should agree on shared purpose involving community-tested goals and outcomes all want to achieve. Key decision makers should be at the table when needed, in fact or by real delegation, to avoid long waits to confirm agreements.

Online collaboration software, such as Web-based discussion boards, wikis, and shared project work spaces that provide multiple group working tools, can spur collective creativity, reduce the number of face-to-face meetings needed, and make meetings more productive due to online progress in the interim. But the best online collaboration tools will not help if the people using them work under "command and control" leaders. Community collaborations will most likely succeed if decision makers adopt "facilitative leadership" or "network leadership" styles, in which they empower their staff to openly contribute knowledge from their organizations and make joint decisions with their colleagues from other organizations as needed to keep the process moving forward. One of the goals of an organizational balanced scorecard is to learn from the evidence of performance data to improve the organization's strategy. With a community balanced scorecard, that becomes a goal of *mutual learning* between the collaborators, and ultimately *community learning* to improve the strategy to achieve the community's most important goals for better health outcomes and a better quality of life.

THE COMMUNITY RESULTS COMPACT: A TOOL FOR ADDING STRONG ACCOUNTABILITY AND COMMITMENT TO A COLLABORATIVE STRATEGY

A *community results compact* (CRC) makes collaborators' commitments to a shared community goal explicit, and establishes clear accountability for what each collaborator is expected to achieve. The idea for CRCs in public health is borrowed directly from the "quality of life compacts" of Truckee Meadows Tomorrow (www. truckeemeadowstomorrow.org), an innovative civic organization in the Reno, Nevada, region. CRCs can be useful for any collaborative approach to community-focused performance management. A balanced scorecard is not required. But CRCs are an especially good fit for a community balanced scorecard, and can be a valuable tool to strengthen CBSC implementation.

The basics of a CRC are simple: A CRC is applied to a desired community outcome no single organization can achieve on its own, such as *reducing the childhood obesity rate.* That outcome is a "lagging indicator" of community health status. Each collaborating organization commits to specific actions it will take and specific *leading indicators* it will measure and report to hold itself accountable for achieving results expected to contribute to the longer-term lagging outcome.

When a community results compact is applied to a community balanced scorecard, then the CRC also expresses the commitments of collaborators to agreed-upon strategies for accomplishing the desired outcome, represented as a strategy map for the issue or scorecard "theme" addressed. The actions and performance measures represent scorecard initiatives and leading indicators each collaborator is best positioned to implement. Targets for indicators and timelines for actions enable the collaborators to hold each other accountable for meeting their commitments and achieving short-term results along the way to collectively achieving the outcome. The following sample scenario demonstrates how a CRC could be applied to a theme of a public health community balanced scorecard.

The Process Begins

A coalition of community partners reviewed health status data and accompanying research on the effects of childhood obesity provided by the county health department and came to the alarming conclusion that local children were on pace to live shorter and more disease-filled lives than their parents if current trends continued. Further research on best practices by the health department and community conversations hosted by the public libraries led to recruitment of more partners needed to address this issue successfully (for example, public school leaders), and more interested stakeholders, including youth from the most affected parts of the county. The enlarged coalition convened to develop a strategy map, which they called a "community challenge map," to address the problem, which had two main logic chains leading to the following two strategic objectives:

- Increase age-appropriate activity levels
- Reduce caloric intake with better nutrition

Accomplishing both of these strategic objectives was assumed to lead to achieving the top-level objective to *"reduce the rate of childhood obesity,"* reflected in the following outcome target set for the community:

- Reduce the percent of children screened in public schools as obese, as defined by body mass index, by half in five years

The health department then negotiated specific action plans and targeted performance measures with several of the largest, most important collaborators for a "Community Resource Compact on Childhood Obesity." Also, a local public relations firm was recruited to join the compact, and several teenagers involved in community conversations formed a youth group to join. That led to the following actions and metrics for these collaborating organizations and community groups.

The Public Relations Agency

A pro bono communications study was conducted based on the strategy map and identified key target market segments among children, youth, and parents by demographic, economic, and geographic characteristics. The firm proposed messages on eating and activities for each target group, and vehicles for message delivery. The vehicles ranged from point-of-sale brochures and displays, to social networking Web sites, blogs, and listservs, to face-to-face community engagement activities, to nutritional mentor programs. The firm engaged volunteer youth to develop the name "Movin' on Down" for the communitywide program. *Metrics were developed and targeted for the percent of each target market segment "hit" in a given year for each key message.*

School District

Schools reviewed curricula and food choices for opportunities to increase physical activity and provide better nutrition. They produced wallet cards and pendants with messages for students of different ages connected to the broader

"Movin' on Down" program. Displays and brochures with photos of portion sizes for appropriate caloric intake were posted at points of service in cafeterias. Menus were modified to increase fresh fruit and vegetables—many from locally sourced producers—and emphasize lower fat and sodium choices. High-sugar drinks were phased out of school vending machines. *Metrics included the number and percent of low-sugar vending machines in schools, percent of school sites providing minimum levels of healthy food options, sales of fresh versus prepared food in cafeterias, student nutrition quiz results on portion size and healthy food guidelines, and percent of children participating in appropriate physical activity.*

After-School Programs

The large institutional after-school providers in the county (for example, YM/YWCA, local chapters of national charities and service clubs) all signed the Community Results Compact, then smaller providers signed on. They agreed to support greater activity and healthier eating using USDA food guidelines translated into kid-friendly language and formats. *Metrics included the number of improved participants' self assessments of eating behavior and quarterly average weight loss of children in a program for two or more quarters.*

Parks and Recreation Departments

The departments of each city in the county collaborated on youth focus groups and nonuser surveys to identify barriers to use of park and recreation facilities. They developed actions to overcome barriers, such as a Web- and phone-text-based "buddies" program for teens teaming up to share rides to workout facilities and provide mutual support to maintain exercise regimens. *Metrics included total attendance at recreation activities, number of children using fitness facilities, and standard fitness tracking for participants.*

Sleek Geeks

A group of high school students developed several Web-based supports for Movin' on Down, including social network sites to support better nutrition and physical activities after school, peer-to-peer support connections for eating or exercise, and map hacks accessible on cell phones and PDAs with locations of fast food restaurants with "better choices" on their menus and noting the items with "less bad" nutrition. *Metrics included number of children participating in the Movin' on Down Facebook site, percentage passing food and exercise quizzes on Web pages, and ratings by children of how much the Sleek Geeks' Web sites and online tools helped them eat better and exercise more.*

PTAs: Parents As Partners

Most school PTAs in the county sponsored community forums on how parents can "lead by example" to encourage better eating and more physical activity by their children. The PTAs also developed and distributed "Way to Grow" brochures with tips for busy parents on providing healthier snacks and meals, and on building more activity into family outings, from parking at the far end of the shopping center lot to challenging youth to beat the "10,000 steps a day challenge" using 10-dollar pedometers paid for by PTA fundraisers. *Metrics included the number and percent of parents participating in Movin' on Down programs, results of parent quizzes on food and exercise, and measures of changes made by families in response to the programs.*

County Health Department

The health department played a number of roles to help implement the Movin' on Down strategy, from providing staff support to a volunteer steering committee to providing technical assistance on nutrition to schools, church groups, PTAs, and restaurant owners. The department also was the "scribe" for detailed action planning and the information clearinghouse for reporting on the CBSC strategy and the CRC, including progress against timelines and targets for all strategic initiatives and performance indicators. The department maintained and advertised a Web site (www.movinondown.org) tracking actual obesity percentages of screened children against targets in the CRC and other metrics of children's activity and achievement of weight targets by age, geographic district, and demographic categories. *In addition to hosting the overall metrics of Movin' on Down, the department had some metrics of its own related to children identified as obese or at risk who visit the department's clinics.*

Starting Small and Expanding CRCs

Community results compacts need not be as comprehensive as this sample to help a local health strategy succeed. Just two or three well-positioned collaborators can start to make a difference. Then it's smart to publicize early successes of a small compact to get more collaborators in the community to sign on, building more commitment and accountability for improving results, and strengthening the power of the overall community health strategy.

Chapter 19

Creating the Conditions for Quality Improvement

Sarah Gillen, MPH, and Jennifer McKeever, LCSW, MPH

THE ENVIRONMENT FOR QUALITY IMPROVEMENT IN PUBLIC HEALTH

With a national voluntary accreditation program for local, state, and tribal health departments on the horizon, public health agencies are looking within to identify opportunities to improve their capacity and programs in order to succeed once the national program is launched. Numerous efforts are taking place at the local, state, and national levels to create an environment for quality improvement that will support governmental public health and its partners in systematic efforts to improve public health practice.

An initiative that is helping to create a practice and culture of quality improvement is the third phase of the Multi-State Learning Collaborative: Lead States in Public Health Quality Improvement (MLC), which involves local and state participants, such as governmental public health agencies, public health institutes, public health associations, healthcare providers, and universities from 16 states as well as national partner organizations. The first phase of the initiative explored the use of accreditation as a quality improvement process and helped shape the recommendations that established the Public Health Accreditation Board (PHAB), the nonprofit group that will administer the voluntary national accreditation program. The second phase of the project explored best practices for teaching and implementing quality improvement practices at the state and local level. The states participating in the third phase are cultivating an environment for quality within a community of practice as well as spreading momentum for quality improvement throughout the country.

The MLC project has identified several factors that facilitate the creation of an environment that supports quality improvement practice in public health. This chapter will illustrate these factors and opportunities for incorporating them into the culture and work of an organization in order to improve public health practice.

Topics to be addressed in this chapter include:

- Creating buy-in for quality improvement—engaging leadership and staff participation

- Frameworks that support the systematic adoption of quality improvement within an organization

- Providing support for quality improvement practice—training and resources

- Communicating about quality improvement successes and challenges

CREATING BUY-IN FOR QUALITY IMPROVEMENT— ENGAGING LEADERSHIP AND STAFF PARTICIPATION

In order for quality improvement efforts to take root throughout an organization, quality improvement initiatives require support from a variety of leaders, ranging from the executives to managers to frontline staff. This section of the chapter will discuss the opportunities for creating capacity for quality improvement by engaging leaders, management, and staff, via teams or collaboratives, as well as the community.

Executive Leadership

Executive leaders set the tone and work ethic for the organization that they lead. In public health, executive leaders have an opportunity to integrate quality improvement efforts into the fabric of the organization as a means of reinforcing the organization's commitment to improving the population's health. Clear and consistent messaging describing quality improvement expectations from the organization's executive leaders and management support the establishment of a culture of quality improvement within the organization. These expressions demonstrate that seeking continuous quality improvement for the organization and its programs is simply part of how the organization conducts its business.

Practical opportunities for the executive and senior leadership team to express quality improvement as an integral way of doing business in an organization include:

- Articulating quality as part of the organization's core values

- Incorporating quality improvement skills in job descriptions

- Discussing professional and program improvement opportunities during regular performance reviews

The role of the executive and leadership team within an organization can at times be delicate in terms of creating a nonthreatening and positive environment for quality improvement practice. As improvement efforts become organized, it is essential for executive leadership to avoid creating unsupported mandates and establishing unrealistic expectations. When executives and leaders become partners in the quality improvement efforts of their organization, participating staff members feel that their efforts are supported and valued. Together, senior leaders and staff within the organization can define the problems or challenges they face reaching the goals and objectives of the organization, as well as identify potential resources and solutions.

Quality Improvement Idea

Instructions for submitter:

Please use one idea per form.

Complete section 1.

Complete section 2. In simple terms summarize the current problem or condition and describe the change(s) you are recommending.

Complete section 3. It is your responsibility to research the benefit(s) and/or impact of the idea. List those benefits.

Complete section 4. Fill in the date sent to the supervisor.

Give the original form to your supervisor and a copy to your performance and accountability liaison.

Submitter: complete items 1–4

Submit this proposal to your supervisor and a copy to your performance and accountability liaison

1. Name		Date
Division	Telephone ( ) ext.	Immediate supervisor

2. Idea title:
   Description: Describe the process you want to change and how you want to change it. Attach additional pages and/or materials as needed.

3. Expected improvements:
   This idea will improve customer service/operations in the following way(s):

4. Submitter:
   Date sent to immediate supervisor and performance and accountability liaison.

Figure 19.1   Washington's staff feedback/Quality Improvement Idea form.

Washington state has participated in the MLC throughout all three phases of the project. Performance improvement efforts in Washington illustrate a tremendous commitment to quality between the state and local health departments. Also, within these departments, Washington has demonstrated that the organizations' leaders and all levels of employees collaborate to improve the practice of the organization. The form shown in Figure 19.1 demonstrates this commitment to collaboration. Via the Quality Improvement Idea form, staff members within a state or local department have the opportunity to present suggestions to senior leaders regarding areas within the organization that could benefit from concentrated quality improvement efforts.

As demonstrated above, staff members at different levels of the organization play critical roles helping to facilitate momentum and spread of quality improvement initiatives. Management and frontline staff have the ability to spread enthusiasm for quality improvement by collaborating with their peers and providing peer support for improvement efforts. Program and team leaders within an organization have the ability to identify resources such as time, expertise, and funding to support the quality improvement efforts. Managers should support their staff by creating time for quality improvement efforts in the workload of those involved. They may also facilitate and provide direction in relation to the strategies of the organization's participants in quality efforts.

Quality Improvement Teams and Collaboratives

A core ingredient for quality improvement practice is getting the right team of people to the table to problem-solve and test solutions together. A collaborative team to conduct quality improvement efforts may be formed by bringing together multiple individuals within an organization or by creating a collaborative of teams from multiple organizations.

Tips on forming strong quality improvement teams include:

- Pick a champion (internal or external) that can lead the team

- Define roles of various team members (for example, note takers, researcher, data cruncher)

- Establish expectations of the group (frequency of meetings/expected attendance, location, logistics)

- Establish goals and principles of the project

- Identify content experts both internal and external to the team that can help advise potential interventions that may lead to improvement

It is important that team members make a commitment to participating in the process and being present at all meetings. Depending on the complexity of the target being addressed, the team might need to be multidisciplinary to ensure that individuals with understanding and content knowledge of the issue being addressed are contributing to the thought process.

Forming teams and collaboratives to do quality improvement fosters peer learning among participants, which leads to quick leaps toward innovation. Innovation can be spread quickly when multiple team members and collaboratives are working to advance the field of practice in a target area. Teams and collaboratives also reinforce a supportive environment for quality by spreading enthusiasm and ownership for quality within an organization or multiple organizations.

During the second phase of the MLC, Michigan formed a learning collaborative among four local health departments that worked individually within their health departments and together as a group to identify strategies for improving their capacity. The health departments each formed a team that addressed unique target areas for improvement. The four teams met together on multiple occasions in an effort to share lessons with one another regarding how they were conducting their quality improvement efforts and to share their innovations or movements toward improvement. Now in the third phase of the MLC, the leaders of Michigan's MLC-2 quality improvement projects are now serving as mentors to additional health departments in Michigan that are seeking to improve their practice.

Community Engagement

The nature of public health work is multifaceted and often requires collaboration with partners and community members. As an organization prepares to do quality improvement, it is important to look to key stakeholders that should be at the table. External stakeholders can assist the organization with identifying priorities for improvement. Additionally, external partners might take on a role of helping implement solutions that are tested to achieve improvement. Bringing key partners and stakeholders to the table in this fashion invites their support and commitment to helping the organization and its initiatives improve.

FRAMEWORKS THAT SUPPORT THE SYSTEMATIC ADOPTION OF QUALITY IMPROVEMENT WITHIN AN ORGANIZATION

What gets measured gets done.

—Unknown

The implementation of systematic efforts to improve the processes and programming of the organization can add greatly to the environment that drives the performance of employees and organizational partners. Systematic organizational improvement may be driven by a strategic plan that focuses on results. Additionally, there are several frameworks for improvement that can be used to guide systematic improvement processes that touch on how various systems within an organization function together to achieve the organization's goals and objectives. This section of the chapter will highlight opportunities for embedding quality improvement efforts throughout the organization in a systematic manner to create the environment for all employees to support quality improvement.

Strategic Planning

Creating a strategic plan is an important endeavor toward identifying key activities that will enable an organization to achieve its mission and vision. In-depth strategic plans that include a framework for measuring the progress and impact toward implementing activities provide a backbone on which the organization can conduct quality improvement to assure that its programs are meeting the organization's goals. In addition to outlining the strategies, goals, objectives, and activities of an organization, a strategic plan may also include an evaluation plan that involves activities that test and measure improvement.

Organizational Improvement Frameworks

In addition to using a strategic plan as a tool to guide quality improvement efforts for an organization, there are numerous organizational improvement frameworks that look at multiple facets of organizational process. Adopting an organizational improvement framework such as the Baldrige Criteria for Performance Excellence or balanced scorecard (both of which are discussed in greater detail in Chapters 5 and 18) provides opportunities to engage employees from all corners of the organization in a process that continuously assesses the organization's performance. These frameworks assess the organization's strategic planning capacity as well as leadership, customer service, financial processes, knowledge management, workforce development, process management, and measurement of results.

The Florida Department of Health (DOH) joined the MLC in the second phase of the project. Florida has a long history in public health of utilizing organizational frameworks for performance management and quality improvement practices and, as a result, has seen significant health and process improvements. The County Health Department (CHD) Performance Improvement Process provides a set of key indicators for CHDs to measure, improve, and compare performance, provides a statewide view of performance on an annual basis to guide statewide initiatives, ensures that there is a quality improvement process in every CHD, and promotes collaboration throughout the organization. The "County Performance Snapshot," shown in Figure 19.2, is a reporting tool used by Florida's local health departments, contains standards and measures framed around the Results category for Florida's Sterling Criteria (similar to Malcolm Baldrige Criteria), and include:

- Product and Services Outcomes
- Customer-Focused Outcomes
- Financial and Market Outcomes
- Workforce-Focused Outcomes
- Process Effectiveness Outcomes
- Leadership Outcomes

The Miami–Dade County Health Department is the largest of Florida's 67 CHDs, and eighth largest in the United States. The CHD has utilized the Sterling Criteria for Organizational Excellence as the basic framework of their performance improvement initiatives and, as a result, has made significant improvements in the areas of strategic planning, customer satisfaction, and human resource focus. The CHD has been the recipient of two Governor's Sterling Awards—one in 2002 and a second award in 2006.

PROVIDING SUPPORT FOR QUALITY IMPROVEMENT PRACTICE—TRAINING AND RESOURCES

Training

Creating the environment and attitudes for quality improvement requires giving staff the training and access to information and resources that are needed to

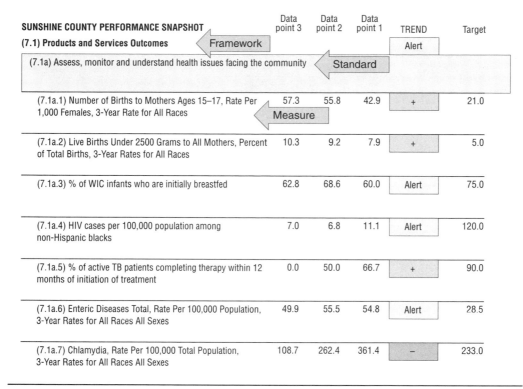

SUNSHINE COUNTY PERFORMANCE SNAPSHOT (7.1) Products and Services Outcomes Framework	Data point 3	Data point 2	Data point 1	TREND Alert	Target
(7.1a) Assess, monitor and understand health issues facing the community Standard					
(7.1a.1) Number of Births to Mothers Ages 15–17, Rate Per 1,000 Females, 3-Year Rate for All Races Measure	57.3	55.8	42.9	+	21.0
(7.1a.2) Live Births Under 2500 Grams to All Mothers, Percent of Total Births, 3-Year Rates for All Races	10.3	9.2	7.9	+	5.0
(7.1a.3) % of WIC infants who are initially breastfed	62.8	68.6	60.0	Alert	75.0
(7.1a.4) HIV cases per 100,000 population among non-Hispanic blacks	7.0	6.8	11.1	Alert	120.0
(7.1a.5) % of active TB patients completing therapy within 12 months of initiation of treatment	0.0	50.0	66.7	+	90.0
(7.1a.6) Enteric Diseases Total, Rate Per 100,000 Population, 3-Year Rates for All Races All Sexes	49.9	55.5	54.8	Alert	28.5
(7.1a.7) Chlamydia, Rate Per 100,000 Total Population, 3-Year Rates for All Races All Sexes	108.7	262.4	361.4	–	233.0

Figure 19.2   County performance snapshot of Florida's performance improvement system.

support their quality improvement work. Quality improvement practice is still relatively new to public health. Efforts have been made in recent years to adapt quality improvement tools and training materials from other industries in a manner that is relevant to public health. Participants in the MLC have found that multiple forms of training are needed to engage local and state health departments in quality improvement practice. Many states in the MLC have conducted widespread learning sessions to provide training on core concepts related to quality improvement. See the sample agenda in Figure 19.3 from a training workshop offered in Florida during MLC-2.

In addition to large plenary-type training meetings, "on the spot" or "just in time" training for teams that work on quality improvement projects is also needed. As teams are working through their quality improvement projects it is important to have access to content experts that can inform the quality improvement techniques being used, as well as content experts on the public health issue that is being addressed.

Incentives

Earlier in this chapter we identified that leaders should be careful to avoid creating an "unfunded mandate" in terms of expecting staff members and teams to conduct quality improvement work without providing the appropriate resources

Statewide Performance Improvement Training
Hilton Tampa Airport Westshore
May 8, 2009

Time	Quality tools			
9:00 a.m.	*Opening Plenary Session—Tampa Bay Ballroom* **Steven Woolf, MD, MPH,** Virginia Commonwealth University "Making the Most of Clinical Preventive Services"			
10:00 a.m.	Break			
	Tampa Bay Ballroom	*Westshore 3 & 4*	*Westshore 5 & 6*	*Palm Board Room*
10:15 a.m.	**Roland Martinez** Miami–Dade CHD *Identifying Key Processes*	**Betty Serow** DOH Office of Planning, Evaluation & Data Analysis *Problem Solving Using QI Tools*	CHD Panel Presentation Pinellas CHD, Sarasota CHD, St. Lucie CHD *Creating an Efficient Clinic*	**William Boyd,** CDC *How Can Patient Flow Analysis Assist in Evaluating Service Delivery?*
11:45 a.m.	Lunch	Lunch	Lunch	Lunch
1:15 p.m.	**Roland Martinez** *Getting to the Core of Process Mapping*	CHD Panel Presentation Pinellas CHD, Sarasota CHD, St. Lucie CHD *Creating an Efficient Clinic*	**Stacy Baker** Public Health Foundation *Getting to the Heart of Tough Problems*	**William Boyd** *How Can Patient Flow Analysis Assist in Evaluating Service Delivery?*
2:45 p.m.	Break	Break	Break	Break
3:15 p.m.	**Roland Martinez** *Getting to the Core of Process Mapping*	**Stacy Baker** *Getting to the Heart of Tough Problems*	**Betty Serow** *Problem Solving Using QI Tools*	
4:45 p.m.	Adjourn	Adjourn	Adjourn	Adjourn

Figure 19.3   Agenda from statewide training conducted by the Florida MLC project.

to problem-solve and seek innovation. Incentives are very important to helping participants in quality improvement efforts feel that there is a value and sense of priority for their work. Incentives may come in the form of funds to support purchasing books and materials that aid the initiative or perhaps in the form of technical assistance or consultant support. The incentives do not need to be large investments, but should address the costs that team members will experience when conducting quality improvement activities.

COMMUNICATING ABOUT QUALITY IMPROVEMENT SUCCESSES AND CHALLENGES

One key component to creating an environment for quality improvement is communicating lessons learned, successes, and challenges related to improvement efforts. By communicating improvements and struggles, peers are able to spread learnings from the hard work that has been done to test and analyze opportunities for process improvement. Enthusiasm for improvement is infectious among peers and colleagues within an organization, and also the organization's stakeholders.

Acknowledging Failure and Opportunities for Growth

There may be times when quality improvement efforts are not hugely successful and do not lead to huge gains in efficiencies. Nonetheless, communicating these findings provides an opportunity for colleagues to understand that they are working in a safe environment that values the spirit of continuously learning about the work of the organization. When the MLC-2 project team from Florida shared its efforts to conduct a collaborative addressing chronic disease with the larger MLC collaborative, the team noted that sometimes failures or challenges in conducting quality improvement provide the greatest opportunities to learn and excel. Now in the third phase of the project, the central office is using the lessons learned in the previous collaborative as it rolls out a new and improved collaborative process with additional health departments.

Celebrating Small Victories and Incremental Steps toward Process and Health Improvements

Developing a spirit of enthusiasm for the hard teamwork that goes into quality improvement projects is very important to creating momentum in order to get to the finish line and foster sustainability of the effort. Celebrating small steps toward understanding process improvement helps participants believe in the process. Success can come in many forms when it comes to conducting quality improvement work—it is important to use many forms of communication to celebrate success and innovation.

Potential Opportunities and Methods for Communicating and Disseminating Quality Improvement

There are many ways to share information with colleagues, partners, and stakeholders about the hard work that has been accomplished conducting quality improvement efforts. In the second phase of the MLC project, several states used storyboards to communicate information from their quality improvement projects with peers within their state. The storyboards provide an opportunity to succinctly document the aim of the project and quality improvement activities that were conducted, and represent data and information that were used to measure improvements, as well as the outcomes of the project. Storyboards are an excellent tool for quality improvement participants to spread the details of their accomplishments and lessons learned with their peers.

In addition to the storyboards, several MLC states have hosted a session called a "learning congress" or "showcase" meeting that brings together public health practitioners and stakeholders from throughout the state in a one-day session where the findings of recent quality improvement projects are shared and discussed.

These forms of communicating about quality improvement efforts provide opportunities to spread enthusiasm and innovation. The enthusiasm and quest for innovation are infectious, and motivate additional peers to step back and look at new opportunities for improving the public health practice of the organization.

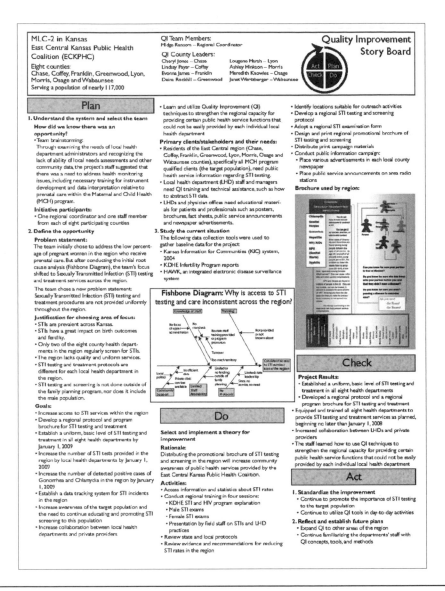

Figure 19.4   Storyboard created by the Kansas MLC project.

SUMMARY

Much of creating the environment for quality improvement work is getting people engaged to seek improvement and change within an organization. The following are suggestions that were outlined in this chapter:

- Support from executive leaders in the form of setting the tone and expectation for quality as well as providing resources that support quality improvement work.

- A promising method for engaging employees in quality initiatives is to use teams or collaboratives that enable groups of employees to problem-solve and test solutions together. The most important thing is to enable folks to get started.

- Making quality a systematic component of how the organization conducts its business helps engage staff at all levels within the organization. This can be done in the form of creating metrics for the organization's strategic plans—or in greater depth by adopting a framework for organizational improvement such as Baldrige or a balanced scorecard.

- Providing resources in the form of training and incentives is essential to helping teams access the information and support needed to conduct quality improvement efforts.

- Communication is key to spreading innovation and enthusiasm.

Chapter 20

Performance Management in Action—The Role of Leadership

Leslie M. Beitsch, MD, JD

INTRODUCTION

By virtue of a long career in public health practice, it has been my privilege to visit numerous local and state health departments across the United States. Invariably these visits were a true learning experience. Each health department was impressive in its own right, showcasing one or more innovative, high-quality programs.

Recent surveys by the National Association of County and City Health Officials (NACCHO) and the Public Health Foundation (PHF) confirm the findings of my informal "convenience sample" survey. Most health departments have representative exemplary programs—meaning there are clear examples of high performance. Stated most positively, this research found that, generally, health departments have quality improvement (QI) activities taking place. However, they tend to be informal and localized to specific programs or areas. Examined more critically, public health agencies lack formal performance improvement initiatives. Moreover, rarely do organizations have quality improvement activities widely disseminated; they tend to be localized in pockets of the agency.

Given the positive aspects of this information, while noting the current public health limitations, leadership plays a critical role in the potential transformation of health department performance management (PM) capacity. The steadily evolving external environment is trending toward a national accreditation system for public health departments. The bedrock foundation of this voluntary accreditation process is to foster improved public health performance and quality. Yet, even without the push–pull of accreditation, leaders and funders alike want health departments to maximize their performance and contribute to improved community health outcomes.

This chapter offers reflection and guidance that may assist a health department leader as they embrace the challenge of developing a formal quality improvement system in their agency.

ESTABLISHING A QUALITY IMPROVEMENT CULTURE

Savvy public health veterans can recall numerous failed "new" proven methods introduced during the course of their careers. More cynically, these fads represented the "flavor of the month," and were introduced by well intended but naive past administrations. Even when the ideas had genuine merit, resistance to change throughout the organization crippled implementation. How does leadership avoid being victimized by ancient history and surmount these obstacles?

Senior Leadership Sets the Tone

A necessary prerequisite (necessary but insufficient) is that leadership must walk the quality improvement talk. Espousing the language of QI without actually modeling the behavior will increase skepticism and call leadership commitment into question.

W. Edwards Deming introduced 14 principles fundamental to the formation of quality organizations. See Figure 20.1 for a full listing of Deming's *14 points*. An important precept embedded in many of them is the recognition that employee involvement—nay ownership—is the linchpin to success. Leadership can set the tone by demonstrating inclusion—intentional engagement of all levels of the organization in reaching decisions affecting the entire health department. Mere gestures and symbolism will short-circuit your efforts.

Ensure that quality improvement is a regular agenda item in meetings of senior management. Rotate reporting at these gatherings so that all senior staff comprehend that it means them, too. Be willing to share the steps you have taken to improve quality within your immediate areas of responsibility.

Building a Formal Structure

Systemwide quality improvement does not occur randomly. A formal organizational structure designed to serve the purposes of the quality improvement

1. Create and publish a company mission statement and commit to it.
2. Learn the new philosophy.
3. Understand the purpose of inspection.
4. End business practices driven by price alone.
5. Constantly improve the system of production and service.
6. Institute training.
7. Teach and institute leadership.
8. Drive out fear and create trust.
9. Optimize team and individual efforts.
10. Eliminate exhortations to the workforce.
11. Eliminate numerical quotas and MBO focus on improvement.
12. Remove barriers that rob people of pride of workmanship.
13. Encourage education and self-improvement.
14. Take action to accomplish the transformation.

Figure 20.1   Deming's 14 points (abridged).
Source: The W. Edwards Deming Institute (www.deming.org).

initiative should be erected as early as feasible. The actual structure is less important than having one, in particular one that reflects how the health department typically conducts its business. In short, it could be combined with other standing committees, or could be a separate committee altogether. Work of this committee (often called a *quality council*) should feed into the regular senior management meeting structure. Alternatively, the quality council could be seated as the senior management committee itself.

In order to fully incorporate the teaching of Deming and other quality pioneers, formal mechanisms must be put in place within the structure to capture the knowledge and support of the frontline employee. Likewise, senior management must also be cultivated. To accomplish this top–down and bottom–up, one organization I recently worked with established the executive management team as the "boundary setters" for a larger quality council that included all levels of employees within the health department. This approach gave the executive committee authority to set the ground rules (the "what" of QI) while continuing to empower employees to determine the "how." This successful strategy resulted in the development of acceptance and ownership of QI by executives within the health department as well as staff providing direct services.

Mentoring Others

Admittedly, the success of any QI program implementation is multifaceted and complex. But a great deal is dependent on both the formal structure and the right leadership. The selection and mentoring of champions to guide key aspects of the initiative is crucial. Leadership in all organizations is divided into formal leaders (those who possess titles and job descriptions of leadership positions) and informal leaders (individuals recognized by others for their wisdom, regardless of rank within the organization). If you do not already know, learn the identity of these latter individuals. Nurturing the formal and informal leaders as champions and placing them in positions of responsibility for QI committees or as heads of QI teams expands the potential for broader acceptance and buy-in agencywide. Part of the mentoring process is coaching these leaders—share with them individually what you are trying to accomplish and why. In addition, provide them with the necessary tools and training to take an active role in the introduction of a performance management program.

Combining the notion of garnering leadership support with engagement of employees at all levels within the health department is a further demonstration of organizational commitment to QI. General acceptance and less skepticism are likely to follow. Be alert for the myriad soft signs, especially body language: more head nodding, fewer scowls, and less arm-crossing during staff meetings.

Health Department Transparency

In an information vacuum, rumors and innuendo will replace facts. Freely revealing information routinely fills the void that would otherwise likely be replete with errors and misinterpretations (or worse). This is just as true for a health department as any other organization. Research from the balanced scorecard revealed that only five percent of employees were familiar with key organizational strategies to achieve objectives. This magnitude of organizational disconnect can dramatically reduce the likelihood of successful rollout of any new program. In the commercial world, failed product introduction may lead to bankruptcy or plummeting share value on Wall Street. In government, it leads to inefficiency and lowers workers' job satisfaction.

One Midwestern state health department regularly published its executive management team meeting minutes on their intranet. In a world where many people complain about access to too much information, most staff did not feel the need to review the minutes. However, many did, and this modest commitment became more than a symbolic gesture to inform employees agencywide. Just like staff meetings and newsletters, it became another way of establishing a genuine QI culture and modeling the behaviors leadership wished to implement.

A Southern state with a rapidly developing QI reporting system (quadrant 3 of the Turning Point model) takes transparency to the next stage. Employees who are the owners of the various processes and metrics within the reporting system directly enter the data they are responsible for. Any employee of the health department can access their own data as well as any other metric via the agency intranet on a 24/7 basis. With this transparent approach there is never any mystery about performance versus expectation.

Marketing Quality Improvement

Communicating the importance of QI is one component of a successful marketing effort. Pursuing the intentional strategy of transparency just mentioned is one aspect of this communication. Marketing also includes the selling of the product. In this case the products are QI and performance management. Getting the word out and creating a "buzz" are essentials of selling any concept. Leadership must take an active role in creating the marketing buzz and regularly reigniting it. Consider the example of the Shameless Commerce Division of National Public Radio's *Car Talk* as a source of inspiration.

QI and performance management, thoughtfully presented, can actually sell themselves. In my experience, few employees, public health employees in particular, actually come to work to do a poor job. True, they want to be paid for their efforts (typically modest pay), but they take inordinate pride in their labors. Sometimes they lack the tools, resources, or training to perform optimally. QI, properly introduced, will assist them in reaching higher levels of performance within the constraints they face daily. Who doesn't want to achieve better results with a similar amount of effort?

One important caveat must also be acknowledged, and it may require convincing leadership and senior management: employees must be empowered with the authority to do their jobs well (back to Deming's 14 points).

In short, marketing quality improvement requires reminding everyone why they entered public health as a career in the first place—to improve the health of the community. Little additional coaxing may be necessary, provided leadership stays on task and remembers to walk the talk. Keeping the word out there during staff meetings, establishing QI teams and committees will help keep QI fresh on their agendas. Yielding power in order to actually gain it may prove to be the most cumbersome obstacle for leadership and the employees alike.

Leadership Role in Structuring a Performance Management Framework

Thus far I have been using the terms quality improvement and performance management interchangeably. Let me step back for a moment to offer some clarification. Generally, quality improvement approaches are utilized to strengthen performance within a program or process. When there is a systematic effort to improve performance, using QI methods across an entire organization in numerous programs and processes, it is termed performance management. Some practitioners call the use of QI tools and methods within specific programs or processes "little QI." At the enterprisewide level, the purposeful use of QI to manage overall organizational performance is sometimes referred to as "big QI," or performance management.

It is a pivotal role of leadership to establish the structure within the health department that supports performance management. As mentioned in the chapter introduction, although quality improvement is practiced in most health departments (the good news!), it is not incorporated into a formalized performance management system (the opportunity). An earlier chapter in this handbook (Chapter 5) describes Baldrige and other national quality awards. Baldrige, along with balanced scorecard and the Turning Point model, are some examples of big QI, or performance management systems.

Defining the Governance

In order to accomplish the goals of big QI certain functions need to be facilitated through a formalized structure. Somewhat paradoxically, it is less important what the structure looks like than that it exists and is a good fit for the health department. As an example, it was noted earlier that governance of QI could be placed under the auspices of a quality council. Whether the council would be the executive management team or a subsidiary body with a clear charter is itself a leadership decision.

Determining the Rules of Engagement

Consistent with the principles of transparency and marketing discussed previously, the respective roles of each committee in the performance management framework should also be laid out in clear terms. In the earlier section about establishing a QI culture, an allocation of responsibilities was described whereby the senior executives served as the boundary setters while the newly formed quality council determined the strategies to address the priorities identified by senior management. The choice of roles is a local decision that should respect historical patterns at your health department, with sensitivity to what has proven effective within the culture of the organization.

In addition to reaching conclusions regarding which committee will do what, and where authority is vested, an overall QI plan should be written and disseminated. In essence, this brief document should detail in broad terms the decisions for the questions just outlined. It should state the purpose of the QI program and its proposed activities. Basically, it should be a short, easily understood document. Sharing it will promote collective accountability to ensure full implementation.

Addressing All the Elements

The Baldrige performance management system consists of seven criteria:

1. *Leadership.* How upper management leads the organization, and how the organization leads within the community.

2. *Strategic planning.* How the organization establishes and plans to implement strategic directions.

3. *Customer and market focus.* How the organization builds and maintains strong, lasting relationships with customers.

4. *Measurement, analysis, and knowledge management.* How the organization uses data to support key processes and manage performance.

5. *Human resource focus.* How the organization empowers and involves its workforce.

6. *Process management.* How the organization designs, manages, and improves key processes.

7. *Business/organizational performance results.* How the organization performs in terms of customer satisfaction, finances, human resources, supplier and partner performance, operations, governance and social responsibility, and how the organization compares to its competitors.

Other performance management systems offer similar domains (see Figure 20.2). In setting the dimensions of the enterprisewide health department performance management plan, whether or not you subscribe to the Baldrige approach, all the Criteria should be addressed somewhere in the structure of the plan and the allocation of individual and committee responsibilities. A high-flying, fully functioning quality organization is dependent on all of these areas being considered thoughtfully.

Keeping All Eyes on the Prize

Frequent and regular attention to the QI agenda is a necessary leadership prerequisite to the achievement of QI objectives. Having set forth a QI plan, established a framework, and appointed committees will not alone ensure that the actual work is done. Follow-up and its management are essential. A simple and straightforward approach is to make QI/PM a standing agenda item (that does not

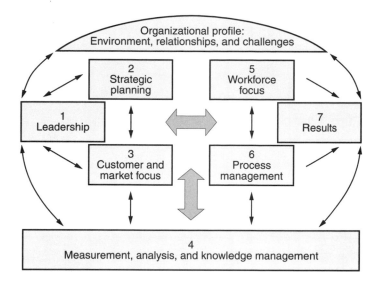

Figure 20.2   Florida Sterling Council Criteria for Performance Excellence framework: a systems perspective.

get tabled) in the executive management team meetings. Updates should also be included in the regularly scheduled meetings of mid-level management as well as frontline employees.

As noted in the section on establishing a QI agency culture, it is up to leadership to walk the talk. Consistent attention and follow-through will do more to signal leadership intentions than just rolling out the program and making a big splash. Doing both is even better!

Alignment of QI/PM and Agency Priorities

Rather than being separate or additional work, QI/PM are tried and proven means to accomplish key agency objectives. Although in its most mature form a performance management system should include virtually all programs and activities within the health department, resources should initially be dedicated to areas of high priority.

One way to assure that priorities are not overlooked in the frenzy of activity that sometimes accompanies a thousand flowers blooming is to intentionally structure alignment into the major work products of the health department. Figure 20.3, adapted from work done at the Florida Department of Health, depicts the outline that ensures that key metrics are reinforced throughout departmental activities. Even annual performance appraisals should be modified to reflect agency priorities and their achievement.

If alignment is pursued aggressively, everything from each individual's annual review all the way to mission, vision, and values—and all in between—will line up. Emphasizing the common use of measurement objectives can simplify this task. In other words, try not to use different metrics for each of the efforts outlined

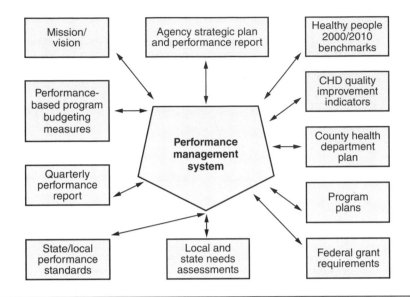

Figure 20.3 Interrelated measurement components for a public health system.

Source: L. Beitsch, C. Grigg, K. Mason, and R. Brooks, "Profiles in Courage: Evolution of Florida's Quality Improvement and Performance Measurement Systems," *Journal of Public Health Management Practice* 6: 31–41.

in Figure 20.3. In fact, using the same key metrics consistently will focus attention on alignment and achievement.

Ensuring Workforce Development

Deming in his work pointed out quite forcefully that management is typically the problem in organizations, and that workers are the solution. Even if you do not completely buy this pejorative against management, there is little room for disagreement that the workforce is essential for the development of a formal quality improvement system in the health department.

Earlier, the section on culture addressed the crucial concept of employee involvement. Intimate knowledge of the problem—and perhaps more importantly, the solution—is most accessible by those closest to the issue or process itself. As imperative as empowerment may be, workforce training in QI enables empowerment to be actualized.

Although most people have individual learning styles that meet their needs, experience now suggests that the adult learner model is most effective with employee teams for gaining acceptance and use of QI tools and methods. This approach utilizes "just in time" teaching. Employee teams are constituted by leadership to address specific issues (an agency priority perhaps). Training is offered to the teams and then applied immediately to the problem at hand. Optimally, teams have coaches available to assist them when subsequently they reach the inevitable roadblock. Some health departments with resources available have been able to "embed" coaches who can provide ongoing teaching as the need for additional tools arises.

The approach just described is somewhat resource-intensive and does not provide training to all staff at one time. This means leadership needs to plan for ongoing training until all employees have had an opportunity to participate in a team. While this may appear inefficient, immediate use of tools by teams addressing health department problems leads to learning that is retained. Retention is further assured by ongoing use through multiple QI cycles (rapid-cycle improvement).

Leadership has an additional task: that of freeing up time for QI teams to perform their work. This includes time for QI teams to meet and to perform out-of-group homework like data collection. Expecting staff to do their usual assignments (without adjustment) and to fulfill their roles on QI teams may result in resistance that threatens success.

Maintaining and Sustaining QI Despite Constraints

The daily challenges of working in a resource-constrained environment often result in retrenchment. One example is the natural tendency to reduce travel and training budgets in an effort to maintain current staffing levels in the programs. In the near term this logic appears unassailable. But to escape the inevitable vicious cycles of downward-spiraling budgets, it sometimes is necessary to make investments when they can least be afforded. QI and PM fall into this category. Without investments in time and training, the downstream (temporally) dividends of efficiency and cost savings can not be realized. Unfortunately, it often takes considerable time for investments to yield these payoffs.

A health department I have worked with for many years temporarily discontinued key aspects of its QI program in the aftermath of 9/11. The program had been nurtured and expanded under several directors. At the time it was difficult to argue against the wisdom of a brief shift in emphasis. The short pause, however, turned into an extended break, and after a few years the entire program had to be virtually rebuilt from the ground up. Sadly, much of the institutional memory was also erased. This example emphasizes three key points:

1. There will always be crises in public health. If we allow them to interfere with our ongoing commitment to constant efforts at self-improvement, then we will seldom achieve our long-term objectives.

2. Shifts in leadership can jeopardize hard-fought gains. For the full benefit of QI/PM to be reached, efforts have to be extended over time and grow within the agency.

3. Although it goes by many names, regardless of its moniker QI/PM is not a fad. Moreover, as seen in myriad other industries, it is gaining emphasis. Like any other activity fully instituted within the health department, it must receive ongoing support from leadership to be sustained.

It is a rare health department that does not face continued funding obstacles, especially in the current economic downturn. The majority of budgets comprise staff salary and benefits. This makes staff time as scarce as general revenue. During the early phases of QI/PM implementation a common lament by employees is that they lack time for QI. This viewpoint, also logical, is premised on the belief that QI is an "extra" job, and most employees already have more than enough to do. Yet until QI is incorporated into their roles, the efficiencies and improvements are not likely to be realized. In order to sustain and nurture QI, often early in the QI introduction, leadership will have to free up time for teams to pursue QI work. Later, as the benefits are recognized by employees themselves, this juggling may occur more organically.

SUMMARY

Leadership has an instrumental role to play in the health department implementation of a successful performance improvement system. Primarily, leadership oversight is focused on big QI, the enterprisewide performance management component. Several dimensions of the leadership role were presented. The major caveats are highlighted below:

- Leaders establish the organizational culture of the health department with respect to QI/PM.

  - Engagement of the entire workforce of the health department at all levels is an imperative.

- Selling the concepts of QI to staff need not be arduous; virtually all employees are searching for a way to perform their jobs better.

  - Marketing should be intentional and designed.

  - Personally following QI/PM principles speaks loudly and boldly as a communications tool.

- Leadership sets forth the formal structure of the PM system and defines the elements of engagement (the "what" of QI).

  - Delegated authority is granted to committees, teams, and employees to determine the "how."

  - Regular and frequent follow-up of QI/PM is necessary to keep efforts on track.

- Management and leadership must align QI/PM activities with organizational strategic plans and key priorities.

  - QI processes should focus on health department priorities.

  - Planning products and metrics should mutually reinforce one another.

  - As many measurements as possible (for grants, funders, and targets) should be complementary.

- The workforce should all receive QI training, and an adult learner model is recommended.

- Investments in QI/PM should not wane or recede during public health or budgetary crises if the effect is to be sustained.

Chapter 21

Roles and Responsibilities of Teams

Grace L. Duffy and John W. Moran

INTRODUCTION

Building teams has never been optional. The great heroes, no matter how self-sufficient, have a core of trusted associates around them when times get tough. Red Adair, the famous Texas oil field engineer of the late 1900s, didn't shut down oil rig fires by himself, New York City police and firefighters all pulled together after 9/11, and Warren Buffett, the hero of Wall Street, checks his sources before buying and selling companies.

Leaders are successful because we know how to work with others. Teams come in many different flavors, forever changing based on the goal of the situation. Every day situations happen that draw us together to use our common knowledge and skills for improvement and support. These situations become unifiers of people, uniting us in unique ways. People working together to make improvement within an organization is a concept that has been around for as long as organizations have existed.

Good teams require good leaders who value their employees' opinions, are not threatened by them, and reward workers when appropriate. Good leaders serve as coaches, not commanders. We realize, too, that we all benefit when teams for which we are ultimately responsible accomplish good work. We value our employees' opinions, and facilitate rather than control problem solving and decision making.

Over the last two decades, team members have been given more autonomy within teams as public health organizations and providers struggle to become more effective. The concept of teams has been adapted to the requirements of the not-for-profit and local government structure. Formal teams came into existence in the 1960s with the influence of global work methods. The Japanese concept of *quality circles*, individuals from the same work unit working together to improve their products and output, was very popular in the 1970s. Since then, the idea of groups of employees meeting together to solve problems affecting their functions and service areas has become increasingly common. Team members have been told that their opinions count and that they will be recognized for their good work individually and as part of the team. Successful teams today are effective because individual expectations are met, and not at the expense of the organization or the community.

The department's expectations are met, too, when a team is successful. Local health departments formulate teams for a variety of reasons. Mostly teams are asked to solve problems so an organization can become more effective or efficient. More recently, with the pressure to reduce levels of management, teams have been given further authority and accountability for critical processes within departments. Several other chapters in this handbook reference the benefit of team involvement in problem solving, decision making, Lean Six Sigma projects, data analysis, and other areas critical to serving community needs.

Some of the most dramatic examples of teams improving processes involve simple problems. These are problems that are well understood—and perhaps better understood than by management—by the average employee, the employee closest to the problem. One example is the staff of the Orange County, Florida, Health Department immunology team who banded together to support the front desk clerical workers during heavy client appointment periods. Frontline workers, supervisors, and department specialists all scheduled time at the front desk to provide adequate capacity to answer questions, deliver test results, assist in medical referrals, and cover telephone calls. As a result of this two-week effort, the stress of the assigned clerical personnel performing front desk and other required client support activities was significantly reduced. Workload was rebalanced to better use the skills available within the department for the long term. Turnover in the clerical staff was reduced to zero for the six-month period under study, and morale within the department improved markedly.

This example shows the impact of employees and other team members banding together with a common goal. The situation—whether a crisis or just a good idea—provides an environment for growth. When teams are successful, they improve employee morale and ultimately contribute to a culture that helps keep employees satisfied with their work environment. This positive attitude helps maintain a low turnover rate within the organization because individuals feel they have contributed, added value, and made a difference.

Individually, when people change their attitude at work, their personal lives are affected. Personal relationships developed by the team members in Orange County Health Department have remained strong two years after the project was finalized and process changes integrated into the daily operations of the department.

Building teams means creating the opportunity for people to come together to share concerns, ideas, and experiences, and to begin working together to solve problems and achieve common goals. There are some significant risks we take as leaders when we encourage the use of teams within our department. Involving others in decision making takes time. It is easier in the short term to make choices on our own. Many of us fear the overwhelming wave of opinion and input that comes with supporting a team environment. Some of us are concerned about being confronted with evidence of our own fallibility, or we just don't see teams as worth the time. Many of us have heard stories where instituting teams within the organization caused severe disruption. How do we circumvent these potential pitfalls and support the positive outcomes teams can offer?

MANAGEMENT'S ROLE IN SUSTAINING TEAMS

Teams are essential to the client-driven and process-focused organization. Other chapters in this text address the ongoing need to involve community partners in our efforts for continual improvement. Figure 21.1 contrasts the characteristics of the traditional (stuck) organization with the organization (moving) now required for competitive success. Zenger, et al., in their work of the mid 1990s, *Leading Teams*, talk about the 180-degree change that has occurred in organizations. Organizations have radically altered direction in several ways to address heightened competition and economic pressures.

The stuck organization in Figure 21.1 represents the traditional top-down silo approach to management. When the rate of change was slower, we were able to look inside the organization for stable processes, long-term successful trends, and consistent management practices. Now that the rate of change has escalated, the organization must be constantly "moving" toward bigger, better, and faster ways of meeting community and client expectations. The organization has moved from being internally driven to customer- and community-driven, from functionally focused to process-focused, from management-centered to employee-involved.

Why is this so? Because the global economy has become totally interdependent. One organization can no longer live in its own world without considering the impact of what is going on around us. We are forced to anticipate customer needs, forced to consider the impact of processes that overlap all areas of the supplier-to-company-to-client service chain, forced to consider the valuable input to be gained from employees and partners.

If teams are essential to the new organization, skilled leaders are essential for effective teams. The executive in such an organization has a role that, like a fulcrum, must balance the load and support its weight. Leadership of the team environment is the very core of success. The executive and senior management team can be the life or death of teams in the organization. Critical elements of executive leadership are:

- Special training and skills in team leadership and support to reduce the risk of failure in the eyes of the individual teams and the organization as a whole

The stuck organization	The moving organization
Internally driven	Customer/community driven
Functionally focused	Process focused
Management centered	Employee involved

Figure 21.1   Contrasting the stuck and the moving organization.

Source: J. Zenger, et al. *Leading Teams: Mastering the New Role* (New York: McGraw-Hill, 1994).

- Senior management support, attention, and training for the first-line team leaders

- Increased visibility of executive management in team activities and review meetings

- Clear charters from senior management for the roles, responsibilities, and authority of teams, especially where teams overlap established reporting structures

- Making it explicit to first-line team leaders that their assignments are more than just an additional duty in their daily assignment

Without skilled leadership at all levels, teams can easily flounder, go too far or not far enough, lose confidence, or simply lose sight of the assigned goal. People who contribute to the direction and focus of the department with their ideas and suggestions feel a greater sense of ownership and involvement. Not only is the quality of work better, but also as workers are more committed and involved, employees stay longer and commit at greater levels.

Many line and mid-level managers have been eliminated from organizations as an expense reduction, and yet this segment is an essential link in any improvement process. It is the middle manager that encourages the first line to share the things they learn about the organization, customers, services, costs, community, trends, and anything else that allows them to contribute ideas for improvement. Make it easy for senior and middle managers to contribute to improvement efforts. Acknowledge the contributions of teams in your organization.

H. J. Harrington writes in *Quality Digest* (2002), "top management is essential to getting any improvement process started, but middle management keeps it going. If top managers truly accept their roles as planners and direction-setters, they distance themselves from day-to-day problems facing their departments, which means it is middle managers who actually run their organizations and ensure that they continue to improve."[1]

Leaders must not ignore the valuable transition middle managers serve in the team environment. Top leadership must focus toward the outside client and partners and yet remain supportive of the internal employees who keep the organization going. Executives set the direction; middle managers take that direction and make it happen with the first line.

The executive's role in a team environment is complex. Using the senior and middle management structure to cascade team behaviors from the executive office to the first-line supervisor and line worker enhances this role. Figure 21.2 lists some behaviors suggested by Harrington to maximize the effectiveness of the senior management team.

A key part of any change process is cascading sponsorship. Without a concentrated effort directed at transforming the senior management team, creating the team environment throughout the organization will fail. Employees at all levels of the organization must feel motivated to participate in the team environment. The role of the sponsor is a pivotal one within a team culture.

The team sponsor is the leader who supports a team's plans, activities, and outcomes. Characteristics exhibited by an effective team sponsor may include:

- Developing close working relationships with and understanding of their clients
- Focusing on the big picture and managing it
- Focusing on process rather than actions
- Recognizing continuous improvement as well as meeting targets
- Rejecting requests to make decisions that should be made at lower levels
- Providing role models for first-level managers and employees
- Maintaining honesty
- Sacrificing departmental performance when necessary to improve total organizational performance
- Proactively stimulating upward communication
- Sharing data openly at all levels
- Practicing consensus decision making whenever possible
- Communicating priorities and holding to them
- Establishing networks that identify potential negative trends
- Placing a high priority on problem prevention
- Treating everyone as equally important
- Demonstrating the importance of meeting schedules and getting the job done without compromising quality
- Handling negative situations with a smile more often than with a frown
- Being a good listener

Figure 21.2   Executive behaviors for encouraging middle management team support.
Source: H. J. Harrington, "Creating New Middle Managers," *Quality Digest* (August 2002): 14.

- Believes in the concept/idea
- Possesses sound business acumen
- Is willing to take risk and responsibility for outcomes
- Has authority to approve needed resources
- Is listened to by upper management

A good team sponsor goes out of his or her way to create a motivating environment in which teams can prosper. See Table 21.1 for a list of characteristics exhibited by an effective team sponsor.

A basic principle in relationships is that one person can not motivate another. Motivation comes from within and is a consequence of one's environment. This environment may consist of past experiences, the present situation, competency to do the job, working conditions, degree to which one feels empowered to act on behalf of the department, and so on. Each person has a unique set of needs that, if fulfilled, helps them feel motivated. An effective leader provides an environment in which teams may feel motivated.

Table 21.1 Team participant roles, responsibilities, and performance attributes.

Role name	Responsibility	Definition	Attributes of good role performance
Champion	Advocate	The person initiating a concept or idea for change/improvement	• Dedicated to see it implemented • Absolute belief it is the right thing to do • Perseverance and stamina
Sponsor	Backer, risk taker	The person who supports a team's plans, activities, and outcomes	• Believes in the concept/idea • Sound business acumen • Willing to take risk and responsibility for outcomes • Authority to approve needed resources • Upper management will listen to her or him
Team leader	Change agent, chair, head	One who: • Staffs the team, or provides input for staffing requirements • Strives to bring about change/improvement through the team's outcomes • Followers entrust to lead them • Has the authority for and directs the efforts of the team • Participates as a team member • Coaches team members in developing or enhancing necessary competencies • Communicates with management about the team's progress and needs • Handles the logistics of team meetings • Takes responsibility for team records	• Committed to the team's mission and objectives • Experienced in planning, organizing, staffing, controlling, and directing • Capable of creating and maintaining channels that enable members to do their work • Capable of gaining the respect of team members; a role model • Is firm, fair, and factual in dealing with a team of diverse individuals • Facilitates discussion without dominating • Actively listens • Empowers team members to the extent possible within the organization's culture • Supports all team members equally • Respects each team member's individuality

Continued

Table 21.1   *Continued.*

Role name	Responsibility	Definition	Attributes of good role performance
Facilitator	Helper, trainer, advisor, coach	A person who: • Observes the team's processes and team members' interactions and suggests process changes to facilitate positive movement toward the team's goals and objectives • Intervenes if discussion develops into multiple conversations • Intervenes to skillfully prevent an individual from dominating the discussion, or to engage an overlooked individual in the discussion • Assists team leader in bringing discussions to a close • May provide training in team building, conflict management, and so on	• Trained in facilitating skills • Respected by team members • Tactful • Knows when and when not to intervene • Deals with the team's process, not content • Respects the team leader and does not override his or her responsibility • Respects confidential information shared by individuals or the team as a whole • Will not accept facilitator role if expected to report to management information that is proprietary to the team • Will abide by the ASQ Code of Ethics
Timekeeper	Gatekeeper, monitor	A person designated by the team to watch the use of allocated time and remind the team when their time objective may be in jeopardy	• Capable of assisting the team leader in keeping the team meeting within the predetermined time limitations • Sufficiently assertive to intervene in discussions when the time allocation is in jeopardy • Capable of participating as a member while still serving as a timekeeper

Continued

Table 21.1   *Continued.*

Role name	Responsibility	Definition	Attributes of good role performance
Scribe	Recorder, note taker	A person designated by the team to record critical data from team meetings. Formal minutes of the meetings may be published to interested parties.	• Capable of capturing on paper, or electronically, the main points and decisions made in a team meeting, and providing a complete, accurate, and legible document (or formal minutes) for the team's records • Sufficiently assertive to intervene in discussions to clarify a point or decision in order to record it accurately • Capable of participating as a member while still serving as a scribe
Team members	Participants, subject matter experts	The persons selected to work together to bring about a change/improvement, achieving this in a created environment of mutual respect, sharing of expertise, cooperation, and support	• Willing to commit to the purpose of the team • Able to express ideas, opinions, suggestions in a nonthreatening manner • Capable of listening attentively to other team members • Receptive to new ideas and suggestions • Even-tempered, able to handle stress and cope with problems openly • Competent in one or more fields of expertise needed by the team • Favorable performance record • Willing to function as a team member and forfeit "star" status

To do this, Russell Westcott, coauthor of *The Quality Improvement Handbook*, suggests using the six R's:

1. *Reinforce.* Identify and positively reinforce work done well.

2. *Request.* Information. Discuss team members' views. Is anything preventing expected performance?

3. *Resources.* Identify needed resources the lack of which could impede effective performance.

4. *Responsibility.* Clients make paydays possible; all employees have a responsibility to the client, internal and external.

5. *Role.* Be a role model. Don't just tell; demonstrate how to do it. Observe the team's performance. Together, critique the approach and work out an improved method.

6. *Repeat.* Apply the above principles regularly and repetitively.[2]

It is not just senior leadership who sets the stage for a motivating environment. One of the major roles of all team members is the perpetuation of a positive and future-focused organization. The development of a team culture creates the climate in which motivation can grow. Since those within the organization always notice the senior management team, their behaviors are critical to the establishment of effective team behaviors throughout the company. In a truly effective team environment, all team players exhibit behaviors that reinforce positive team outcomes. Figure 21.3 identifies a number of techniques that have proven to be effective team motivators.

- Catch team members doing something right and positively reinforce the good behavior in that specific situation.

- Use mistakes as learning opportunities.

- Reward team leaders and members who take risks in changing, even if they sometimes fail.

- When discussing situations, listen closely to the team leader or member. Respect their opinion, even if it must be modified.

- Acknowledge the team's reason for action, but don't agree to it if it's inappropriate.

- When giving performance feedback, reveal reactions after describing the behavior needing change, not before it.

- Encourage members to make suggestions for improving. Always give credit to the team or member making the suggestion.

- Treat teams with even more care than other business assets.

Figure 21.3 Techniques for effective team motivation.

TEAMS COME IN DIFFERENT FORMS

A team is a group of individuals organized to work together to accomplish a specific objective. An organizational work group may not necessarily function as a team. However, a team may comprise members of a work group. When a group comes together in a synergistic whole to accomplish a common goal, those individuals become a team.

A team cares about achieving common goals. Teams are formed with the understanding that improvement can be achieved using the skills, talents, and knowledge of appropriate individuals.

There are a number of different roles required in the effective deployment of teams in the workplace. Table 21.1 describes the major roles including team champion, sponsor, leader, facilitator, and member. Other roles such as scribe and timekeeper may be rotated between team members to allow for individual growth opportunities. Many organizations also rotate the responsibilities of team leader and facilitator, providing critical training and reinforcement to the team members before assigning accountability for those roles.

Teams are used in many different organizational situations. As workers become more skilled in their activities and decision-making abilities, additional responsibility is added to their assignments. Work teams may have close supervision from first-line management where self-directed or cross-functional teams may be given a high level of autonomy and accountability for critical outcomes within the department.

Several different types of teams are described below.

Departmental or Work Team

A departmental team is composed of persons having responsibility for a specific process or function and who work together in a participative environment. The departmental team is a permanent group generally reporting to a single, common management. Employees as a group assume added responsibility for solving problems and making improvements within their own department or function. The team leader is generally the one responsible for the function or process performed within the work area.

Improvement Team

Process improvement teams (PITs) focus on creating or improving a specific business process. A PIT may attempt to completely reengineer a process or work on incremental improvements. If addressing a major improvement, the team is usually cross-functional, with representatives from a number of different functions. Managers often assign a problem to a temporary group of employees selected for specific skills or characteristics related to the issue or improvement.

Cross-Functional Team

People from different functions or departments meet regularly to address mutual problems or issues, hence the term "cross-functional." Process improvement teams will often become cross-functional if the objective of the PIT is to effect a major improvement or change.

In some organizations, cross-functional teams carry out all or nearly all of the functions of the organization. In such cases the organization resembles a matrix- or project-type organization. Organizations, in attempting to eliminate internal competition among functional groups, have adopted cross-functional teams for many areas, for example, administrative support, information systems, and facilities management.

The smaller the organization, the more employees are required to work together, often backing each other up as needs arise. Each employee develops a set of overlapping skills in several technical areas. In recent times larger organizations have come to recognize the value of such smaller, cross-functional teams. These flexible teams can move more quickly than larger groups by reconfiguring themselves to meet changing needs.

Project Team

A project team is formed to achieve a specific mission. The project team's objective may be to create something new, for example, a new product or service, or to accomplish a complex task such as upgrading the client profile database.

Typically, a project team employs full-time members on temporary assignment for the duration of the project. The project team operates in parallel with the primary department functions. The project team may or may not be cross-functional in member composition depending on its objectives and competency needs. Often the project leader may be the person to whom the ultimate responsibility for managing the resulting project outcome is assigned.

Self-Managed Team

A self-managed team is an intact work group that handles most daily operational issues with minimal supervision. Often called high-performance work teams, these teams offer employees broader accountability and process ownership. The members often select their own team leaders.

Because of the level of empowerment afforded, careful planning and training is key to a successful self-managed team. Self-managed teams must be enabled first or they are simply leaderless groups of individuals. Initiating self-managed teams is easiest in a new function with little established history. Transforming a traditional work culture to self-management is a difficult process and may be quite disruptive to the organization.

Virtual Team

Virtual teams are groups of two or more persons often affiliated with a common organization or a common purpose. Team members may not be from the same company or organization. The virtual team either partly or entirely conducts their work via electronic communication. Virtual teams may or may not be cross-functional in skills or reporting structure. These teams may or may not be self-managed. Typically, the virtual team is geographically dispersed.

ESSENTIAL CHARACTERISTICS OF ALL TEAMS

No matter what form teams take, there are common characteristics of all successful teams. The organization must focus on integrating these characteristics into the work environment *before* implementing the team concept. Much is written about these components of effective team-building, so only the basics will be identified here.

John Zenger[3] includes the following as some crucial characteristics for members when first initiating a team environment:

- Common goals
- Leadership
- Involvement
- Self-esteem
- Open communication
- Power to make decisions
- Planning
- Trust
- Respect for others
- Conflict resolution

These characteristics are major contributors to high employee morale. They also positively influence customer satisfaction, whether internal or external. The same skills leaders are required to use work well at all levels of the organization. Figure 21.4 summarizes many of the characteristics and elements of dynamic and successful teams.

LEADING TO GET THE WORK DONE

A team can not function effectively unless the members individually function well. The performance of each person acts as a catalyst to the others. It goes back to the cliché about the whole being more than the sum of its parts. Synergy is critical in realizing the benefits of a team environment.

Effective teamwork supports three of the most important motivating factors in the workplace. For most people to feel involved in their jobs they must be:

- Excited about the work
- Fully committed to the work outcomes
- Qualified to do the work

Good leadership generates happy and productive people. Leaders are the lifeblood of the attitude within an organization. How the workforce sees the leadership behaving sets the stage for what happens throughout the organization.

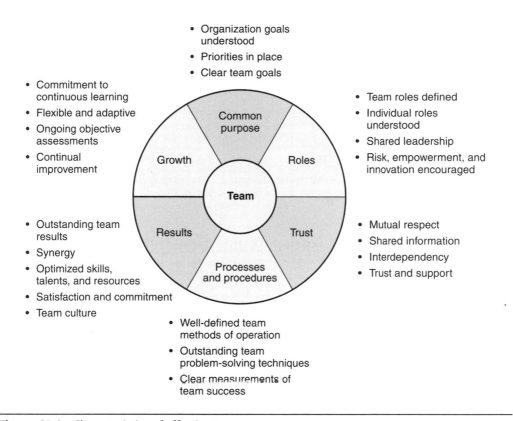

- Organization goals understood
- Priorities in place
- Clear team goals

- Commitment to continuous learning
- Flexible and adaptive
- Ongoing objective assessments
- Continual improvement

- Team roles defined
- Individual roles understood
- Shared leadership
- Risk, empowerment, and innovation encouraged

- Outstanding team results
- Synergy
- Optimized skills, talents, and resources
- Satisfaction and commitment
- Team culture

- Mutual respect
- Shared information
- Interdependency
- Trust and support

- Well-defined team methods of operation
- Outstanding team problem-solving techniques
- Clear measurements of team success

Figure 21.4   Characteristics of effective teams.

As leaders, we focus on two main areas: tasks and people. The more we provide an environment in which our people can excel, the less effort we, as leaders, need to personally put into the tasks. Create good people, get them working together with the right direction, resources, and authority, and the tasks will get done in a way that delights the client and other important partners.

The best approach leaders can take is to:

1. Reassure

2. Challenge

3. Empathize

4. Inform

5. Explain

6. Direct

7. Guide

8. Delegate

Supporting an effective team environment requires all of the above approaches. For people to work comfortably in teams we must answer yes to each of these three questions:

1. Do the employees really want to be here?

2. Is the objective something worth doing?

3. Does the employee really want to do this task?

If the answer to these three questions is yes, then we can safely start expending resources to provide support, training, leadership, and recognition to the teams and feel confident that improvement and change will be the result of their efforts.

MAXIMIZING TEAMS DURING IMPROVEMENT AND CHANGE

Maintaining a strong team environment is difficult in quiet times. It becomes a full-time job during times of revolutionary improvement and change. The senior leader becomes the ultimate coach. Change reduces productivity, which affects profitability. Teams become distracted by surrounding pressures and lose focus. Some get angry, some try to grab power, some simply retreat into their own shells. Everyone looks to the top to "fix" the discomfort. Even the people who are excited about change and are willing to help don't always agree on the next plan of action.

Trust becomes critical when change escalates. Just when the industry wants innovation, the human response is to entrench into what we already know. Many of us fear the unknown. Trust is best built by letting individuals know "what is ahead" whenever possible.

Conventional team-building techniques may not even be enough. Powerful, energizing leadership is required to help handle the increased pressure of change. The best time for growing trust is when people are being tested or challenged. Only then do we get a chance to really prove anything. Will we keep our word? Are we consistent in our behavior? Are we fair in implementing policies and recognition? Are we visible and involved when the teams need us? Will we put ourselves at risk for the sake of the teams and the company?

Teamwork always carries an element of risk, even in the best of circumstances. If teams do not trust their leadership, the risk factor climbs so high it becomes a barrier to cooperative effort. Individuals start looking out for themselves at the team's expense, doubting that the group will adequately protect them.

The actions of senior leadership can either encourage or destroy the trust required for an effective team environment. We must not become careless with small actions. Take every chance to create a climate of trust. Actions such as sharing information, following through on commitments, keeping people informed, and helping teams see how their actions directly support bottom-line results will encourage a climate of trust.

Some major "trust busters" have been identified by Jeff Dorman & Associates.[4] See Table 21.2 for a summary of their suggested indicators of potential team destroyers and corrective approaches.

Table 21.2 Trust busters and team destroyers.

Indicator	Symptom	Corrective approach
Purpose of the team is no longer linked to strategic goals of the organization.	The team is excluded from corporate planning. It may not understand its role within the greater organization.	Keep team informed of changes in strategic goals. Involve teams in deploying organizational changes and improvements.
Management commitment and personal involvement have slipped.	Team leadership is unable or unwilling to use a team approach and does not encourage the use of team-building activities. He or she often uses a "command" decision style rather than a "consensus" decision style. The leader does not share his or her power or leadership responsibilities.	Leadership training for all team leaders and supporting managers. Provide strong executive support to those leaders who exhibit team behaviors and reward the same in their employees.
The team is facing a hostile or indifferent environment.	The team's climate discourages members from feeling comfortable, from being direct and open, and from taking risks.	Establish and maintain a strong climate of trust in the company. Reward trusting behavior at all levels of leadership.
Assigned members lack needed knowledge, skills, experience, or attitude.	Team members are not qualified, professionally or socially, to contribute to the team and thus do not help it to achieve its goals. Team members do not have the specific skills sufficient to meet their assigned task responsibilities.	Initiate or expand a systematic process of skills analysis, training, and development in technical and communication skills for teams and their leaders.
Team coaching is not available or is inadequate for the new tasks.	In order not to upset team members, neither group nor individual errors or weaknesses are addressed directly enough so they are eliminated.	Train team leaders and managers in addressing and correcting issues on a timely basis. Support their efforts.
Team leadership is inadequate to help the team meet objectives.	The team may not understand its objectives, and if it does, it may not believe they are worthwhile. It may set targets that are either uninspiring or unreachable. Team members' performance may be reviewed only infrequently.	Work with senior leadership to establish clear charters for team objectives. Establish review processes to keep targets and progress in view of all involved parties.
Team building is nonexistent or inadequate.	Teams that are required to work together compete rather than collaborate. Because teams do not meet to compare agendas, their priorities may conflict.	Establish and maintain a cycle of communication and team reviews. Train all teams and leaders on meeting skills.

Continued

Table 21.2   *Continued.*

Indicator	Symptom	Corrective approach
The team process is ignored or improperly managed.	Problems that are faced by the team are not solved effectively and efficiently.	Hold team leaders and facilitators accountable for addressing team problems.
Members are not behaving as a team.	Team members are not committed to the aims and purposes of the team and are reluctant to expend personal energy on meeting the team's goals.	Look for barriers to team commitment. Use senior management to reinforce and recognize good team behavior.
Team members are unsure of what's expected of them.	Team members' roles are not clearly defined, efficient communication procedures have not been developed, and administrative procedures are not supportive of the team's efforts.	Train and implement team facilitators to help teams define roles and responsibilities. Take personal interest in the roles of individual team members.
Recognition and reward for work done well is nonexistent or inappropriate.	Team members do not generate new ideas, perhaps because risk taking is not encouraged and rewarded by the organizational climate.	Restructure the organization's reward and recognition system to support the new, more effective team environment.

USING CONFLICT TO STRENGTHEN TEAMS

Conflict is a recognized stage in the team development process. Scholtes, Joiner, and Streibel describe the four phases of team development (forming, storming, norming, and performing) in *The Team Handbook*.[5] Since conflict will happen during most change processes, we might as well benefit from it.

Conflict between team members can occur at any of the stages, but is more likely to surface during the *forming* and *storming* stages. Conflict is common and useful. It is a sign of change and movement. Conflict is neither good nor bad. The effort should not be to eliminate conflict but to refocus it as a productive rather than destructive force. Conflict can be a vital, energizing force at work in any team. When conflict occurs within or between teams, do not ignore it. Address the conflict, use it to find the friction that change has created within the team, and use problem-solving techniques to resolve and improve the situation. See Chapter 14, "Basic Tools of Quality Improvement" and Chapter 15, "Advanced Tools of Quality Improvement," for more on problem solving and team decision-making tools.

Leaders, with guidance from a facilitator if needed, can help transform a conflict into a problem-solving event by:

- Welcoming differences between teams and team members

- Listening attentively with understanding rather than judgment

- Helping to clarify common goals among the conflicting parties

- Acknowledging and accepting the feelings of the individuals involved

- Offering support to the parties in resolving the differences

- Reinforcing the value of each of the parties to the organization as a whole

- Creating appropriate means for communication between those involved in the conflict

SUMMARY

Nurturing a team environment is one of the major success factors of any growing organization. Just as the entrepreneur must reach out to partners as his or her business expands, so leaders in larger organizations must develop a climate of trust within the whole team to maintain competitive results.

The benefit of teamwork is available at any level within the organization. The executive team is one of the most visible, while teams at the line-worker level may provide the best return on investment. The techniques for initiating, maintaining, and rewarding teams are pretty much the same at all levels. Choose the right people, train and mission them appropriately, support and recognize them. Certainly this is easier said than done. The value of the effort is well worth it, however. No one can lead a large and complex organization alone. We need each other to succeed in this environment of rapid change and improvement.

Chapter 22

The Reality of Teams in Resource-Constrained Public Health

William Riley, PhD, and Helen Parsons, MPH

The purpose of this chapter is to review how to build and sustain quality improvement (QI) teams in public health departments, where resources are often constrained. The role of leadership will also be addressed because it is a key factor in whether QI teams successfully complete their aims. The three sections of this chapter begin with an overview of teams and team characteristics. The second section discusses implications and suggestions for how to build successful QI teams in public health departments while the third section focuses specifically on QI teams in public health.

TEAMS

Teams exist everywhere in the healthcare sector. In public health, teams are used for virtually every activity carried out in health departments, including community, clinical, and management-focused activities. While the science of public health is expanding rapidly, the application of that knowledge to public health practice is limited by the effectiveness and efficiency of teams charged with putting that knowledge into practice. As new management techniques and technologies are developed, especially quality improvement methods, public health teams must be appropriately trained to successfully implement these new approaches.

A *team* is defined as two or more persons who interact interdependently and adaptively toward a common goal and have each been assigned specific roles or functions to perform.[1] A QI team is defined as a group of individuals who work together to deliver services for which they are mutually accountable.[2] Although a remarkable amount of research has been conducted to determine how teams function, it has been difficult to clearly define exactly what teamwork is.[3] Teams have the potential to offer more adaptability, productivity, and creativity than any one individual can offer,[4] yet their failures can have equally deleterious effects, including missed deadlines and low productivity.[5]

A QI team has special features that differentiate it from typical work teams. A work team usually resides within one department, often consists of members of the same discipline, involves ongoing functions of the organization, and is formal in that it appears on an organizational chart. A QI team, on the other hand,

Table 22.1   Comparison of work teams versus quality improvement teams.

Work team	Quality improvement team
• Within one department	• Cross-departmental
• Focused on one discipline	• Interdisciplinary
• Ongoing	• Single purpose
• Formal association	• Informal

is typically cross-departmental, interdisciplinary, serves a single purpose, and is more informal in nature.

Table 22.1 compares the distinctive features of a work team and QI team. It is helpful to keep these characteristics in mind when a public health manager decides to create a team for improvement.

Deming's 14 Points

W. Edwards Deming, one of the creators of QI methods, developed numerous concepts for how to create and sustain quality improvement teams. These concepts have been proven effective in private industry and have relevant applications to public health. Deming's 14 points, which characterize successful quality improvement teams, are as follows:[6]

1. *Create a constancy of purpose for improvement of services and outcomes.* Deming suggests a radical new definition of an organization's role. It will only achieve its mission through innovation and constant improvement.

2. *Adopt a new philosophy.* Americans are too tolerant of poor service. Deming advocates a new approach in which mistakes and negativism are unacceptable.

3. *Cease dependence on inspection.* In manufacturing, American firms typically inspect a product as it comes off the production line. Defective products are then reworked. In effect, a company is paying workers to make defects and then to correct them. Quality comes not from inspection but from improvement of the process.

4. *End the practice of awarding business on price tag alone.* Purchasing departments customarily operate on orders to seek the lowest-priced vendor. Frequently, this leads to supplies of low quality. Instead, they should seek the best quality and work to achieve it for any one item with a single supplier in a long-term relationship.

5. *Improve constantly and forever the system of production and service.* Improvement is not a one-time effort. Management is obligated to continually look for ways to reduce waste and improve quality.

6. *Institute training.* Too often workers have learned their job from another worker who was never trained properly. Initial orientation and ongoing training of public health team members is important to break this cycle.

7. *Institute leadership.* The job of a supervisor is not to tell people what to do or to punish them but to lead. Leading consists of helping people do a better job.

8. *Drive out fear.* Many employees are afraid to ask questions or to take a position, even when they do not understand what the job is or what is right or wrong. The economic loss from fear is high, and staff must feel secure to achieve better quality and productivity.

9. *Break down barriers between staff areas.* Departments are often competing with each other or have goals that conflict. They do not work as a team so they can not solve or foresee problems. Worse, one department's goals may cause trouble for another.

10. *Eliminate slogans, exhortations, and targets for the workforce.* These never helped anybody do a good job. Let people put up their own slogans.

11. *Eliminate numerical quotas.* Quotas take account only of numbers, not quality or methods. They are usually a guarantee of inefficiency and high cost.

12. *Remove barriers to pride of workmanship.* People are eager to do a good job and distressed when they can not. Too often, misguided supervisors, faulty equipment, and defective materials stand in the way.

13. *Institute a vigorous program of education and retraining.* Both management and the workforce will have to be educated in the new methods, including teamwork and statistical techniques.

14. *Take action to accomplish the transformation.* It will take a special top management team with a plan of action to carry out the quality mission. Workers can not do it on their own, nor can managers.

Each of these points should be taken into consideration as public health departments start the process of developing QI teams within their organizations.

Stages of Team Development

Teams go through predictable stages of development, from their initial constitution until they perform effectively. Table 22.2 identifies the four stages that teams typically experience: *forming, storming, norming,* and *performing.*[7] A description of these four stages and how they apply to QI projects follows. While not all teams go through these stages, the table provides a helpful model to understand how a QI team in public health progresses over time.

Table 22.2   Stages of team development.

Stage	Description
Forming	Team members may have ambiguity and confusion when initially brought together for the purpose of the QI project.
Storming	There may be conflict between team members involving disagreement over what to accomplish, how to accomplish it, lack of progress, or domineering behavior.
Norming	Open communication is established between team members and the team starts to confront the task at hand.
Performing	The team works productively and effectively on achieving the QI project.

Forming. When a team is forming, members cautiously explore the boundaries of acceptable group behavior. A team leader can help build trust during this stage by providing clear direction and purpose for the project, involving members in developing plans, and establishing ways to work together. QI teams often select their roles—facilitators, recorders, and timekeepers—as an initial step for establishing effective working relationships.

Storming. Storming is often the most difficult stage for a team. During this stage, team members may argue, become defensive, create factions, or try to establish dominance. All these behaviors can create increased tensions and stress among team members. In order for leaders to overcome the storming stage, they must develop and implement agreements about how decisions are made and who makes them.

Norming. During this stage, the initial resistance fades and team members get used to working together. This happens because team members grow to accept each other and establish ground rules (norming) for their roles. Conflict tends to reduce as relationships become more cooperative and less competitive, resulting in a greater sense of team cohesion.

It is important for a leader to bring the team into the norming stage; otherwise the team members will remain inert in the storming stage. As teams resolve differences, there is more time and energy to devote to work.

Performing. In this last stage, the team members have settled their disputes and become more comfortable with each other. They better understand the work and what is expected of them. The team becomes effective and productive.

Many QI tools and techniques have been developed to assist teams as they progress through these four stages of development. A QI team can become stalled in a stage of group formation and unable to achieve the performing stage. To prevent this from occurring, and to facilitate a team moving to performance, it is important for a public health leader to understand the stages of group formation and help teams move through these stages expeditiously.

CREATING SUCCESSFUL QUALITY IMPROVEMENT TEAMS IN PUBLIC HEALTH DEPARTMENTS

Effective team performance is necessary to successfully design and implement quality improvement (QI) projects in public health departments. QI projects always require teams of people to identify a process to improve, study the process, conduct tests of change, and implement a new process. Distinguishing factors between teams that effectively conduct a QI project and teams that fail are the level of team skills and effectiveness of the team leadership. QI projects often do not achieve the intended goal because they fail to adopt basic team skills. The following discussion will identify and discuss best practices to help QI teams in public health departments succeed in each of the four stages of team development.

Recommendations for the Forming Stage

In the forming stage, it is important for a QI team to have leadership support from all management levels in the public health department, and that the appropriate individuals are selected to participate on the team.

Five factors have been identified that explain how teams are critical to success in quality improvement initiatives.[8] These factors should be considered in a public health department when a team enters the forming stage.

1. *Visualizing process problem.* Quality problems are often not visible to individuals at senior management levels, but the impact of these problems can be experienced by the entire organization. It is the individuals doing the work who are most aware of problems that have become systemic in nature and that require systemic solutions. The farther one is from the front line of care, the more removed one is from seeing day-to-day problems. Thus, if we wish to identify quality problems, we need individuals on our teams who are close to the problem and understand its manifestations and nuances.

2. *Frontline staff.* Frontline public health staff are usually those who are most knowledgeable about the process and its context. To understand a process, it is essential to have team participation from individuals who have the best, most detailed understanding of the process.

3. *Improvement ideas.* Individuals at the front lines often have the most feasible suggestions for improvement. Not only do the frontline staff understand the process best, they are also the most valuable source of improvement ideas.

4. *Support from all levels.* Addressing quality problems requires the support of all individuals in the organization, not simply those at senior level. Identifying and proposing solutions to quality problems is key to quality improvement efforts, but unless those involved in solution implementation understand fully the rationale for the effort, implementation is likely to fall short.

5. *Empowerment.* High-functioning teams empower people by providing opportunities for meaningful participation in problem identification and problem solving.

These five factors help a team in the forming stage because they clarify team membership and purpose. They also ensure that those individuals who are most familiar with the process are included in the analyzing and improvement of that process.

Recommendations for the Storming Stage

As teams progress through the forming stage, it is inevitable that members will encounter some resistance to change, have conflicting views with other team members, or not agree on a course of action. A number of QI methods and techniques have been developed to help teams move through this storming stage. During storming, public health QI teams can become stalled and fail to progress to the norming stage. The following five factors can help teams to overcome this phase of team development:

1. *Brainstorming.* Brainstorming is the method for a team to creatively generate a high volume of ideas by creating a process that is free of criticism and judgment.[9] Using this method, teams can open new ways of thinking when a team is stuck.

2. *Nominal group process.* The nominal group process allows the team to participate equally in a process and prevents one person from dominating a discussion or imposing a point of view. This technique is performed by generating a list of issues, problems, or solutions to be prioritized and allowing each person on the team to rank these issues by priorities.[10]

3. *Develop a team charter.* A team charter is useful in referring the group to ground rules for acceptable and unacceptable individual and team behavior as well as how decisions will be made (consensus or majority rule).

4. *Assigning and rotating roles.* At least three roles should be selected and designated for each work session: facilitator, timekeeper, and record keeper. These three roles should be rotated within the team in order to maintain a sense of fairness within the group.

5. *Team etiquette.* Create ground rules for team etiquette. Such ground rules are not necessary in every QI team, but can be useful if difficult conversations are anticipated. Such ground rules include the following: a) raise your hand and be recognized by the facilitator before speaking, b) be brief and to the point, c) make your point calmly, d) avoid personal agendas, and e) listen respectfully.

Recommendations for the Norming Stage

In the norming stage, QI teams in public health departments have established, accepted ground rules and working relationships that create a sense of team cohesion and reduce tension. Five factors that help effective QI teams in public health departments progress from the norming stage to the performing stage include:

1. *Continued leadership support.* Most QI teams consist of frontline staff and mid-level managers. When such teams conduct a project, they need top leadership support and interest from the beginning of the project, through implementation of the recommendations, until completion. Without this continued leadership support and commitment, the project can lose momentum and there is a much higher chance that project drift will occur.

2. *Training in QI methods and techniques.* This is a workforce capacity issue. Extensive training of QI teams is not a prerequisite to successful projects. While teams need to have people with the necessary knowledge and skills to facilitate the QI project, this can be accomplished in a variety of ways including the "training the trainers" approach, videoconferencing, collaboration with other health departments, or drawing on resources from state health departments and public health professional associations such as the National Association of County and City Health Officials (NACCHO), the Public Health Foundation (PHF), and Turning Point.

3. *Interdepartmental teams.* All QI teams endeavor to improve on organizational processes, and most processes in public health are interdepartmental, which means they involve more than one department.

4. *Availability of resources for QI teams.* An effective QI team in a public health department needs time to conduct the improvement and technical assistance to guide the team. Neither of these resources (time and technical assistance) should be barriers to a public health department. Studies have shown that QI teams can successfully perform with limited financial and technical assistance as long as they are given sufficient time to perform their tasks.[11]

5. *Identify a repetitive process.* QI teams often fail to achieve successful results because a problem has been identified that may not be appropriate for the method. QI techniques are more suitable for activities that are repetitive in nature such as registration, scheduling, reporting, producing, monitoring, and surveillance. Repetitive activities lend themselves more easily to identifying a clear beginning, process steps, and ending.

Recommendations for the Performing Stage

It is necessary for a team to enter the performing stage in order to successfully complete a QI project in a public health department. There is no set time frame for how long is required for a team to pass through the first three stages of group development. While a group typically progresses through these three stages, the quicker it happens, the faster the team gets to the performing stage, and the greater the likelihood that the team will successfully achieve its aim. If a team takes a long period of time to go through the first three stages or relapses from the performing stage back to an earlier stage, the probability of failure is higher. The following recommendations are useful to ensure that teams to not revert back to the previous stages:

1. Use collaboratives to partner in getting technical assistance training.

2. Create multi-county partnerships to support a quality improvement department.

3. Leadership commitment and support are needed at all levels to ensure success. It is not an efficient use of resources for a quality improvement project to not achieve its aim, have competing priorities, or show poor alignment of agency priorities with community needs.

4. Build internal workforce capacity.

5. Make quality improvement a part of everyday work. Quality improvement must be continuous and integrated into everyday operations, not just an add-on.

Once the performing stage has been achieved, teams are in a position to efficiently and effectively address specific areas of quality improvement within their organization.

Discussion

How can QI be implemented successfully in public health departments where resource constraints are a fact of life? Public health departments are adept at networking to achieve population improvement goals, and QI methods and techniques help to maximize efficiency and effectiveness. The ordinary QI team is a complicated creature where members must work out personal differences and find strengths on which to build.[12] Resolving the team pressure is as important as improving processes.

QI AND TEAMS IN PUBLIC HEALTH

Public health professionals are particularly adept at applying new QI methods and techniques to public health processes because of the strong emphasis on team functioning and extensive use of team facilitation skills. Several QI methods and techniques are used to help generate group consensus, which is the very essence of public health. QI teams are the primary vehicle through which problems are analyzed, solutions are generated, and change is evaluated.[13] Teams are used for most activities carried out in public health departments, and as quality improvement methods are introduced into agencies, successful use of these approaches is dependent on appropriately staffed, well-functioning teams.

Using the science of improvement in public health departments can help teams to achieve optimal efficiency and effectiveness by creating value and minimizing waste in the delivery of public health services. QI helps teams to understand how processes work, and to redesign processes to work more efficiently. Major types of waste can be identified and eliminated including rework, bottlenecks, waiting, redundancy, poor focus, and work unrelated to the health department mission.

Perhaps the best example of QI is found in the Toyota Production System, which has been described succinctly by several authors.[14] With four basic assumptions that underlie its success,[15] Toyota has integrated teamwork and QI into making it one of the most successful organizations in the world:

1. The organization is guided by a long-term philosophy

2. The right process will produce the right results

3. Value is added by developing personnel and partners

4. Use continuous improvement to drive organizational learning

Public health departments are ideally suited to adapt these four assumptions in order to achieve teamwork and continuous improvement usually resulting in better outcomes. Table 22.3 shows examples of how these four assumptions can be incorporated into public health departments with minimal effort or resources.

Effective quality improvement teams engage in "double loop learning,"[16] which is learning about how to continually improve operations coupled with learning about learning. For example, in a large public health learning collaborative supported by the Robert Wood Johnson Foundation, 33 local health departments and one tribal government in Minnesota participated in training, design, and implementation of QI projects where they learned about quality improvement by conducting a quality improvement project.[17] This approach to learning reflects a basic practice for healthcare leaders to link operations and learning at the site where work is done.[18]

Leading Teams in Resource-Constrained Health Departments

Leadership is an essential feature for QI teams in public health. In a study of 20 high-performing microsystems in various healthcare settings, it was found that leadership at all levels of the organization was necessary to successfully implement QI initiatives. This improvement revolved around three fundamental processes:[19] 1) building knowledge (learning), 2) taking action (doing), and 3) reviewing

Table 22.3   Application of Toyota's four assumptions for teamwork in public health departments.

Assumptions	Examples in public health
Guided by long-term philosophy	Healthy People 2010, mobilizing
The right process will produce the right results	Redesigning the process for WIC clinic appointment scheduling
Add value to the organization by developing people and partners	Workplace capacity assessment, networking for smoking cessation campaign
Organizational learning driven by continuous improvement	Participating in QI collaboratives and preparing for public health accreditation

(reflecting). Effective leaders in public health realize that they need to continually learn to gain understanding of that which they wish to change. Effective leaders also seek to engage every person at the level and place of his or her own work in doing his or her own work and improving outcomes.[20]

An important distinction has been made between team performance (the outcomes of team's actions) and team effectiveness (how the team interacts).[21] Management for better results in public health departments can be reliably obtained only through fundamental improvement by the leaders. Public health leaders become the champions of improving population health, the ultimate driver of all public health activities.

A management framework for understanding quality is very applicable in public health departments.[22] This quality triangle consists of three components (shown in Figure 22.1):

1. *Quality.* This is the understanding that quality improvement is defined by the mission of public health, which is to achieve a healthy population. This mission and commitment are a focus of every member of the public health department, pursued every day.

2. *Scientific approach.* Interventions and quality improvement projects are based on evidence and the best science available.

3. *All one team.* Believing in people, treating everyone (staff, clients, partners, and stakeholders) with dignity, trust, and respect.

The model is simple and can be easily reproduced on a flip chart. When faced with a difficult problem, teams can work their way around the triangle looking for a critical point that may be forgotten. Using this triangle also reinforces the notion that the elements are interdependent. Taken separately, they are not as powerful as when used together.[23]

This public health quality triangle has several implications. First, quality and productivity are two sides of the same coin, not opposing forces. There is concern experienced in public health departments that quality improvement is one more task to perform in schedules that are already overloaded, and will reduce productivity. This viewpoint is largely invalid. In countless settings, applications of quality improvement methods and techniques have been shown to improve outcomes, decrease costs, and heighten staff empowerment. While staff training and organizational learning are needed in the early stages of introducing quality improvement methods into an organization, the returns on the investment are substantial.

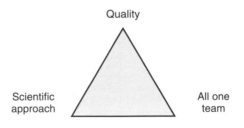

Figure 22.1   Public health quality triangle.

Moving Forward

Most public health professionals are trained in their own discipline, with little knowledge of process design or improvement. In fact, many health professionals are process illiterate.[24] Deming makes an important distinction between "professional knowledge" (for example, the science and art of public health) and "profound knowledge" (the science and art of process improvement),[25] which helps explain how to integrate QI into public health department teams. These skills can be acquired and applied by public health departments as a way to continually improve the performance necessary for achieving increased population health status. Implementing QI teams in public health departments is a proven method from other industries to analyze current processes and identify improvement that could lead to better efficiencies and waste reduction. Keeping all of these concepts in mind in the development of a QI project in local public health will ensure that the team is setting itself up for success.

Chapter 23

Using Influence to Get Things Done

Barbara Volz, MEd, MPH, CCPS

Teamwork is the ability to work as a group toward a common vision, even if that vision becomes extremely blurry.

—Author unknown

WHAT IS INFLUENCE?

Any discussion of using influence to get things done must first begin with an understanding of what influence is. Influence. Leadership. Power. People tend to use these terms interchangeably, without giving thought to their meanings. So what *do* they mean and how does one know if one has any of them? Merriam-Webster defines "influence" as *the power to direct the thinking or behavior of other people,* usually indirectly. Robert Kreitner and Angelo Kinicki describe "power" as a *"social influence process in which the leader seeks the voluntary participation of others in an effort to reach goals."* According to Dwight Eisenhower, *"Leadership is the art of getting someone else to do something you want done because he wants to do it."*

Plainly, as Mintzberg says, power and influence are interchangeable forms, and drawing distinctions between the two adds little to gaining an understanding of them. Influence is the power to change people's behavior; power is the ability to influence people's behavior. Whichever term one uses, whether one says one is leading people or influencing them, it is clear that people's behavior is being guided. And leadership can be seen to be the use of power or influence to accomplish a goal.

ORGANIZATIONAL STRUCTURE

Every organization has a structure to which it adheres. Within the organization there is a formal power structure based on legitimate power, which is the power of position within the organization. People higher in the structure make decisions affecting the behavior of people lower in the structure. Typically, when we talk about power within an organization we are talking about this power of position: the hierarchy that makes the formal decisions in every organization's life. But in addition to the formal power structure there is also an informal power structure. Sometimes it is based on tenure; sometimes it is based on expertise, or on personality. But in every organization there are people who can affect the actions of others because of who they are, not because of their position in the hierarchy.

Every organization has both types of power structures, and in order to make changes effectively within an organization both power structures must be taken into account. Nothing can be accomplished working outside of either system, and in fact both systems need to be used to make permanent, effective change.

The fastest way to lose credibility and influence is to ignore or, worse yet, try to circumvent the formal power structure. The very first rule of getting things done is never to do anything without your boss's knowledge and permission. On the other hand, it can be catastrophic to overlook the informal power structure. The legitimate influence structure is obvious: everyone answers to a supervisor; every employee is constrained by the organization's rules and by their supervisor's decisions. But every rule, every decision, depends on the employees to carry it into effect. It is vital to identify those persons within the organization who influence how well the supervisor's decisions are made operational. These informal power brokers at times can have a greater ability to make things happen, or to prevent them from happening, than those in the formal structure.

So a person needs the support of both the formal power system and the informal power system in order to succeed in making long-term change. The formal power structure can mandate change, but if the informal structure resists, permanent change is impossible. The informal power structure may want change, but as long as change is opposed by the supervisor, or is against the rules, change is not going to happen.

GAINING INFLUENCE

So how does influence work? It is not mysterious. We all influence one another's behavior every day. If Susie wears a new blue shirt and everyone tells her how nice she looks, Susie is being influenced to wear the shirt again. So influencing others is something we all do. Is it honest to influence other people, or is it manipulative? Such a value judgment depends on the situation: what is the goal of the manipulator? how is it being accomplished? Yes, influence can be used dishonestly, but as a general rule people can not be influenced to do things they are not already disposed to do. And most instances of influence are either insignificant, such as Susie's shirt, or positive.

The process of gaining influence is actually the process of becoming a good leader. One begins with a vision and a dedication to making that vision reality. When other people see that one believes in what one is doing and that one is dedicated to accomplishing the goal, then other people become more likely to commit to that goal also. People do what you need them to do to accomplish your goal because it is now their goal, too. Antoine de Saint Exupéry said, "*If you want to build a ship, don't drum up people together to collect wood and don't assign them tasks and work, but rather teach them to long for the endless immensity of the sea.*"

Before other people will commit to what you want done they have to believe that what you want is worth doing and that there is a possibility things could be different. How much easier it is to do something that everyone agrees needs to be done! But you are the example, and if you act disinterested, no one else is going to care either.

Others must also see you as trustworthy. If you do not do what you say you will do, then people will have no inclination to do what you want them to do. No one wants to follow someone who will turn around and stab them in the back at the first opportunity, or give up part of the way through. Everyone is familiar with the coworker who wants to be in charge and volunteers for things, and then does not follow through with the task. Such a person quickly loses any ability to garner support.

Another important aspect of influencing others is respect for the people with whom you are working. People need to believe that what they say matters, that their opinion is being heard. This does not mean you have to give people what they ask for; it does mean you have to listen to them and let them see that you take them seriously.

All of these things must be in place before one can influence or lead others to make change. It does not matter whether one's power derives from the formal structure or the informal structure, these are the underlying elements required to become a leader—to get other people to do what one wants them to do.

DEVELOPING A COLLABORATIVE APPROACH

If one has the legitimate power of the organization, one can simply dictate what is to happen. But experience shows that dictating has severe limitations. For one thing, if one simply commands that something be done, it is likely to be done only when one is watching. Anyone who has raised children is familiar with this phenomenon: a rule is set down, but if a parent is not diligent in enforcing it, the child soon ignores it. And for another thing, attempts at dictatorial management will quickly run afoul of the informal power structure: messages don't get delivered, supplies are unavailable, and so on.

With collaboration, on the other hand, everyone is involved in deciding what needs to happen and how it should be done. And because they can feel that their opinion counts, they are more likely to abide by a decision even when they do not get their way. Robert Hargrove says that, *"Collaborative people are those who identify a possibility and recognize that their own view is not enough to make it a reality."* When collaboration happens, cooperation follows. Little happens without the assistance of other people, so collaboration is key.

However, collaboration is not something that magically happens. Collaboration requires a lot of up-front work and time spent talking face-to-face with people and listening to their ideas. Collaboration establishes a working relationship among a group of people; cooperation follows as they work toward common goals. This work continues during any project as a team is built, conflicts are resolved, and goals are accomplished.

CONFLICT MANAGEMENT

No discussion of leadership or collaboration and cooperation is complete without some words about conflict. Conflict is inevitable. Seldom do all people agree on all things. The key to managing conflict is to embrace it whenever possible. Better ideas can grow out of conflict if no one becomes entrenched in a viewpoint and respect for all is maintained. It is important to make sure that everyone's viewpoint is heard and taken into consideration and that ways are sought to make the proposal more attractive for those who are having difficulty with it, even if you are not going to be able to accommodate them.

To do this, it is important to seek out the potential dissenters and find out what their potential interest in a project would be. If their viewpoint can be taken into consideration, then this should be built into the project. If not, then they should hear why things are not going to be done their way. In this way they at least can feel that they were respected enough to be heard.

MAKING IT OPERATIONAL

People often want to know whether followers believe in their leaders. A much more relevant question is whether the leaders believe in their followers.

—John Gardner, former Secretary,
U.S. Department of Health, Education, and Welfare

The next question is how to go from the theory of influence to the fact of getting something concrete and real actually done. What follows is one example of how to do this taken from a project on quality; there are many other ways.

The first step in any project is to determine who needs to be involved in what you need to do. This in itself may require some time and effort and talking to others to determine who would be affected.

The next step—and this is vital—is to have face-to-face contact with everyone you can identify as an interested party. Talk to them about the proposal: explain to them what the plan is and solicit their input. Let them know that you care what they think and how they feel about the project. Once they understand how the proposal will impact them, they will have their own outcomes they will be advocating for. The goal is to have *their* outcomes advanced by *your* proposal. After you understand their positions, you will be able to improve your proposal so that the interests of as many people as possible will be served in a positive way while keeping the proposal's central purpose intact.

A good idea at the end of this step, if it is feasible, is to have a group meeting where remaining differences and objections can be ironed out in a collaborative way. The people who have bought into the central goal of the proposal will help you win over those who are holding back, and the final result will have the feel of a consensus. Everyone will be looking at the project as *their* project.

From this point onward, frequent individual and group meetings will be important. Everyone needs to be kept informed as to progress and problems so they can celebrate the one and help overcome the other.

In this particular instance it was decided to assess our organization and determine our strengths and needs. Our organization is small, about 20 people. So, in order to build a collaborative process, it was decided to involve as many people as possible in the project. It was hoped that if a collaborative process was used, cooperation would follow. If your organization is small, include everyone; if it is large, be sure to get both the formal and informal power leaders involved, even if you know they are not going to agree!

It requires an excellent facilitator to make the assessment process go smoothly. We were fortunate to be able to have someone from outside our organization to lead our process. This allowed us to avoid preexisting biases either for or against any inside issues. The assessment, if properly conducted, should give you a good picture of what your organization does well and what needs work.

Once we had the results from our assessment tool, we were able to incorporate those results into a strategy for change. We utilized our supervisors, as a group of legitimate power holders who met regularly, to determine which items would have the most impact if they were addressed. If your organization does not have a comparable group, form one. Using the information gained from the assessment tool, lead the group through the development of an influence diagram or an inter-relationship digraph (Figure 23.1).

Our interrelationship digraph guided our organization in deciding where to start. Since the assessment tool happened to illuminate more than one weak point in our organization, the digraph helped us form an idea of which areas were most significant. In order to engage the informal power system, we also discussed the criteria for deciding on a project. For example, what does the group think is

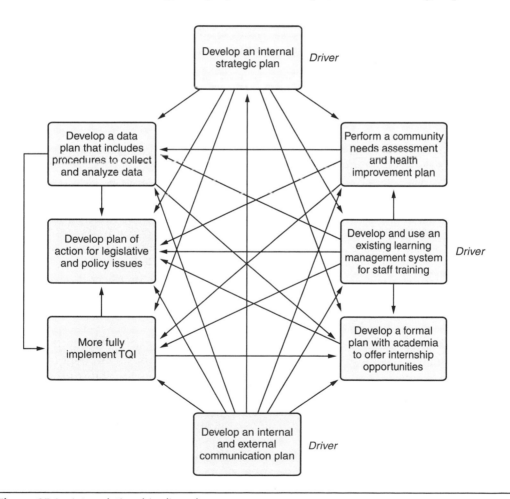

Figure 23.1 Interrelationship digraph.

	1—Not important	2—Important	3—Somewhat important	4—Very important	5—Extremely important
Working toward accreditation					
Improving our ability to do everyday tasks without stress					
Better/more community engagement					
Building staff morale					
Low-cost project					
Does not require a lot of time					

Figure 23.2   Likert scale chart for ranking priority of improvement actions.

important? Does the group want to focus on certification, on internal communication or morale, or perhaps on community perception? When four to six criteria have been chosen, they can be presented to the entire staff of the organization for ranking using a Likert-type scale (Figure 23.2).

We used e-mail as the easiest way to get a response in a short period of time. The grid was disseminated to everyone in the organization quickly, with a request for input. Everyone was asked to rate the choices and e-mail them back. This showed what the staff was interested in improving. You will want to choose the criterion with the largest number of votes that most closely matches what the majority of people are telling you is important, so look for the mode. This procedure is basically a voting procedure, so the number that best describes what the majority wants is what you will use. You could ask the management staff to decide which one they thought was most important, but that is not a collaborative approach and ignores the informal channels of power.

The next step for us in our collaborative approach was to apply the criteria for a good decision to the weaknesses spotlighted by the assessment tool. Build a separate grid for each identified weakness; this allows the staff to think about how the criteria apply to the various weaknesses. Ask the staff to rate how they view working on this area of weakness in terms of the criteria that have been determined to lead to a good decision, using an assessment tool such as shown in Figure 23.3, for example.

The two grids (Figures 23.2 and 23.3) then can be combined in order to make a decision grid (Figure 23.4). The supervisors have determined the criteria for a good decision, and the staff have decided what they think is the most important

Goal	0—Very poor Does not meet this goal	1—Fair Meets this goal	2—Good Meets this goal well	3—Very good Meets this goal well
Working toward accreditation				
Improving our ability to do everyday tasks without stress				
Better/more community engagement				
Building staff morale				
Low-cost project				
Does not require a lot of time				

Figure 23.3   Tool for assessing ability to meet organizational goal.

	Accreditation	Tasks	Community	Morale	Low cost	Little time	Totals
Weights	3	5	4	5	4	3	
Data plan	(3) 9	(1) 5	(2) 8	(0) 0	(0) 0	(0) 0	22
Community needs assessment	(3) 9	(1) 5	(3) 12	(2) 10	(0) 0	(0) 0	36
Strategic plan	(3) 9	(3) 15	(3) 12	(3) 15	(2) 8	(1) 3	62
Policy and legislative activities	(2) 6	(0) 0	(0) 0	(0) 0	(3) 12	(1) 3	21
Staff training	(3) 9	(2) 10	(3) 12	(3) 15	(0) 0	(0) 0	46
Work with academic institutions	(3) 9	(0) 0	(1) 4	(0) 0	(3) 12	(0) 0	25
Communications	(3) 9	(3) 15	(3) 12	(3) 15	(3) 12	(2) 6	69
TQI plan	(3) 9	(2) 10	(1) 4	(1.5) 7.4	(1) 4	(0) 0	34.5

Figure 23.4   Decision grid for priority actions.

thing to work toward. Both the formal, or legitimate, channels of power and the informal channels of power have been engaged—everyone has had a chance to provide input into the decision process. So choosing the area on which to focus the organization's first efforts should satisfy every group.

CONCLUSION

If your actions inspire others to dream more, learn more, do more, and become more, you are a leader.

—John Quincy Adams

This process of collaboration, while simple at first glance, takes enormous amounts of time and energy. It requires patience, problem solving, and a willingness to believe in the people around you. To not get lost in the process, you must have a clear vision of where you want to go and be able to communicate that vision.

Chapter 24

Orange County Health Department STD Quality Improvement Case Study (October 2005 – July 2006)

James Hinson, Team Leader and STD Department Manager

THE SITUATION

Using the seven-step plan–do–check–act problem-solving model (see Figure 24.1).

Plan

Step 1: Describe the problem

Step 2: Describe the current process

Step 3: Identify the root cause(s) of the problem

Step 4: Develop a solution and action plan

Do

Step 5: Implement the solution

Check

Step 6: Review and evaluate the results of the change

Act

Step 7: Reflect and act on learnings

Snapshot results of this quality improvement project are shown in Figure 24.5, page 341.

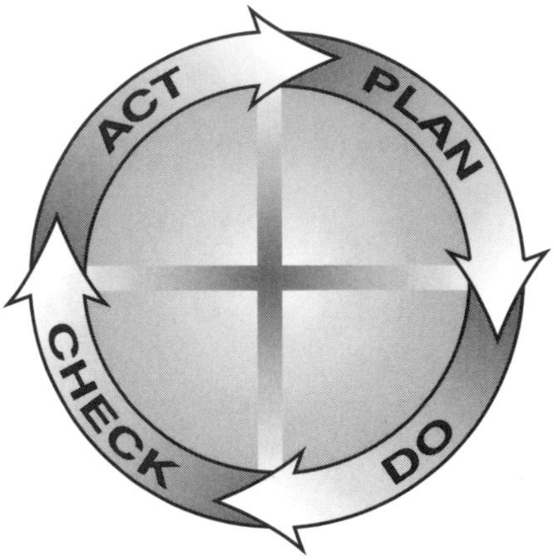

Act:

7. Reflect and act on learnings

Plan:

1. Describe the probelm

2. Describe the current process

3. Identify the root cause(s) of the problem

4. Develop a solution and action plan

Check:

6. Review and evaluate the results of the change

Do:

5. Implement the solution

Figure 24.1   The plan–do–check–act cycle.

Between 2004 and 2005, the Orange County Health Department (OCHD) saw a sharp increase (45 percent) in new early syphilis cases in its jurisdiction, from 136 cases per year to 195 cases per year. Following a trend that was seen in Florida and nationwide, these new syphilis cases were mostly seen in the MSM (men who have sex with men) population. Based on the accelerating rate of increase per year since 2001, the sexually transmitted diseases (STD) team knew that syphilis would grow into a larger epidemic if not rapidly controlled.

Short on staff and already feeling stretched to the limit with statutory responsibilities, the STD team was not sure what more they could do to stop the spread of the disease in their community. Within the unit, turnover was high, resources were limited, and employee satisfaction was low according to a recent departmentwide employee survey.

Due to the urgency of the problem and need for new solutions, the local health department leaders considered the STD unit ideal for piloting a new quality improvement (QI) project, taking productive QI methodology from the private sector and using those tools in the public sector. In years past, OCHD had tried to bring QI to the entire health department by training upper managers in QI methods. However, QI never really "trickled down" to the remainder of departments. Trying a more "bottom up" approach for the STD QI project, the department formed a QI team that consisted mainly of the frontline workers, having a combined 75+ years STD experience. Ultimately, if this model proved successful in addressing the syphilis problem, the health department hoped to expand it throughout the entire agency.

To assist the STD QI team, OCHD provided a hands-on training opportunity and hired a highly-recognized consultant to coach the team in applying QI methods in regular team meetings to address the problem. In order to make time available for the staff involved to be able to meet regularly, OCHD administration was very flexible in allowing the STD department to focus on the higher priorities during the duration of the initiative. Very critical to the success of the QI team activities was for the other STD department staff to help pick up the slack while the project meetings took place, which they did in a magnificent manner.

At the Public Health Foundation–led kickoff meeting, the STD team was introduced to QI tools such as the why tree, affinity diagram, and fishbone diagram. In this initial exploration of reasons for the rising syphilis rates, they came up with several potential root causes, including constant turnover of skilled disease intervention specialists (DIS) workers, lack of training for DIS workers, and OCHD's poor reputation in the MSM community.

STEP 1: DESCRIBE THE PROBLEM

Problem Statement: Early syphilis is increasing in Orange County.

Reason Selected: Surveillance data showed significant increases in early syphilis over the previous four years. If not rapidly controlled, early syphilis could become a larger epidemic, costing the community hundreds of thousands of dollars in health-related costs for early, late, and congenital syphilis cases, in addition to potential costs resulting from syphilis-associated HIV transmission.

Measures of Project Success

1. Reduce new early syphilis cases by 25 percent compared to the previous year (outcome measure).

2. 100 percent of disease intervention specialists (DIS) will test a minimum of four associates per month for syphilis through DIS-initiated fieldwork.

3. Increase the quarterly cluster index to 1.0 on early syphilis cases among MSM.

4. Increase the quarterly contact index on all early syphilis cases, including MSM cases, to 1.41.

The team identified four measures of its success: one outcome measure and three performance measures for processes important to reaching the outcome goal. Two process measures—the contact index and cluster index (process measures related to eliciting partner names and testing at-risk individuals)—were identified as areas for improvement because the team performed below the state average and CDC goals. The third process measure was a new internal standard for "field blood draws," which could be tracked monthly.

Measure	Team baseline (Previous 6 months)	State average (Previous 6 months)	CDC goal
Cluster index	0.51	0.66	1.0*
Contact index	0.84	1.41*	2.0

* Team target

STD Team Members

- Jim Hinson—Team Leader
- Earl Boney—QI Lead
- Anne Marie Strickland—QI Support
- Donna Bouton—Department Administrative Assistant
- Preston Boyce—DIS Supervisor
- Barbara Carroll—Operations Manager
- Shonda Mitchell—Surveillance Supervisor
- Rajendra Hiralal—DIS Supervisor
- Scott Fryberger—DIS Staff
- Isabel Hudson—DIS Staff

Milestones

- Team committed to problem statement
- Identified national and state standards
- Defined measures and targets
- Completed first working/learning session
- Drafted expectations for members on QI team

STEP 2: DESCRIBE THE CURRENT PROCESS

There are six major processes involved in field blood draws: preparation, acquiring vehicle, fieldwork, field recording, blood handling, and post-test procedures.

Before we began doing the process maps, we all had our own way of doing things. Now with these maps we are all on the same page, and can use them to train others.

—Raj Hiralal

Sample Process Map for Field Blood Draws: Preparation

1. Examination of the current process for doing blood draws revealed areas of inconsistent DIS practices and inefficiencies in the way the process was currently carried out (see Figure 24.2).

2. The DIS field preparation process took too much time—estimated as much as two hours each time.

3. The two areas that consumed the most time for field preparation were getting the key to unlock the supply cabinet and getting permission to use a vehicle (involving several permission steps).

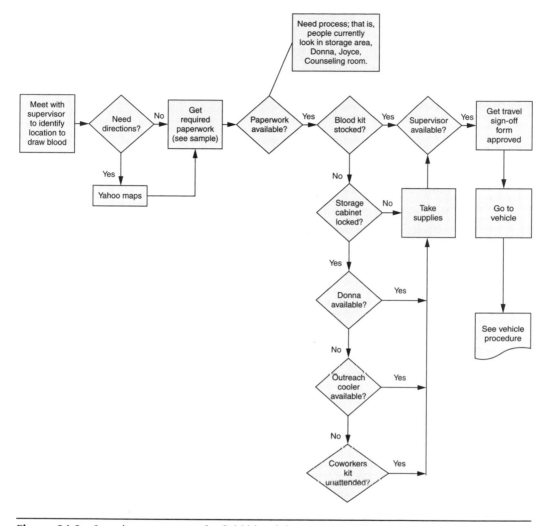

Figure 24.2   Sample process map for field blood draws: preparation.

Milestones

- Completed seven process maps (one overall, six detailed) related to carrying out blood draws.
- Identified opportunities for cutting down time in two major areas of field preparation, as well as improving other processes.

QI Tools Used in This Step

- Process mapping
- Brainstorming
- Discussion

STEP 3: IDENTIFY THE ROOT CAUSE(S) OF THE PROBLEM

Problem. Early syphilis is increasing in Orange County.

Cause-and-Effect (Fishbone) Diagram: Root Causes for Rising Syphilis Cases

1. After conducting an initial root cause analysis examining the possible reasons for the increasing rate of early syphilis in Orange County, the DIS saw that an overlapping issue in various categories was high staff turnover (see Figure 24.3).

2. By delving deeper into the issue, the team concluded that staff turnover affected their performance indicators.

3. The rate of turnover for DIS workers was high at OCHD, where the average length of stay for DIS new employees was six months or less.

The contact index relies on information provided from clients, and this is where the experience of DIS workers helps in pushing the contact index up . . . It takes some time and exposure to develop these relationships [with clients].

—Scott Fryberger

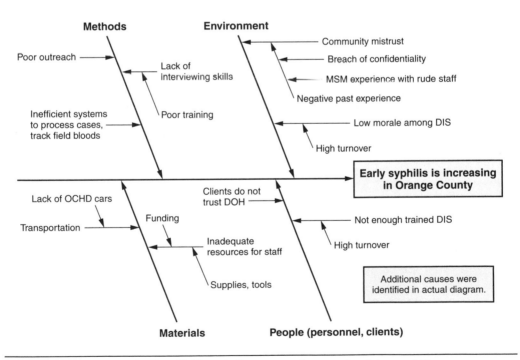

Figure 24.3   Cause-and-effect (fishbone) diagram: root causes for rising syphilis cases.

Initial Fishbone Diagram for Staff Turnover

The STD QI team located most of their turnover problems in four main areas (see Figure 24.4):

1. Lack of useful training

2. Low morale

3. Work environment (including space and interpersonal issues)

4. Lack of good candidates

Milestones

- Completed initial fishbone diagram showing major causes of the syphilis problem, and identified that staff turnover was underlying most of these causes

- Created detailed fishbone and affinity diagrams on staff turnover with coworker input

- Decided to focus on staff turnover and programmatic processes that are within departmental control

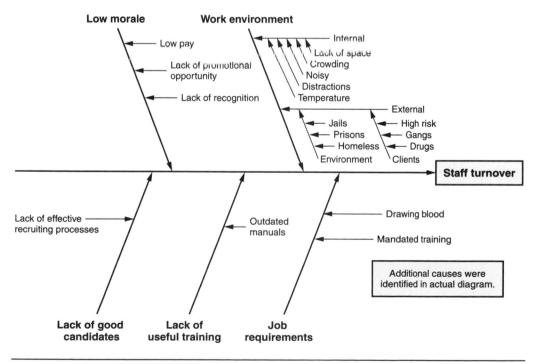

Figure 24.4   Initial fishbone diagram for staff turnover.

- Repeated a department SWOT (strengths, weaknesses, opportunities, and threats) analysis to take stock of what they had accomplished since the last analysis and identify strengths they could use to address future STD unit needs

QI Tools Used in This Step

- Brainstorming
- Affinity diagram
- Management survey
- SWOT analysis
- Fishbone diagram
- Process maps/drill-downs
- Priority-setting matrix

STEP 4: DEVELOP A SOLUTION AND ACTION PLAN

To tackle staff turnover, the team found that there were multiple areas members could work on. Because of this, they had to focus their attention first on the areas they felt were most important. Through multivoting, the team determined that the three most important areas to address were the following (from most to least important):

- Training
- Finding good candidates
- Low morale

In addition, the team set aside time in weekly meetings to improve the processes that were hindering the unit's success.

Sorting Activity: "Lack of Useful Training"

Identified cause from fishbone spine	What is to be done first?*	What do we control?
Can't do job = Skill	2	Y
Accountability	3	Y
Gossip	4	Y
Logical decision making	5	Skills needed = Y (learned)
Internal customer service	1	Y

* Result of multivoting on priority to address. Lowest number = Highest priority.

C/I/C Chart: Staff Turnover

Things within our:		
Control	Influence	(Have) Concern
• Gossip	• Hiring	• Salary
• Training	• Interdepartmental relations	
• Recognition		
• Process		

Control and influence was an important concept introduced to the team by the team's consultant, which helped the team prioritize what causes they could most directly affect.

Milestones

- Analyzed maps of current processes to pinpoint areas for improvement

- Identified three priority areas for action plan to address root causes of turnover: lack of useful training, lack of good candidates, and low morale

- Analyzed each area of the fishbone and categorized potential solutions within the team's control or influence

- Selected strategies the team could easily control that would affect programmatic processes or environment

- Submitted proposal for additional vehicles

- Requested help from HR and outside organizations on behavioral interviewing

- Submitted proposal to human resources to increase salary grade

- Collected information on strategies effective in other jurisdictions

- Reviewed evidence and recommendations for controlling syphilis in MSM populations

QI Tools Used in This Step

- Multivoting
- Sorting tool
- Control/influence/concern chart

STEP 5: IMPLEMENT THE SOLUTION

The team implemented changes by dealing with easily addressed problems first. Among their first successes, they reorganized space and made supplies more readily available to decrease preparation time for field blood draws.

Next, the team implemented several other solutions such as enhanced DIS training and coaching, recognition of staff accomplishments, obtaining vehicles for the unit, increasing the base rate of pay for DIS, and creating a consistent process for data gathering.

Action registers helped the team track progress.

Sample from Action Register: "Lack of Good Candidates"

Action	Owner	Due date	Comments
1. Improve interview/ hiring process	Jim/ Barbara	2/16	To include: review "people first" HR support database for information/ job-specific description/requirements/ and so on, qualifying questions, interview questions
2. Conduct informal survey of current field staff	Scott	3/2	Ask how DIS found out about job, what would make them stay

Milestones

- Changed assignments for orientation training and initiated regular case review sessions for continuous on-the-job learning

- Health department approved unit request for three new vehicles

- DIS workers sent to national STD meeting for training

- Implemented new interviewing process for DIS candidates

- Trained newly hired people using improved process maps

- Clarified and eliminated unnecessary steps in procedures:

  - Centralized location of forms

  - Made supply cabinet unlocked for all DIS

  - Eliminated use of certain forms in the preparation process

- Reorganized space for better work environment

- Started recognizing DIS workers for their work and contributions

- Increased base rate of pay for DIS 10 percent

QI Tools Used in This Step

- Action register

STEP 6: REVIEW AND EVALUATE THE RESULTS OF THE CHANGE

1. By the end of the nine-month project, new early syphilis cases leveled off and began to decline (see Figure 24.5). During the same period, syphilis increased in Florida peer counties.

2. 100 percent of DIS conformed to minimum blood draw standards for the last two months (see Figure 24.6).

3. Achieved cluster index above CDC standard for four consecutive quarters (see Figure 24.7); attributed by team members to better interviewing skills.

4. Contact index target was improved but target not met—needs additional action (see Figure 24.8).

Milestones

*   Gathered data and charted progress on the indicators

*   Revisited fishbone diagram on turnover and identified that most causes had been addressed, or were being addressed, by the team

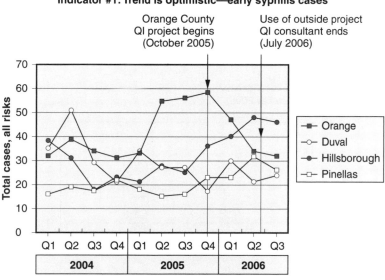

Figure 24.5   Total reported early syphilis cases by quarter, 2004–2006: Orange County compared to peer counties* in Florida.

Source: Syphilis data: Florida Department of Health, STDMIS system; 2006 data for all four counties provided as of 10/13/2006.

* Peer county designation created by Community Health Status Indicators (CHSI) project, HRSA, 2000, based on population density, size, and poverty levels. CHSI data notes are available at http://www.communityphind.net/CHSI-CompanionView.pdf.

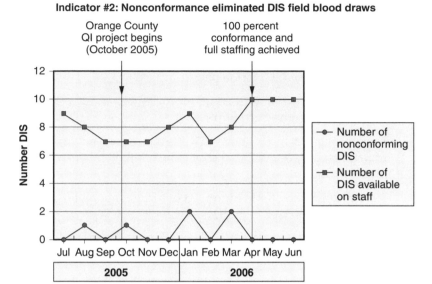

Figure 24.6 Staff nonconformance to OCHD standard for field blood draws (each DIS testing ≥4 associates per month for syphilis through DIS initiated fieldwork) and DIS staff available, by month.

Source: DIS data: Florida Department of Health, supervisor and staff teaching.

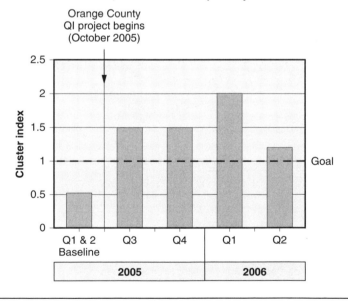

Figure 24.7 Cluster index, early syphilis: MSM Orange County, by quarter.

Source: Florida Department of Health.

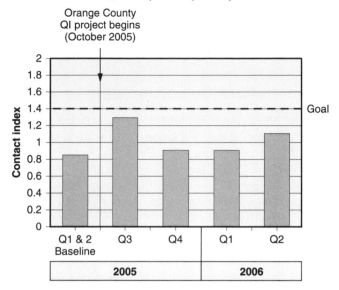

Figure 24.8   Contact index, all early syphilis: Orange County, by quarter.
Source: Florida Department of Health.

QI Tools Used in This Step

- Control chart
- Fishbone diagram

STEP 7: REFLECT AND ACT ON LEARNINGS

The community is more accepting and receptive to our team because of the improvements we've made within our unit.

—Jim Hinson

Secondary Effects of QI Effort. In addition to advances made in their indicators, the team also reported the following successes that grew out of the QI initiative:

- Stopped DIS staff turnover (a root cause)
  - Zero DIS left the unit in the first half of 2006; six had left in 2005.
  - Fully staffed for the first time in group memory.
- Improved morale and teamwork
  - Increased job satisfaction: STD employee satisfaction surveys show an 18 percent increase in 2006 compared to the last survey in 2004 (significant at the $p = .05$ level).
  - More cohesiveness and trust in team.

– Better morale and teamwork translated into a better ability to work with the community.

- Team success strengthened OCHD ability to request other project funds

Implementing QI

Since this was the health department's first QI initiative using this approach, the team learned what support needed to be in place for a successful project. While some team members had previous QI training, most learned the new methods by carrying out the project. One of the most important assets was having a consultant who could be neutral, provide expertise from other fields, and help keep the team focused. The team also identified other practices and expectations they saw as necessary to successfully carry out the QI process; however, they also found that establishing these practices and expectations proved to be a challenge.

Some *challenges* identified by the team:

- Dedicating staff to full attendance at all team meetings

- Staying focused on priority issues

- Scheduling subject matter experts for process drill-down documentation

- Using quality tools effectively

- Securing embedded consultant with required support skills

Other Team Lessons

The project gave the team many other insights, such as:

- Most useful tools: affinity diagram, fishbone diagram, process mapping

- Biggest surprise: the problem is not necessarily what you think it is

- Maintaining focus on quantitative measures requires discipline and time commitment

- Barriers and gaps must be documented for action

- QI projects must be aligned to organization's goals

Milestones

- Completed evaluation using interviews, quarterly questionnaires, and data review

- Recognized team members with letters of commendation from the local health officer, certificates of accomplishment, and a placard with team members' photos in the lobby

- Shared successes through agency presentations, newsletters, and milestone meetings

- Other units became interested in QI and requested project participation

LOOKING BACK—FALL 2008

Two years have passed since the Orange County Health Department (OCHD) undertook the STD improvement project. Like many health departments, Orange County is facing challenges of funding, manpower, scarce resources, and increasing community needs. OCHD senior management remains committed to quality improvement as the path to increased community service and organizational performance, and the vision of "A healthier future for the people of Florida." Orange County Florida has a population of over one million residents, and over 40 million visitors a year come to the area attractions, including Disney World, Universal Studios Florida, and the convention center. With this large, transient population, consistent monitoring of STD incidence is imperative to achieve appropriate plan–do–check–act processes and control STDs.

As the Winter Park Health Foundation project was having its successes, two other STDs were increasing in Orange County, as well as statewide—chlamydia and gonorrhea. These bacterial infections, while easily treatable, many times go unrecognized (asymptomatic) by an infected person, thus leading to medical complications and spreading of the diseases in the community. Seeing this increase, STD management moved more manpower toward this growing issue, especially focusing on infected pregnant females. During 2007 in Orange County, over 1200 pregnant females had chlamydia or gonorrhea. Increased effort was placed on assuring that these medically at–risk individuals were adequately treated, and an effort made to notify their partners of possible exposure and infection so they could seek evaluation and treatment and not reinfect the pregnant female, in order to have a favorable outcome of a healthy baby and mother. Though this movement of personnel caused efforts with syphilis to be somewhat lessened, the lessons learned during the project served to help the STD department to look at the increasing STD situation in Orange County in a different manner, and to begin to take steps to manage the increasing numbers of STDs using tools and methodology learned in the syphilis initiative.

One example of action taken was that the STD clinic flow was analyzed, and the decision was made to focus on that process to increase the number of clients that could be seen, as well as improve client satisfaction. The entire clinic process was mapped, with improvements initiated at many stages of the operation. The clinic went from 22.5 to 37 hours of availability to the public for care, thus providing the opportunity to see more clients. Staff morale improved with alternative flexible work schedules, and revenues have increased. The waiting area and intake areas are being renovated to a modern, professional appearance. The result of using the QI process is that persons with or exposed to STDs have a better chance of getting rapid, quality care, and the community will be healthier with this opportunity to reduce the spread of STDs, thus helping us reach our vision.

Critical to the improvements has been the continual support of senior management in providing the necessary resources to meet the growing demands of the program. Six vehicles are now available to the DIS field staff. DIS morale has improved. Ongoing surveys are showing that client satisfaction is improving, and the results of using the QI tools as presented by the Winter Park Health Foundation (WPHF) have well served, and will continue to be used by the OCHD STD program.

The return on the initial investment of time and resources to train staff in the use of QI tools has more than paid for itself in the continuation of use of the tools in the different processes in the program, providing a proven process that permits optimal resolution to our challenges.

Seeing the success that this initiative had with the STD program, the Orange County Health Department launched an internally funded major quality initiative to improve septic system permitting in Spring 2008. This project achieved the following outcomes.

Wins for the Program Process Action Team (PPAT)

- Date-stamping of all paperwork received.
- Comment form kept in each green folder and utilized.
- Green folder labeled with re-host number for tracking.
- Updated instructions (in process).
  - Spanish and English versions (in process)
- Immediate line locator input by clerical staff.
- Workload rebalancing for management file reviews.
- SharePoint site established for project documentation.
- Adjusting front counter hours at Mercy Drive location to meet state guidelines (8–4). Shorter hours allow staff to address paperwork requirements before end of day.

OCHD embarked on the development of a departmentwide quality system in Fall 2008. The department has again retained the embedded consultant involved in the 2006 STD and 2008 septic system permitting improvement team activities. The consultant is tasked with coaching senior leadership, the department QI coordinator, and selected teams in the skills necessary to become totally self-supporting in their quality and performance improvement efforts.

OCHD is committed to the use of quality tools and techniques to provide an ever-increasing level of service to the public health community in Orange County, Florida. The team outcomes, community acceptance, fact-based decision making, and improved morale resulting from OCHD quality efforts have convinced senior management in the department that quality improvement is a core element of their organizational culture.

Chapter 25

The Minnesota Public Health Collaborative for Quality Improvement

Dorothy Bliss, MPA, Debra Burns, MPA, Kim McCoy, MS, MPH, and William Riley, PhD

INTRODUCTION

The Minnesota Public Health Collaborative for Quality Improvement (QI Collaborative) is a partnership between the local Public Health Association, the Minnesota Department of Health (MDH), and the University of Minnesota, School of Public Health. The goal of the QI Collaborative is to institutionalize quality improvement practice throughout the public health system in Minnesota. The work of the collaborative is guided by a steering committee that includes representatives of each of the partner organizations.

The QI Collaborative was initiated in 2007 as part of the Multi-State Learning Collaborative funded by the Robert Wood Johnson Foundation. Participation in the Multi-State Learning Collaborative was seen by MDH and local public health leaders as a significant opportunity to strengthen Minnesota's performance improvement framework. From April 2007 through March 2008, the QI Collaborative facilitated eight quality improvement projects across the state, involving a total of 33 local health departments and one tribal government. The work of the QI Collaborative is grounded in the *model for improvement*[1] and loosely based on the Institute for Healthcare Improvement *Breakthrough Series*.[2]

Projects were solicited through a statewide request for applications. Four of the eight projects selected were single-county projects and the others involved multiple counties. Each of the projects focused on a different target area and thus had a unique aim statement and unique measures.

METHODS

Each project team that participated in the QI Collaborative included local public health staff, a graduate student and faculty member from the School of Public Health, and MDH staff. Some teams also included key community stakeholders such as healthcare providers and human services officials. A local public health professional served as the lead staff person for each of the project teams. Most of the team members were new to quality improvement.

The QI Collaborative initially sponsored three videoconference training sessions led by quality improvement experts from the School of Public Health. Teams were taught the model for improvement and the plan–do–study–act cycle as well as tools such as root cause analysis, process mapping, control charts, and run charts. Teams worked together during the training sessions to define their problem and aim statements, develop performance measures, and plan their improvement process. Additional training was provided to teams via monthly, one-hour conference calls, which also included project status updates and general sharing of challenges and successes.

In addition, teams submitted monthly reports to document their progress. The reports briefly documented the changes that were implemented by the teams and the quality improvement tools that were used in the process.

In the time periods between the monthly conference calls, project teams were busy implementing their plan–do–study–act cycles. They conducted rapid tests of change, evaluated the results, and then returned to the planning phase of the cycle until the change was ready for full-scale implementation.

RESULTS

Six of the eight projects exhibited breakthrough improvement. The other two projects showed incremental improvement and are ongoing. See Table 25.1 for an overview of the eight projects.

Overall, the QI Collaborative has had a positive impact on the Minnesota public health community in a variety of ways:

- *Strengthened collaboration between local, state, and academic partners in Minnesota.* The QI Collaborative was particularly helpful in strengthening the relationship between Minnesota's public health practice community and the University of Minnesota, School of Public Health. It also provided opportunities for graduate students to gain practical experience working with a local health department.

- *Spread quality improvement across the state.* Over 230 people representing MDH, local public health, and the School of Public Health were trained in the model for improvement, the plan–do–study–act process, and other quality improvement tools. Evaluation results indicate that participants are using their QI skills in a variety of ways. They are also sharing their skills with colleagues in other departments and agencies.

- *Produced process improvement that has statewide relevance.* Several of the project teams developed improved processes that have the potential to improve statewide public health performance:

  - The project on the timeliness of personal care assistant reassessments improved their on-time reporting from 62 to 100 percent. The project was initiated largely in response to new legislation that will penalize local health departments for late reporting.

Table 25.1   Overview of eight Minnesota Public Health Collaborative projects.

Topic	Aim	Outcome
Appointment participation	Improve appointment show rates at WIC clinics	Varied by department, but little improvement overall. Team members agreed to explore root causes of the problem and try again.
Latent TB treatment	Decrease staff time spent documenting treatment of latent tuberculosis infection by 10 percent	Time spent charting TB cases was *reduced by over 17 percent.*
Health alert network	Reduce staff time devoted to HAN testing	Staff time devoted to HAN testing was *reduced by 70 percent.*
Dental varnish	Provide dental fluoride treatment to at least 20 children	*104 children received dental fluoride treatment.*
Mental health screening	Increase social-emotional screening of children and adolescents	*169 children were screened* and 46 were referred to treatment. The next phase of the process will focus on triage.
Data integration	Improve immunization rates by integrating data from WIC, immunization registry, and child/teen checkups	Immunization rates increased three percent in WIC clinics and six percent in non-WIC clinics.
Personal care assistant reassessments	Improve timely completion of personal care assistant reassessments	On-time completion of personal care assistant reassessments *increased from 62 percent to 100 percent.*
Workforce competency assessment	Increase Leadership Council understanding of public health competencies	Leaders with at least an intermediate understanding of public health competencies *increased from 28 percent to 61 percent.*

- The project on staff time devoted to documentation of treatment of latent TB infection created an electronic record to supplant the myriad of paper forms that were required.

- Another county reduced the amount of staff time spent on health alert network (HAN) testing by 70 percent. Since all local health departments are required to test the HAN on a regular basis, the findings of that project are widely relevant as well.

LESSONS LEARNED

Many local public health departments operate with a small number of staff who are charged with meeting all of the public health needs of their communities, from immunizations to nutrition counseling to mold mitigation. Not surprisingly, staff time required was the biggest challenge in implementing these quality improvement projects. It is difficult to prioritize quality improvement in the midst of multiple competing interests that require immediate time and attention. Other challenges cited include lack of quality improvement knowledge and experience, and skepticism on the part of staff and leaders about the value of quality improvement methods. However, evaluation results demonstrated that these challenges were overcome by the learning and success derived from the collaborative.

Following are recommendations from the project teams:

- Focus on a well-defined and discrete project that is completely within your control.

- Successful quality improvement requires a strong, sustained commitment from leadership and team members.

- Dig deep to identify the true cause of a problem and be open to a range of possible solutions.

- Quality improvement is about improving *the process*, not the people.

All teams have expressed enthusiasm for a continued investment in the quality improvement effort. They were actively engaged in the process and excited by the results of their efforts. Local public health department participants were particularly surprised by how quickly they achieved improvements in their processes and outcomes. This rapid success was a key incentive for continued progress at state and local levels.

For further information about the QI Collaborative, contact Kim McCoy in the Office of Public Health Practice at the Minnesota Department of Health at kim.mccoy@state.mn.us or 651-201-3877.

Minnesota Public Health Collaborative for Quality Improvement

Central and Northwestern Minnesota Counties
August 2007 – May 2008

Life happens: helping clients keep WIC appointments

The Situation

When a mother misses a WIC appointment, it can leave a gap in a whole range of preventive health services that she and her children receive. They miss out on not only food vouchers, but nutrition education as well. Opportunities for parenting education, referrals for home visits, immunizations, dental varnishing, and information regarding other community resources are also lost or delayed by missed appointments. Missed appointments create scheduling issues for local health departments by leaving holes in the appointment schedule, especially at off-site clinics where staff do not have access to other work duties. On the other hand, missed appointments create appointment "crunches" when rescheduled appointments are squeezed into already full WIC clinic dates.

The central Minnesota local public health directors group had often discussed these challenges, yet none of them had tried a systematic approach to improving WIC "kept appointment" rates. When the MLC-2 quality improvement grant was announced, they agreed that this would be a good opportunity to see if something could be done to improve the situation for everyone.

Becker County, in northwestern Minnesota, also recognized the problems with missed WIC appointments. They had already begun making some changes to ensure that clients would not miss out on services, but saw that the MLC-2 grant could provide more structure to their effort and a chance to learn from other counties. Becker and the counties in central Minnesota combined their similar proposals to form a single QI project with the hope of learning from each other.

Aim Statement

By February 29, 2008, increase the rate that clients keep their appointments at Women, Infants, and Children (WIC) clinics.

The Minnesota Public Health Collaborative for Quality Improvement is a partnership of the Minnesota Department of Health, the University of Minnesota, and the Local Public Health Association.

The counties started with **surveys** of those who missed their WIC appointments as a way to identify and categorize the barriers clients faced. They agreed upon a common definition of "missed appointment" so the data could be compared. A **fishbone diagram** (Fig. 1) was created to group the causes of missed appointments (People, Machinery, Equipment, Methods, and Materials), and it revealed a number of issues related to missed appointments, including:

- Transportation issues, location of WIC clinic
- Forgetting appointments, having a conflict with work times
- Finding the WIC process too difficult

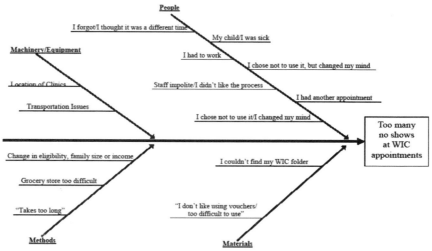

Fig. 1

Team Members:

Joyce Mueller, Crow Wing County Public Health
Ronda Stock, Becker County Public Health
Marlene Hufford, Isanti County Public Health
Janelle Schroeder, Kanabec County Public Health
Sylvia Cook, Mille Lacs County Public Health

Bonnie Paulsen, Morrison County Public Health
Sherry O'Brien, Stearns County Human Services
Heidi Brings, Todd County Public Health
Cindy Pederson, Wadena County Public Health
Wendy Kvale, MDH PHN Consultant
Dorothy Bliss, MDH Principal Planner
Sandra Potthoff, UMN Faculty Advisor
Abiola Fashanu, UMN Graduate Student

2

Each participating county collected survey data for one month and then compared responses. The group then **brainstormed** a range of potential interventions.

Each county also created a **process flow diagram** (Fig. 2) of their scheduling and reminder process.

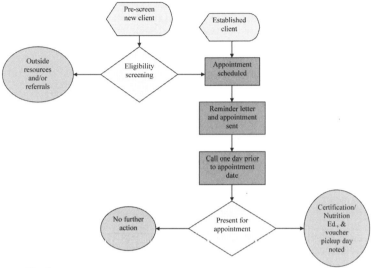

Fig. 2

 Although defined as a single project for the purposes of the grant, the group agreed that it would be more meaningful if each county chose and implemented the interventions most appropriate to their settings. Each county tried one or more strategies, including reminder phone calls, postcards, transportation vouchers, calendars, and stickers. These interventions were implemented for six months.

 Some counties had already implemented a reminder protocol and maintained a fairly high rate of kept appointments. Other counties experienced an initial increase in kept appointment rates, but those increases have not been maintained. One reason identified in this phase of the project was that although reminder phone calls can be helpful, and cell phone numbers have been requested, clients may change their cell phones frequently for a variety of reasons, including cost.

The participating counties sense a need to return to the planning phase of this cycle to consider other possible root causes of missed appointments and to consider alternative interventions. Some plan to continue surveying clients about missed appointments.

The testing of new reminder protocols in general is seen as having enriched the WIC clinic process and has been experienced as positive by many of the counties, which plan to continue various interventions where possible (depending on expense).

Lessons Learned

The QI process led to positive actions on the part of the local health departments involved in the project, changes they believe have improved the WIC clinic experience and relationships with clients and the general public. Many of the counties had experimented with different reminder interventions, but had not developed a systematic method of testing and sharing those strategies with other local health departments in the region. None of the local health departments had tried creating a flow chart to understand the WIC clinic process. The QI project facilitated communication and increased understanding among these counties of both quality improvement and WIC clinic issues.

The aim of the project was to improve WIC kept appointment rates. Although this goal was not reached, the use of QI tools was found to be helpful and the knowledge gained can be applied as needed to improve quality in all public health programs.

For more information about the Central/Northeast Minnesota QI project, contact Joyce Mueller, Crow Wing County Public Health, joyce.mueller@co.crow-wing.mn.us, 218-824-1087.

Support for this project was provided by a grant from the Robert Wood Johnson Foundation®.

Minnesota Department of Health
Office of Public Health Practice
85 East Seventh Place, Suite 200, Saint Paul, MN 55101
Phone: 651-201-3880 Fax: 651-201-3881
Email: ophp@state.mn.us

4

**Minnesota Public
Health Collaborative
for Quality
Improvement**

*Minnesota Counties Computer Cooperative
August 2007 – May 2008*

Taking It to Bits: How Developing an Electronic Record Improved Communication in Latent TB Clinics

The Situation

Latent tuberculosis infection (LTBI)* remains a concern throughout Minnesota, due primarily to the increase in immigration from countries where TB is endemic. While many counties in Minnesota have few if any LTBI cases in a given year, larger rural and urban counties have consistently large caseloads. The paperwork for these cases is cumbersome, involving multiple paper reports required by the federal government and the state health department, which ask for much of the same information.

The Minnesota Counties Computer Cooperative (MCCC), a group of counties in southwest, south central, and west central Minnesota developed and shares a software system for tracking public health data. Additions and refinements to the system are made regularly, as members identify areas that would benefit from electronic record-keeping.

When the MLC-2 quality improvement grants were announced, the group considered several possible projects but decided that creating an electronic means of tracking LTBI cases would benefit the most MCCC members *and* potentially improve public health. What they did not expect to get out of the QI process was a new way of structuring TB clinics and communicating with clients.

Aim Statement

Decrease the time spent documenting treatment of patients with latent tuberculosis by 10 percent.

The Minnesota Public Health Collaborative for Quality Improvement is a partnership of the Minnesota Department of Health, the University of Minnesota, and the Local Public Health Association.

---

* Persons with LTBI do not spread the disease, but they are susceptible to developing active TB, which would then pose a public health risk. Keeping track of persons with LTBI and making sure that they receive any needed health services, therefore, is an important public health responsibility.

The first challenge in turning this idea into a QI project was to develop an aim statement that was meaningful and measurable. The group decided to focus on reducing staff time to fill out the TB-related paperwork, expecting that creating an electronic record would have this effect.

A **fishbone diagram** (Fig. 1) identified many of the problems with the paperwork process, including redundancies, multiple terms for the same condition, and staff time. The MCCC also hoped that once the paper trail was changed to an electronic record it would decrease the variation in documentation across all the counties.

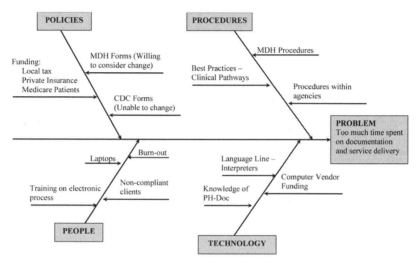

Fig. 1

Team members:

Diane Thorson, Otter Tail County Public Health
Kathy McKay, Clay County Public Health
Kathy Anderson, Clay County Public Health
Karen Nelson, Wadena County Public Health
Local county financial manager, TB nurse, support staff, billing staff, and computer vendor
Luanne McNichols, Minnesota Department of Health
DeeAnn Finley, Minnesota Department of Health
Ayse Gurses, University of Minnesota Faculty Advisor
Schelomo Marmor, University of Minnesota Graduate Student

2

To identify all the data elements that would be needed for an electronic record, the MCCC developed a **process flow chart** (Fig. 2) to show all the steps taken from intake to discharge.

Fig. 2

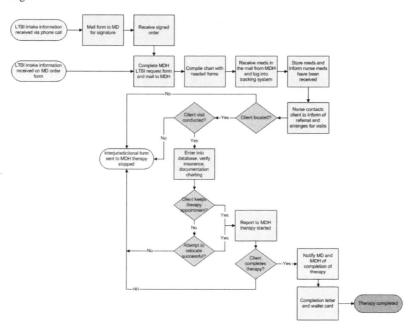

As Otter Tail County, the lead county in the QI project for the MCCC, developed the electronic record, they identified new data elements that would help with data entry and consistency among records. The draft electronic record sample is now in place and being used as of April 1.

The development of the electronic record revealed inconsistencies and redundancies in the paperwork process. It also revealed difficulties in gathering information from individuals with latent TB, many of whom are foreign-born (see lessons learned, below). After making changes and using the electronic format, the initial analysis revealed that the time spent charting TB cases was reduced by over 17 percent (aim was 10 percent).

3

With this success, the goal now is to finalize the electronic record format and then implement throughout the MCCC counties. When ready, they will use web-based training tools to disseminate the new process and train staff.

Lessons Learned

Using the QI process as a way to look more closely at not just the paperwork but the process of collecting data on latent TB cases and working with clients, Otter Tail County found a number of unexpected benefits and lessons learned.

- As they developed the electronic record, researching best practices related to latent TB, the county stumbled upon a best practice (incentives) and started to use a program they were neither looking for nor aware of: gift cards from MDH for clients who complete TB therapy.
- To help with data collection for the new electronic record, a nursing student from another county developed picture cards for communicating with non-English speaking clients. This new form of communication on TB improved not only the accuracy of information but also the nature of the interaction with clients. It also has helped improve compliance with the required regimen of medication for latent TB.
- In addition to improving communication with clients, staff and the student worker observed that wait times at the drop-in clinic were quite long. The local health department started scheduling specific appointment times and making reminder calls. This has not only improved kept appointment rates but also significantly reduced wait times at the clinics.
- DVD training tools for patient education during visits are now available for use as well.

For more information about the MCCC QI project, contact: Diane Thorson, Otter Tail County Public Health, dthorson@co.otter-tail.mn.us , 218-998-8333.

Support for this project was provided by a grant from the Robert Wood Johnson Foundation®.

Minnesota Department of Health
Office of Public Health Practice
85 East Seventh Place, Suite 200, Saint Paul, MN 55101
Phone: 651-201-3880 Fax: 651-201-3881
Email: ophp@state.mn.us

4

**Minnesota Public
Health Collaborative
for Quality
Improvement**

Carver County, Minnesota
August 2007 – May 2008

Streamlining the HAN Testing Process

The Situation

The Minnesota Department of Health (MDH) requires that each local health department and tribal health service annually test their own health alert network (HAN). During a test, a test health alert is sent to contacts in that jurisdiction. These contacts are asked for an immediate response. The local department logs how quickly those replies come in as a way of measuring how effectively the health alert is getting out. In Carver County, those tests would consume nearly a day and a half of staff time.

The health alerts in Carver County were sent out by email and one fax machine. The fax machine would take several hours to finish transmitting to its preprogrammed list of contacts. When replies came back, also by fax and by email, a staff person was assigned to make a notation of the actual time that each reply was received. Staff would continuously monitor the fax machine and email for incoming responses and record the responses on a detailed spreadsheet – a cumbersome and time-consuming process.

Everyone knew that this was an inefficient process, but they did not have a systematic way of analyzing what was happening or to figure out how to make it better. Carver County public health personnel had started to think that the only solution to this problem would be to purchase expensive tracking and communications software.

When Carver County Public Health staff heard about the opportunity to do a quality improvement project through the MLC-2 grant, they jumped at the chance to learn some new tools to solve this relatively minor but time-consuming problem.

Aim Statement

By March 1, 2008, to decrease staff time dedicated to a HAN testing event by 50 percent.

The Minnesota Public Health Collaborative for Quality Improvement is a partnership of the Minnesota Department of Health, the University of Minnesota, and the Local Public Health Association.

Carver County started by developing a **process-flow diagram** (Fig. 1) to detail the steps in conducting a HAN test, with time estimates for each part of the process, from sending the health alerts to logging the responses.

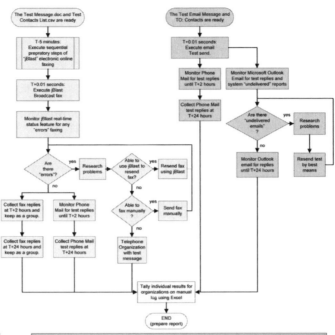

Fig. 1

Team members:

Melanie Countryman, Carver County Public Health
RaeJean Madsen, Carver County Public Health
Deb Hammond, Carver County Public Health
Emily Thompson, Carver County Public Health
Heidi Innaver, Carver County Public Health
Josh Carlyle, Carver County Public Health
LuAnne McNichols, Minnesota Department of Health
Allison Thrash, Minnesota Department of Health
Kathleen Thiede-Call, University of Minnesota Faculty Advisor
N. Pamela Saungweme, University of Minnesota Graduate Student

2

PLAN, cont'd

A **fishbone diagram** (Fig. 2) helped them to pinpoint some possible causes of excess staff time. They noted in particular that it took a long time to log test responses. They used **brainstorming** as a way of identifying possible interventions to decrease the amount of time related to logging test responses.

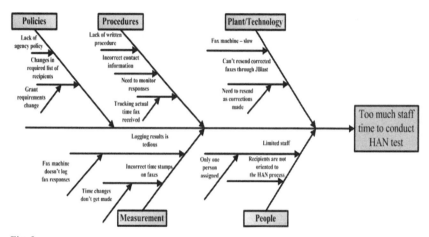

Fig. 2

Another planning step taken was to **survey** other local health departments in Minnesota to see how they conducted HAN tests and what issues they were seeing. Carver County Public Health intended to use the survey results to generate a list of additional interventions to try. The only new intervention that was identified, however, was the purchase of an emergency broadcasting system, which was cost prohibitive. However, the survey did have an added benefit of making connections with other agencies, which can continue into the future.

Carver County Public Health tested several interventions, including:

- Two people logging replies coming in by email and fax.

- Making improvements to the Excel spreadsheet to make it easier to fill out.

- Developing a standard response form which allowed less frequent monitoring of the fax machine and more efficient logging of test responses.

3

Carver analyzed the results of these interventions and discovered that the most significant change came through the revision of the reply form.

Intervention	Result
Two people logging replies	No change in staff time
Streamlined Excel spreadsheet	Decrease of 2 hours
Revised reply form (email and fax) and decreased monitoring of faxes	Decrease of 5 hours
Net decrease in staff time for event:	**70 percent**

Carver County Public Health modified their HAN testing process to incorporate the standard reply form (Fig. 3), developed a written procedure for the HAN testing process, and disseminated their survey findings to HAN staff statewide so that others can benefit from this information.

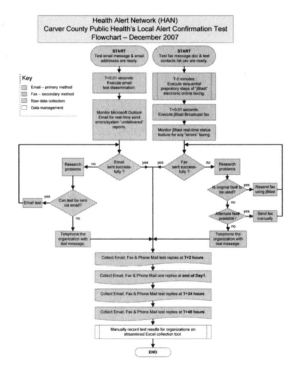

Fig. 3

4

Future plans include improving their management of the HAN contact information and increasing the percent of contacts who respond to the health alert (currently at 65 percent).

Lessons Learned

Carver County's QI project was well-defined and discrete, focused on a process that was completely within their control. That focus helped both with identifying the problem and in implementing a successful solution.

Through the use of QI tools, Carver County Public Health was able to pinpoint the real problem with the testing system – a time-consuming response logging process. As a result of having the problem accurately identified, they were able to implement a successful "low tech" and low cost solution.

For more information on the Carver County QI Project, contact Heidi Innvaer, Carver County Public Health, hinnvaer@co.carver.mn.us, 952-361-1329.

Support for this project was provided by a grant from the Robert Wood Johnson Foundation®.

Minnesota Department of Health
Office of Public Health Practice
85 East Seventh Place, Suite 200, Saint Paul, MN 55101
Phone: 651-201-3880 Fax: 651-201-3881
Email: ophp@state.mn.us

5

Northeastern Minnesota Counties
August 2007 – May 2008

**Minnesota Public
Health Collaborative
for Quality
Improvement**

The Mouths of Babes:
Increasing Acceptance of Dental Varnishing

The Situation

While early childhood caries are the single most common chronic disease of childhood, dental disease is not often recognized by the public as a serious health problem. It is 5-8 times more common than asthma and 80 percent of tooth decay is found in 25 percent of children. Many parents do not appreciate or understand the serious negative impact tooth decay can have on the lives of their children. Dental fluoride varnishing (a protective fluoride coating brushed on a child's teeth every three months) is becoming a key tool in the effort to prevent caries and improve the dental health of infants and children, especially in populations most at risk.

Over 18 local health departments in Minnesota had already implemented dental fluoride varnishing programs at the time the MLC-2 quality improvement grants were announced. However, counties in northeastern Minnesota were just beginning to raise awareness of childhood dental and oral diseases in the community while simultaneously raising awareness among local health professionals of the ease of application, low cost and safety of implementing a dental fluoride varnish program in a public health setting.

The MLC-2 project seemed to create a perfect opportunity to take advantage of a learning opportunity and to bring visibility and credibility to the practice of dental fluoride varnishing in the northeast region. Preliminary efforts revealed that not only was the practice of dental varnishing relatively unknown in the area, but a number of barriers (both internal and external) needed to be overcome to implement the procedure into local public health practice.

Aim Statement

From September 1, 2007 to November 30, 2007, at least 20 children, two months to five years of age and enrolled in the Koochiching County Women, Infants and Children (WIC) Program, will receive a PHN dental fluoride treatment.

The Minnesota Public Health Collaborative for Quality Improvement is a partnership of the Minnesota Department of Health, the University of Minnesota, and the Local Public Health Association.

Koochiching County acted as the lead county in this project. A **force-field analysis** (Fig. 1) helped to identify the driving and restraining forces for implementing dental varnishing, such as:

- resistance to the practice by area dentists and among public health professionals
- the need for education and training about dental health
- a lack of parental knowledge
- preschoolers with dental caries and access issues
- insurance problems
- too few dental health providers to accommodate the underserved population
- culture affecting family's dental decisions
- under-funded public dental services

+ Driving Forces	Restraining Forces -
Serious dental problems in at-risk children →	← Parents don't understand importance of dental health
Passionate regional advocacy →	← Overshadowed by other client needs
Easy to administer →	← Unfamiliarity with procedure
Growing "best practice" in U.S. →	← Lack of staff time
Support from dentists →	← Resistance from dentists
	← Billing/reimbursement problems
	← Lack of long-term funding

Fig. 1

Team members:

Julie Myhre, Carlton-Cook-Lake-St. Louis Community Health Board
Deb Larson, Koochiching County Public Health
Cindi Korpela, Aitkin County Public Health
Terri Allen, Carlton County Public Health
Deb Smith and Bonnie La Fromboise, Fond du Lac Reservation
Ruth Pierce, Itasca County
Mike Duffy, Lake County Public Health
Marie Margitan, Minnesota Department of Health
Kari Guida, Minnesota Department of Health
Jim Hart, University of Minnesota Faculty Advisor
Jan Arleth, University of Minnesota Graduate Student

Koochiching County designed a **process flow chart** (Fig. 2) and implemented a dental varnishing program, intended to reach children 6 months to through age 5, in programs including WIC, Maternal and Child Health (MCH) and Child and Teen Check-up (CTC.)

The other counties in the northeast region have been working to address barriers to beginning a dental varnishing program, including acceptance by county officials, local dentists, and public health staff.

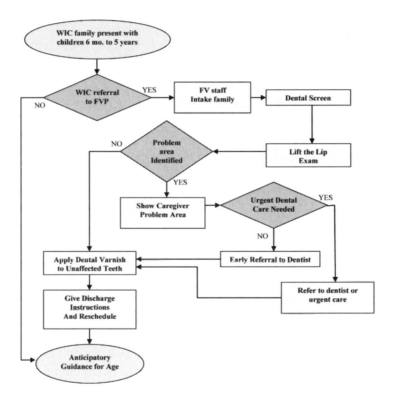

Fig. 2

3

Koochiching County has found that the work flow of the dental varnish program can be affected by the number of staff available to screen and offer dental varnishing to parents for their children, and by the number of staff available to apply the coating to teeth. As more parents come to accept dental varnishing, this process flow may need to be adapted to prevent long wait times.

This quality improvement project is still underway, as the involved counties continue to work toward developing dental varnishing programs.

Lessons Learned

The QI project helped team members to learn how to analyze a new program in its developmental stage and also how to identify real and potential barriers that might occur during implementation. Agencies that had not started a dental fluoride program were able to address those barriers and issues upfront as they moved forward in developing and implementing their own programs.

After learning more about QI, the team realized that they had already been using some QI tools but had not named them as such, i.e., brainstorming, surveys and informal force field analysis.

Participants are very interested in learning more about QI and QI tools. The project also exposed members to some helpful web-based tools (e.g., for doing surveys and creating flow charts) that they can continue to use even now.

While it could be challenging at times, the project also learned that it is possible to carry out a QI project effectively on a regional basis. The focus of the project on dental varnishing helped to engage team members in the project because it addressed a significant concern in the region (access to dental care).

For more information about the Northeast Minnesota QI project, contact Julie Myhre, Carlton-Cook-Lake-St. Louis Community Health Services, 218-733-2862, MyhreJ@communityhealthboard.org.

Support for this project was provided by a grant from the Robert Wood Johnson Foundation®.

Minnesota Department of Health
Office of Public Health Practice
85 East Seventh Place, Suite 200, Saint Paul, MN 55101
Phone: 651-201-3880 Fax: 651-201-3881
Email: ophp@state.mn.us

4

Douglas County, Minnesota
August 2007 – May 2008

**Minnesota Public
Health Collaborative
for Quality
Improvement**

Beautiful Minds:
Early Identification of Child Mental Health Needs

The Situation

In rural Minnesota, the children's mental health service delivery system perhaps can be best described as fragile. Consistently at risk due to the absence of a universal early identification process, inadequate coordination among providers, and a persistent lack of child-adolescent psychiatric services, the system has struggled to meet ever-increasing demands.

The Douglas County Children's Mental Health Collaborative, well aware of the fragility and complexity of the current system, has been challenged in recent years to explore options to both enhance and stabilize the service delivery system. In 2007, facing a significant reduction in funding, the Collaborative partners strategized about how to use their limited funds to redesign the current system, placing a greater emphasis on prevention and early intervention. "Shared care" surfaced repeatedly in local conversations as a model that had proven successful in other communities, including a community served by one of the child-adolescent psychiatrists who also serves Douglas County children.

In the fall of 2007, the desire to find a better system became a necessity when Douglas County experienced a significant decline in the already scarce landscape of child/adolescent psychiatric services due to the departure of one of the only three contracted providers in the area. Now the question of where funds could leverage the most "bang for the buck" to improve the mental health of children and adolescents was far more than theoretical…it had become urgent.

The shared care model emphasizes partnerships among professionals and with families to ensure children and adolescents get timely and appropriate screening, triage, and as indicated, treatment by the most appropriate level of practitioner. Armed with this knowledge and with the support of both the child/adolescent psychiatrists and the primary care providers, the collaborative members developed an ambitious vision for implementing the shared care model as a demonstration project. The timing of the MLC-2 quality improvement grants presented the team with a valuable opportunity to access the tools needed to bring their vision into focus.

The Minnesota Public Health Collaborative for Quality Improvement is a partnership of the Minnesota Department of Health, the University of Minnesota, and the Local Public Health Association.

Aim Statement

By March 2008, 30 children (0-18) in the PrimeWest Health System who are seen by [one of three doctors] in the clinic and diagnosed with a mental health disorder will be involved in an evidence-based shared care model.

One of the first applications of quality improvement (QI) the Douglas County project team made was to scale down their focus to a manageable level. A **fishbone diagram** (Fig. 1) helped to identify specific issues contributing to a lack of standardized social-emotional screening of children in the primary care setting.

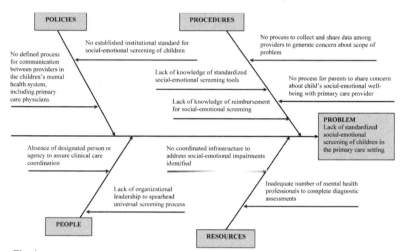

Fig 1

Team members:

Sandy Tubbs, Douglas County Public Health
Dave Stern, Douglas County Children's Mental Health Collaborative
Jeanne Barlage, PrimeWest Health
Mike Woods, Douglas County Social Services
Joyce Crowe, Alexandria Clinic
Sue Ewy, Minnesota Department of Health
Brenda Menier, Minnesota Department of Health
Donna Anderson, University of Minnesota Faculty Advisor
Helen Parsons, University of Minnesota Graduate Student

2

As a result of this analysis, the team chose to apply QI methods to the process for identifying children and adolescents with mental health needs, focusing on social-emotional screening at the child's point of entry into the primary care system.

The current screening process was then documented through a **process flow diagram** (Fig. 2). Gaps in the process were identified and a modified screening process created for one of the Alexandria area clinics. Before implementation, the process flow chart was checked and rechecked and developed in great detail to make sure no part of the process would get lost or omitted.

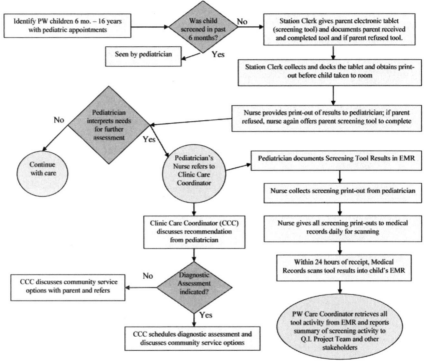

Fig. 2

During a two-week trial of the screening process, parents of a specific population of low-income children and adolescents were given the screening tool at check-in for a pediatrician visit. The results were then compared to a set of standardized indicators. The pediatrician discussed the results of the screening with the parents during the visit.

3

Following the two-week trial, gaps in the screening process were identified during a meeting of all the persons involved in the development and implementation of the screening process, and it was modified to address the identified gaps. This process (plan-do-check-act) was repeated until no further problems in the screening process were identified.

From November 28, 2007 to February 23, 2008, 254 parents of children ages six months to 16 years were offered the screening tool; 169 completed the screening, and 46 children and adolescents were identified has having potential emotional/ behavioral problems and referred to the clinic care coordinator for follow-up.

The clinic will continue to implement the screening tool, potentially expanding its use to 100 percent of the children seen at the clinic. The team will continue to gather data and follow longer-term outcomes for children who are screened to determine the effect of the early screening process on mental health outcomes.

Lessons Learned

Douglas County had a strong mental health collaborative partnership in place before beginning the QI project, which was a key strength in being able to move forward with implementation.

The development of an aim statement was instrumental in narrowing the focus of the project and assuring a clear definition of the desired outcome. The QI tool of process mapping allowed the collaborative partners to break the screening process down into small, very specific steps. The cycle of testing (using plan-do-check-act) reinforced for all involved the importance of assuring that each step of the process is clear and detailed, that all participants are engaged in the process and that everyone understands their critical role in assuring success of the process as a whole.

For more information about the Douglas County QI project, contact Sandy Tubbs, Douglas County Public Health, sandy.tubbs@mail.co.douglas.mn.us , 320-763-6018.

Support for this project was provided by a grant from the Robert Wood Johnson Foundation®.

Minnesota Department of Health
Office of Public Health Practice
85 East Seventh Place, Suite 200, Saint Paul, MN 55101
Phone: 651-201-3880 Fax: 651-201-3881
Email: ophp@state.mn.us

Southwest Minnesota Counties
August 2007 – May 2008

Minnesota Public
Health Collaborative
for Quality
Improvement

All Together Now:
Merging Data to Improve Immunization Rates

The Situation

Information "silos" are frequently acknowledged in government, but rarely addressed. Countryside Public Health – a five-county local health department in rural western Minnesota – recognized that these data silos were not merely an annoyance, but presented a barrier to improving immunization rates in their counties. Public health nurses working in various programs could not confidently make referrals for immunizations because they did not have current information at their fingertips, and parents often did not accurately recollect the immunization status of their children.

The data silos involved include data collected through the federal Women, Infants, and Children (WIC) program, the regional immunization registry (MIIC), and the state's Child and Teen Checkup (C&TC) program. These are all maintained in completely separate systems. The public health nurse would have to look up information from three data sources at the time of a clinic appointment. Experience had shown that kind of effort to be cumbersome and simply not feasible on a regular basis.

About a year before the MLC-2 quality improvement grants became available the system manager for the Southwest Minnesota Immunization Information Connection (SW-MIIC, a 29-county consortium) developed a software application that temporarily merges those three data sets for an accurate, up-to-date report on child immunization status at the time of a client appointment. This innovative application has been in use at Countryside Public Health since the spring of 2006, resulting in increases in immunization rates for four of the five counties.

When the MLC-2 grants came along, the SW-MIIC counties saw an opportunity to use QI methods to test the expansion of this software application into their own local health departments. Since every department runs their programs and clinics a bit differently, and since the consortium includes both small and large departments, the MLC-2 project team wanted to know if the new application would help to increase immunization rates throughout the region.

The Minnesota Public Health Collaborative for Quality Improvement is a partnership of the Minnesota Department of Health, the University of Minnesota, and the Local Public Health Association.

Aim Statement

By March 2008, the WIC children born 11/1/2005 to 2/28/2006 from the participating counties using the merged report will show improvements in DTaP immunization rates and C&TC outreach contacts.

Countryside did some **brainstorming**, studied process flow in the three programs (WIC-MIIC-CTC), and created a **cause and effect diagram** (Fig. 1) that helped them to identify multiple problems with the data silos in their systems, including:

- Different bits of information contained in separate data systems.
- Inaccurate reporting by parents of their children's immunization status.
- Time-consuming efforts by public health staff to look up information in multiple systems; sometimes the choice was between spending time with families or spending time on the computer.

Missed Opportunities
- Not giving all shots that are due (either parent or provider limits # given at one visit)
- Inaccurate assessment of needs
  - shot status not assessed with every visit
  - parents don't get a "Gold" card/don't present with past history/history not in MIIC
  - staff education – staff turnover, lot of information to stay updated on for changes, etc.

Vaccine Supply
- Vaccine shortages
- Storage/handling issues
- Satellite clinics may not have capacity for storing on-site vaccines; low volume clinics where vaccines not routinely stocked

Culture/Beliefs
- Conscientious objectors
- Culture – language barriers, beliefs toward health care
- Not accessing health care because of legal status
- Fear of side effects

Low childhood immunization rates

Systems/Policies
- Shortcomings of MIIC schedule – does not predict all recommended vaccines (Hep A, first influenza, handling of need for re-vaccinations)
- Immunization data slow getting into MIIC
- Patient recall system – not using or not working well
- Under or uninsured population - office charge with shots; difficulties with MnVFC program use
- Clinic hours/parent work schedule – urgent care hours don't include well child exam/ immunizations
- Not established patient

Non-Compliance with Recommendations
- Not following true contraindications
- Provider doesn't recommend a specific vaccine
- Parent doesn't comply with well-child/immunization schedule (lack understanding on importance of vaccine and complications of disease)
- Not meeting minimum intervals (not valid doses)
- Provider using oversimplified schedule – specific brands given on set schedule, may not work with patient's actual history

Fig. 1

2

Countryside then developed a way to temporarily merge three data sets to produce a single report on an "as needed" basis. The merged data is not retained, nor are the original data sets altered in any way. This means that at a client visit, public health staff can accurately check on a child's immunization status and then make the appropriate recommendation and referral to the parent.

To incorporate this merged data set effectively in each program, however, required all CTC, WIC, and immunization staff to agree to adjust their work flow processes (Fig. 2). Creating this buy-in was an important part of the project.

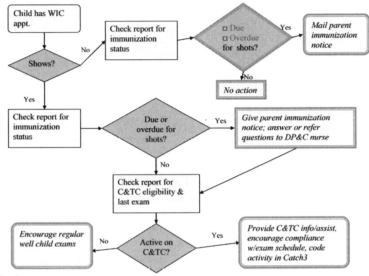

Fig. 2

Team members:

Liz Auch, Countryside Public Health
Sandy Macziewski, Countryside Public Health
Brad Meyer, Nobles-Rock Community Health Board
Genie Simon and Michelle Saffer, Redwood County Public Health
Ann Stehn and Dorie Cogelow, Kandiyohi County Public Health
Mary Rippke, Minnesota Department of Health
Mickey Scullard, Minnesota Department of Health
Donna Anderson, University of Minnesota Faculty Advisor
Selase Morgan, University of Minnesota Graduate Student

3

The counties that make up Countryside Public Health have been using the merged data report for 18 months; other counties in the southwest/southeast region are beginning to try this system in their own settings.

Since 2006, immunization rates for four of the five counties have seen some immunization rates increase. Countryside has also seen increases in the number of children getting in for medical exams. More time is needed, however, to make sure these increases are statistically significant.

Sufficient data are not yet available for the other counties to determine if the process flow changes and the merged data set are having an impact on immunization rates.

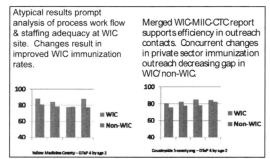

Atypical results prompt analysis of process work flow & staffing adequacy at WIC site. Changes result in improved WIC immunization rates.

Merged WIC-MIIC-CTC report supports efficiency in outreach contacts. Concurrent changes in private sector immunization outreach decreasing gap in WIC/non-WIC.

While Countryside is sharing this system and their expertise with other counties in the southwestern/southeastern region, they do not have sufficient staff time to provide the kind of technical assistance needed to implement it fully. Other counties are, however, continuing to work on making the changes required to utilize the merged immunization data effectively.

Lessons Learned

The QI tools and techniques have helped Countryside demonstrate the importance of *process* for implementing a technology change. Each program had to recognize where in their process the data was needed or would be helpful, and then be willing to alter the process to allow them to incorporate it (e.g., time to run a report). Although Countryside has received requests to share their software, they are quick to point out that it takes more than software to make this information useful for improving immunization rates – it requires active participation and cooperation by all the staff involved in these programs.

For more information about the Southwest Minnesota QI project, contact Liz Auch, Countryside Public Health Service, lauch@countryside.co.mn.us , 320-843-4546.

Support for this project was provided by a grant from the Robert Wood Johnson Foundation®.

Minnesota Department of Health
Office of Public Health Practice
85 East Seventh Place, Suite 200, Saint Paul, MN 55101
Phone: 651-201-3880 Fax: 651-201-3881
Email: ophp@state.mn.us

4

Sherburne County, Minnesota
August 2007 – May 2008

**Minnesota Public
Health Collaborative
for Quality
Improvement**

On Time: Preventing Gaps in PCA Services

The Situation

Minnesota's Personal Care Assistance (PCA) program is designed to support people of all ages with disabilities to live independently in the community. Clients must meet four basic requirements: 1) be eligible for Medical Assistance or Minnesota Care Expanded Benefits or be eligible for the Alternative Care program; 2) be assessed by the country as having a need for PCA services; 3) have a doctor's statement of need for PCA services; and 4) be able to make decisions about their care or have a responsible party who can make those decisions.

It was a great surprise to Sherburne County Public Health, which conducts the PCA assessments in their county, when the Minnesota Department of Human Services (DHS) came out with a report in 2007 that said only 32 percent of PCA assessments statewide were entered into the Medicaid Management Information System (MMIS) on time. Delays in assessment meant delays in recertification, which in turn meant delays in needed services.

Upon further inquiry, Sherburne County Public Health discovered their rate, at 61 percent, was significantly better than the statewide average. But that still left over a third of this vulnerable population with a potential gap in needed services. And Sherburne County was not the only entity concerned about the well-being of their community. Advocates for the physically and mentally disabled had succeeded in getting legislation approved that now requires all counties to increase their rate of on-time PCA reassessments (entered into MMIS) to 100 percent. Counties that do not meet this goal will be assessed a fiscal penalty.

Aim Statement

By February 29, 2008, increase the percentage of Personal Care Assistant Reassessments that are completed on time (i.e., entered into the data system before the beginning date of the new service agreement) from 62 to 80 percent.

The Minnesota Public Health Collaborative for Quality Improvement is a partnership of the Minnesota Department of Health, the University of Minnesota, and the Local Public Health Association.

Sherburne County took immediate advantage of the tools presented at the QI trainings to examine their process for potential changes. They created a map of the current process with a process flow diagram that had more steps and persons involved than they had originally thought.

A **fishbone diagram** (Fig. 1) helped them pinpoint the causes of delays, and identified which ones were within the public health department's control. They saw that many different people and organizations had potential roles in the PCA reassessment and input process, and found that even within the public health department different individuals had different methods for going about the reassessment.

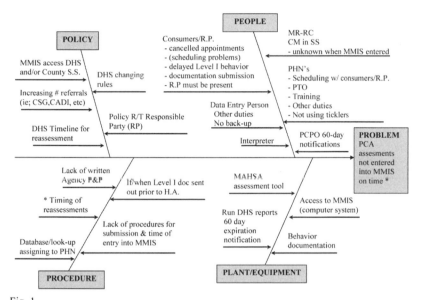

Fig. 1

Team members:

Vonna Henry, Director, Sherburne County Public Health
Kathy Landwehr, Sherburne County Public Health
Kristen Sanders, Sherburne County Public Health
Linda Wolford, MN Department of Human Services
Sue Strohschein, Minnesota Department of Health
Gail Gentling, Minnesota Department of Health
Karen Kuntz, University of Minnesota Faculty Advisor
Mayanka Singh, University of Minnesota Graduate Student

One of the first changes that Sherburne County implemented was to initiate the PCA reassessment process a month earlier – at 60 days prior, instead of 30. They had also realized that if the process got "stuck" at some point (for example, missing one piece of information), it tended to stay there, so they decided to send the necessary paperwork in immediately, even with missing or incomplete information, since the needed information could be added by amending the paperwork later. They created a new **process flow chart** (Fig. 2) for the PCA assessment so that all staff would be following the same procedures.

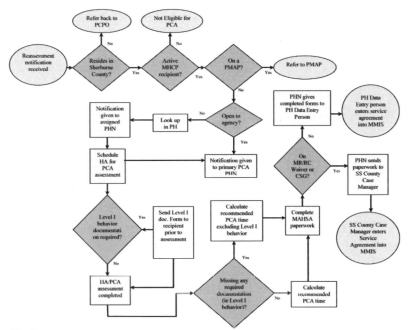

Fig. 2

Sherburne County recently did a manual review of PCA reassessments to determine if they had improved their one-time rate. According to their review, 100 percent of the assessments completed between October 1, 2007 and December 31, 2007 were inputted into MMIS on time. However, Sherburne County is currently waiting for data from DHS to see if their information agrees with Sherburne's findings. Sherburne County wants to make sure they used the same data gathering process that was used in the initial DHS report to assure that the changes in their process did indeed affect the outcome.

3

Even as Sherburne County waits for their data, they are implementing changes within their public health department. The detailed analysis of the PCA assessment process revealed a number of ways in which public health staff could be of more service to clients and families, such as sending them the behavior documentation form prior to the reassessment visit by public health staff.

Lessons Learned

Sherburne County found the QI tools extremely helpful in locating concrete action steps in the midst of a complex and potentially confusing process involving multiple state and local government agencies, advocates, and clients. The cause and effect analysis, in particular, revealed the areas for change that public health could influence.

The initial concern of Sherburne County public health staff to the QI project was that it meant they were not doing a good job. Once they understood that the focus is on the process, and caught the vision for making improvements to the process, they became more enthusiastic. One of the principal concerns now is being held accountable for "fixing" something that has many parts which are not within their control.

Sherburne County also learned that taking a detailed look at one process (albeit a complex one) can yield more than expected. The QI project revealed a variety of (sometimes unrelated) ways that they could adjust what they were doing to better serve the people of their community.

For more information about the Sherburne County Public Health QI project, contact Vonna Henry, Sherburne County Public Health Department, vonna.henry@co.sherburne.mn.us , 763/241-2750.

Support for this project was provided by a grant from the Robert Wood Johnson Foundation®.

Minnesota Department of Health
Office of Public Health Practice
85 East Seventh Place, Suite 200, Saint Paul, MN 55101
Phone: 651-201-3880 Fax: 651-201-3881
Email: ophp@state.mn.us

4

**Minnesota Public
Health Collaborative
for Quality
Improvement**

*Olmsted County, Minnesota
August 2007 – May 2008*

Core Strength:
Improving the Local Public Health Workforce

The Situation

A culture of quality improvement is well entrenched in Olmsted County. For many years county government has focused on improving quality in their services. Within this QI culture, the Olmsted County Public Health Services department used a well-developed performance management system that includes a focus on county-wide workforce competencies. However, the system lacked competencies specifically related to the public health workforce. Without a measurable set of skills, knowledge and attitudes necessary for the practice of public health, managers have been limited in their ability to help employees improve their capacity to provide essential public health services.

Public health managers also could see national accreditation for public health departments appearing on the horizon, and agreed that becoming accredited would be a high priority. Getting ready for accreditation put even more importance on developing a performance management system that would improve the practice of public health.

The MLC-2 project presented a good opportunity to become more intentional and systematic about incorporating a set of public health core competencies into the performance management system, while at the same time making needed improvements to that system.

Aim Statement

By December 2007, 100 percent of Leadership Council members will rate their understanding of public health competencies at 3 or higher (1-5 scale).

The Minnesota Public Health Collaborative for Quality Improvement is a partnership of the Minnesota Department of Health, the University of Minnesota, and the Local Public Health Association.

Olmsted County first created a **logic model** (Fig. 1) that not only identified their ultimate goals (improved public health system performance and improved population health), but also clarified how the QI project fit into their vision and what other elements needed to be addressed. One of those needs was to identify a set of public health core competencies that could be incorporated into the performance management system for public health. They then had managers self-assess their proficiency in the selected core competency domains.

Target Group	Project Plan			Outcome Plan		
	Activities *What we do*	Inputs *What we invest*	Outputs *What we deliver*	Outcome Statement		
				"Learning" →	*"Action"* →	*"Conditions"*
	Activities, Tasks	Resources	Deliverables	Short-Term	Intermediate (Impact)	Long-Term (Impact)
"Phase One *Leadership Council*	• Assess LC awareness of PH Competencies • Determine which PH competencies to include in OCPHS performance Management system for leadership positions. • Assess LC proficiency in selected PH competencies	• Steering committee planning, meeting, training development, time • Meeting, training time for LC and CI Committee	• A set of PH competencies specifically deemed to be important to our work at OCPHS, for use in professional development and performance management for all LC positions • A professional development plan for each LC member	• Increased LC understanding of PH competencies and their use in professional development and performance management" **END OF MLC2 PROJECT**	• Adjust process as needed for roll-out to all OCPHS staff	
Beyond Phase One *all OCPHS Staff* **GOES BEYOND MLC2 PROJECT**	• LC members "work" their development plans • Lessons learned from phase one to adjust process as needed for roll out to all staff	• LC time for professional development planning	• A set of PH competencies specifically deemed to be important to our work at OCPHS, for use in professional development and performance management for all positions at OCPHS	• Increased staff understanding of PH competencies	• Increase LC ability to effectively develop PH competencies in their staff	• Increase staff ability to meet specific PH competencies as shown through increased PH competency ratings in performance appraisals • Maximize PH competency within our agency (maintain a competent public health workforce)
				Public Health Outcome	Improved PH system performance Improved population health	

Fig. 1

Team members:

Dawn Beck, Olmsted County Public Health
Marilyn Deling, Olmsted County Public Health
Judy Voss, Olmsted County Public Health
Marty Aleman, Olmsted County Public Health
Pete Geisen, Olmsted County Public Health
Denise Daniels, Olmsted County Public Health
Kathy Dubbels, Olmsted County Public Health
Larry Edmonson, Olmsted County Public Health
Mary Orban, Minnesota Department of Health
Barb Dalbec, Minnesota Department of Health
Jim Hart, University of Minnesota Faculty Advisor
Anthony Mbuthia, University of Minnesota Graduate Student

The next step was to create a **process flowchart** (Fig. 2) of the performance appraisal process to assess it for variation in the process (i.e., how managers were doing it differently) and areas for improvement. The main areas identified were a need for more focus on goal-setting and working on regular, systematic employee development (i.e., not just at the time of the appraisal).

They also **surveyed** managers to gauge their level of awareness of the public health core

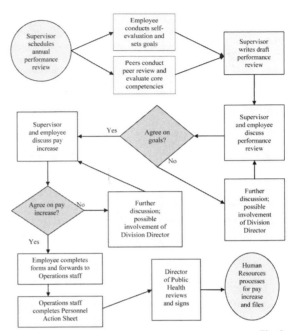

Fig. 2

competencies and found that only 28 percent were aware of public health core competencies and how to use them in professional development and staff performance appraisal.

Olmsted County began to implement changes in the performance management process by:

1) Training supervisory staff in the public health core competencies;
2) Improving the performance management system so that it could effectively use the public health core competencies; and
3) Incorporating the public health core competencies into the improved performance management system.

3

A **follow-up survey** of managers found that awareness of public health core competencies and their use in staff development and appraisals had increased from 28 to 62 percent. Olmsted County plans to use the improved performance management system with managers during 2008 and to continue to evaluate and make changes (if needed), using the **plan-do-study-act** cycle. In 2009 they plan to use the improved performance management system with all public health department staff.

After the improved performance management system is in place, the public health core competencies will be added into the process. Training will be extended to all public health staff, to help them do their jobs in a way that reflects the core public health competencies. Plans also include continuing the self-assessments (e.g., on an annual basis) to determine training and budget needs.

Lessons Learned

Olmsted County discovered that the QI process requires a time commitment, as well as a commitment to being open to learning from the process and a readiness to apply the information learned. It also requires group commitment and collaboration – all the players need to be given a chance to participate so that the process becomes a form of group problem-solving.

Olmsted County found many different QI tools to be effective for assessing problems, and discovered that it was helpful to learn how to apply the different tools in different situations.

Olmsted County also struggled with the complexity of their project. It has a long time frame, of which the MLC-2 grant was just a part. Their project also has a lot of specific terminology which frequently made it difficult to explain, but they ultimately found the QI effort helpful for learning to "tell the story" of their performance management improvement efforts.

For more information about the Olmsted County QI project, contact Marilyn Deling, deling.marilyn@co.olmsted.mn.us; Dawn Beck, beck.dawn@co.olmsted.mn.us; or Judy Voss, voss.judy@co.olmsted.mn.us, Olmsted County Public Health Services (507) 328-7500.

Support for this project was provided by a grant from the Robert Wood Johnson Foundation®.

Minnesota Department of Health
Office of Public Health Practice
85 East Seventh Place, Suite 200, Saint Paul, MN 55101
Phone: 651-201-3880 Fax: 651-201-3881
Email: ophp@state.mn.us

4

Chapter 26

Translating Clinical Quality Improvement Success to Public Health

Bridget K. McCabe, Cathy R. Taylor, and Susan R. Cooper

CLINICAL QUALITY IMPROVEMENT SUCCESS

Some 20 years ago, the healthcare industry began adoption of continuous quality improvement (QI) models used by other complex industrial systems such as airlines and automakers to determine if these techniques could also work for healthcare. From hospitals to ambulatory care settings, organizations across the country are striving to put evidence-based best practices into everyday clinical care. Public health has a rich body of population-based health improvement work to study, for both best practices and lessons learned.

This chapter describes how Tennessee's public health system applied an evidence-based clinical quality improvement approach to improving clinical care in the near term and to decreasing tobacco use at the population level in the longer term. Building on early successes, Tennessee is using the model to educate and support its workforce in developing and implementing other clinical QI initiatives specifically designed to protect, promote, and improve the health of the public. Lessons learned can be used to guide and inform QI efforts in similar venues.

HOW TO BEGIN—THE MODEL WITH WHICH ONE STATE STARTED BUILDING PUBLIC HEALTH SYSTEM IMPROVEMENTS

As with any improvement initiative, a system seeking change benefits from following an improvement model. In Tennessee, we adopted the plan–do–study–act (PDSA) improvement model (Figure 26.1). The choice of this model hinged on two key factors: 1) the leadership had experience with the PDSA cycle in clinical venues, and 2) the cycle is simple in design, easily understood by all levels of staff, and already in use by several groups in the Tennessee Department of Health without their even knowing the formal terminology and theories.

While the PDSA improvement model can be used for projects big and small, Tennessee Department of Health leadership made systems-level quality improvement a top priority. The first step was to start a *broad* planning process with executive staff. The goal of the process was to ensure that the system-level changes are

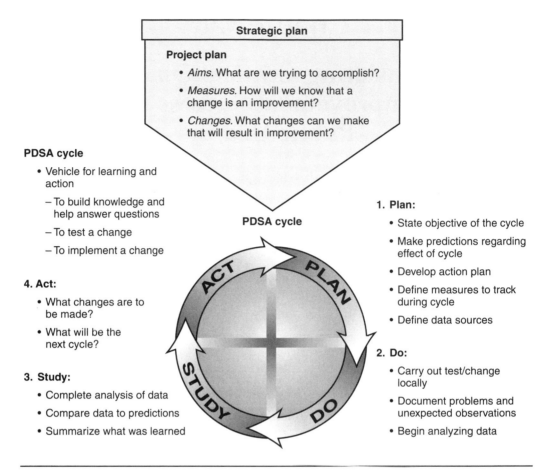

Figure 26.1   PDSA model for improvement.

Adapted from: G. J. Langley, K. M. Nolan, T. W. Nolan, C. L. Norman, L. P. Provost, *The Improvement Guide: A Practical Approach to Enhancing Organizational Performance* (San Francisco: Jossey-Bass, 1996): 10, 60.

consistent with the department's strategic plan and mission. Initially, a leadership group assessed and prioritized the state's public health resources, needs, and challenges. The more specific project planning would be done with a diverse team representing various stakeholders in the process to be changed.

STEP 1. PLAN

1a. Broad Planning

What Could the Public Health System Do Better? In aiming to make improvements, you first have to identify the problem. Often there are too many problems to tackle all at once, so how do you decide? QI projects tend to fall into four categories:

- High impact targets or goals with little effort required (low-hanging fruit)

- High impact targets or goals with significant effort required (high-hanging fruit)

- Low impact targets or goals with little effort required

- Low impact targets or goals with significant effort required

Ideally, QI projects should stick to the first three categories. To build the QI momentum, you will want to start with "low-hanging fruit"—a high impact target with little effort required.

Tennessee's Tobacco Trifecta—An Opportunity to Adopt Successful Clinical QI Practices. For Tennessee, it is no secret that we need significant improvement in many health indicators. Tobacco is the leading cause of morbidity and mortality in the U.S., and Tennessee is one of the highest tobacco-using states in the country. Prior to 2007, the public health system in Tennessee tried valiantly to reduce tobacco use and initiation. However, traditional smoking cessation services were delivered through multiple programs operating independently across the state, each program with its own methods.

In the summer of 2007, Tennessee made history as the first tobacco-producing state to simultaneously adopt smoke-free legislation and increase the state cigarette tax by over 200 percent. With this effort came commitment from the top in the governor's office and the health commissioner's office to support tobacco cessation initiatives across the state. The State of Tennessee Department of Health saw an opportunity—a window opening—to adopt clinical best practices within a framework of continuous quality improvement that targeted both the system and the healthcare provider within the system. We had all of the essential elements that make a QI initiative successful: a will to improve, ideas about alternatives to the status quo, and resources and commitment to execute and make it real.[1]

The Tennessee tobacco cessation initiative was as close to low-hanging fruit as we could hope to find. In addition, we had tremendous support inside and outside the public health system for such an initiative.

1b. Project Planning

With an opportunity for change identified, we developed a project plan and followed the steps of the PDSA cycle.

Forming the Team and Defining the Aims. The tobacco team had representation from all levels of healthcare providers as well as leadership (that is, state commissioner of health and assistant commissioner, who oversees the local health departments) and experts in the following topic areas: tobacco cessation, clinical quality improvement, and data management and information technology. Additional members were added to lend expertise to particular advisory groups that developed from the team. The goal was to have all stakeholders in the process represented.

What Are Our Goals and Specific Objectives? With any new program, a realistic assessment of what you hope to achieve is a good starting point. First we defined our overriding goals: to further reduce tobacco use and initiation in Tennessee over the course of a three-year period. Yet, we know that these goals are long-term and will require years of sustained effort, so to follow the progress of the program, we defined SMART (the mnemonic for *s*pecific, *m*easurable, *a*chievable, *r*elevant, and *t*ime-bound) objectives, divided them into short, intermediate, and long term, and ranked them in priority. For Tennessee's tobacco cessation initiative, we have:

- *Short term.* Assess every patient age 13 and older for tobacco use every clinical visit; for patients with frequent use of clinical services, the tobacco assessment would occur no more frequently than monthly.

- *Intermediate term.* Encourage tobacco-using patients who are not willing to quit to considering quitting at every clinical visit. Assist tobacco-using patients who are willing to quit in entering treatment at every clinical visit.

- *Long term.* Reduce the percentage of Tennessee Department of Health patients who smoke over the course of three years. Reduce the percentage of all Tennesseans who smoke over the course of three years.

Each of these objectives is measurable with the indicators being defined in Section 1c: Measures.

What Prior Knowledge (Best Practices) Can We Apply? Tobacco cessation research has a large body of evidence to support the adoption of standardized, effective clinical practice guidelines, tools, and processes. Such guidelines, however, are not necessarily applicable to special populations like those encountered in the public health setting. In order to make sure our guidelines would be effective, we first went to the Public Health Service–sponsored clinical practice guidelines, then to PubMed for a medical literature review.

Using both the clinical practice guidelines[2] and results of the literature search as the foundation for the Tennessee tobacco cessation program, we developed standardized protocols for each provider category found in the local health departments (for example, physician, nurse, clerk). In standardizing the protocol for the various care providers, we sought a standard (or baseline) level of care for all clients utilizing the public health system. These processes formed the program work steps and the foundation from which we trained and educated the workforce.

We developed protocols for prescribing-level providers (that is, physicians and advanced nurse practitioners) and for non-prescribing-level providers (that is, nurses, dieticians, home visiting paraprofessionals, and front desk clerical staff). The protocols offered a clear, standardized road map as to how each level of provider would offer tobacco cessation services and, if appropriate, counseling. All protocols are complementary. Messages to clients are standardized, cohesive, and frequently repeated for maximum effect.

Significant components of the tobacco cessation program are:

1. Standardized protocols for in-office, short counseling sessions and for treatment with either over-the-counter or prescription medication

2. Increased access to tobacco cessation services with reduced barriers to treatment by dispensing reduced-cost medication at the point of care

3. Automatic referral to Tennessee QuitLine for patients who are ready to quit

4. Efficient data capture through an existing administrative database

5. A structure to evaluate many quick cycles of quality improvement (also called continuous rapid-cycle improvement; see Figure 26.5, page 393).

1c. Measures

How Will We Identify Areas of Success and Areas in Need of Improvement in the Program? For public health programs, measures typically are of three types: process measures, outcome measures, and capacity measures.

Tennessee identified measures to capture both the process and the outcomes for different time frames. We were careful to choose objective measures that reflect systematic clinical performance processes as well as the complex process a patient goes through in attempting to quit tobacco. The program's logic model followed the *transtheoretical model of change*.[3] If we only had a long-term measure, then we would not see much change in the early months or even the first two years of the program. We would not be able to determine if our program worked, or we might wrongly think it did not, if we only looked at early smoking rates.

The process and outcome measures are listed in Figure 26.2. We have yet to set capacity measures as we continue to explore staff expertise (licensed versus unlicensed) and other contributors potentially affecting program outcomes. Currently, we are measuring staffing levels along with patient tobacco use and cessation

---

Process measures

- What percentage of eligible patients (that is, clinical patients ages 13 years and older) are we screening each month? (Also a short-term outcome measure.)

- What percentage of eligible patients (that is, tobacco users) are we counseling each month?

- What percentage of eligible patients (that is, tobacco users willing to quit) enroll in the Tennessee QuitLine and/or start on tobacco cessation medication each month?

- What percentage of tobacco users on tobacco cessation medication return for resupply?

Outcome measures

- *Short term.* Percentage of eligible patients we are screening each month? Each year? Since the start of the program?

- *Intermediate term.* Percentage of tobacco-using patients who change from *not willing to quit* to *willing to quit* each month? Each year? Since the start of the program?

- *Long term.* Percentage of Tennessee Department of Health patients who use tobacco and who smoke (measured annually), percentage of Tennesseans who smoke* (measured annually).

Figure 26.2   Tobacco cessation program measures.

* Center for Disease Control and Prevention, Behavioral Risk Factor Surveillance System data; definition of current smoker is at least 100 cigarettes smoked and currently smokes every day or some days.

behaviors. We are also developing methods to determine optimal staffing for this initiative and for the Tennessee public health system.

How Can We Compare This Program to Another? To be able to compare our results to another program either in Tennessee or elsewhere across the country, we looked at existing surveillance systems and measures. Many measures exist for tobacco and have been conveniently compiled by the Centers for Disease Control and Prevention (CDC). We used, whenever possible, a standardized and validated measure. In the Tennessee tobacco cessation program, tobacco use by patients is captured by three areas of the health department staff: 1) a screening question at the check-in counter, 2) by the patient directly in a patient self-assessment form, and 3) by classification of tobacco use by a healthcare provider. The patient self-assessment utilized questions from *Key Outcome Indicators for Evaluating Comprehensive Tobacco Control Programs* (May 2005)[4] and overlaps with the state's Behavioral Risk Factor Surveillance System (BRFSS) and other statewide surveillance systems. Multiple levels of screening are essential for data quality reviews. A patient, whether a smoker or nonsmoker, should have consistent answers to screening questions and tobacco use questions at each of the three data capture points.

1d. Changes

Some perceive change as an opportunity, while others perceive change as a threat. In Tennessee we are developing a three-part mantra to overcome the biggest hesitations seen when beginning to think about change. Simply stated:

First, *"You eat an elephant one bite at a time."* (African proverb)

Second, *"Don't let the perfect be the enemy of the good."*

And finally, strive for changes that *"Make it easy to do right and hard to do wrong."*

Eating an elephant. If a project appears too large, then divide the project into smaller, manageable parts.

Perfection. Perfection is an aspirational goal; an industry standard is a realistic goal. If you worry too much about getting it completely right, you may never start—don't be concerned about achieving perfection.

Easy to do right. And finally, take any opportunity to remove the potential for human error to enter the system. For example, if a process requires steps A, B, and C in that order, then try to design a system that makes any other order impossible (Figure 26.3).

What Is the Current Process? In viewing how a patient accesses tobacco services at the local health department, we mapped the clinical process by identifying patient contact points during the course of a visit. The patient interacts with three or four different public health staff during any given visit (see Figure 26.4).

The initial process review identified which programs provided tobacco cessation services and which level of staff screened, provided counseling, and/or prescribed medication. The team also assessed best practices for tobacco cessation as they relate to our current system. We asked where we could enhance what we do

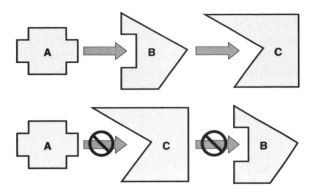

Figure 26.3   "Make it easy to do right and hard to do wrong."

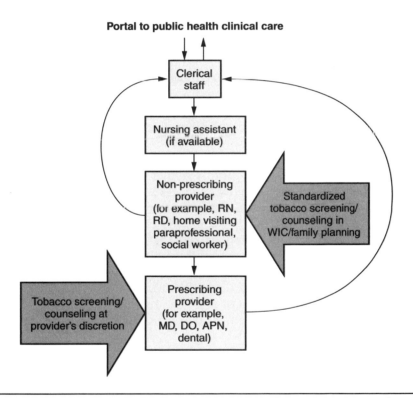

Figure 26.4   Tobacco cessation services within the context of clinical care patient flow in local health department.

well and improve what we do not do well or do not do at all. We discovered that WIC and family planning nursing staff screened for tobacco and provided initial counseling based on a protocol. Primary care clinicians screened some but not all patients, and referrals to the Tennessee QuitLine (an evidence-based tobacco cessation coaching program available free to all Tennesseans) were infrequent.

How Would the Best Practices Fit into Our Current System? We started by identifying the ideal (or standardized) processes and clinical practice guidelines for treating tobacco use. Next, we examined characteristics of health departments across the state that would most impact their ability to completely follow the guidelines. *The numbers and type of staff (that is, prescribing level versus nonprescribing healthcare providers and support staff) at each local health department and the time currently allotted to a clinical visit are the most significant characteristics.*

In Tennessee, there are essentially three categories of local health departments: 1) small one-nurse local health departments with occasional services by traveling physicians, 2) large local health departments with additional primary care services, and 3) large, traditional metropolitan health departments with limited access to on-site prescribing providers and primary care services. Not every health department has access to all level of providers on site. Yet, one strength is the centralized nature of the Tennessee public health system. Tennessee has 95 counties divided into 13 regions: 7 rural regions and 6 metropolitan regions. All rural regions are under the direction of the state health agency, while the metropolitan regions are under contract to the state health agency for statewide programs. Each county has its own local health department supported by a regional office and by larger county health departments within the region.

Knowing the challenges of fitting a standardized process to vastly different categories of health departments, we returned to the process map to identify potential solutions. Each step in the process was written on a sticky note and rearranged for each category of health department. A composite process map representing the potential solution is shown in Figure 26.5; the darker gray boxes and dotted arrows indicate the data capture points.

In addition to the strengths of the top-down, protocol-driven environment of the local health departments, the Tennessee public health system has a single administrative data collection system called the Patient Tracking and Billing Management Information System (PTBMIS). The system captures all patient registration information and demographics, pharmacy inventory and dispensed medication, and all diagnosis and procedures coding. Additional screens can be added to the system to create a hybrid billing and medical information system. Tobacco data are captured from paper forms by the clerical staffs that then enter this data into the administrative hybrid system (PTBMIS).

STEP 2. DO

The tobacco initiative was piloted in August 2007. Over the first 18 months of the program, we reviewed the data quality and gathered baseline data for all measures. Since data for the tobacco cessation program are collected at the point of care through the state's centralized data system, we have near daily access to the data to show how well we are doing with regard to our measures. Process measures are collected and reviewed on a monthly basis. More specifically, short-term and intermediate-term measures are collected and reviewed on a monthly basis while the long-term outcome measures, though collected each month, are reviewed over the course of a year (see Figure 26.2).

Each quarter, we have attempted to set an agenda with regard to a particular measure, either within a region or across the state, and follow a rapid cycle

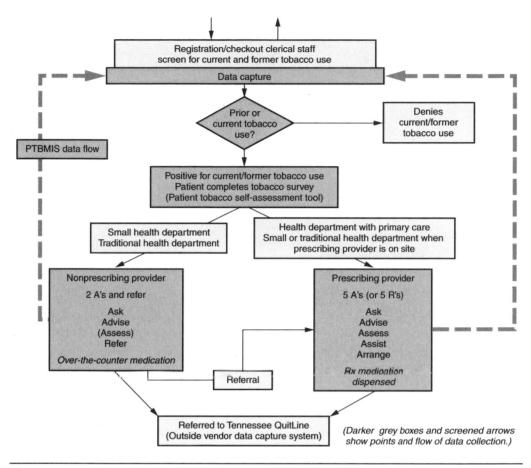

Figure 26.5   Composite process map of best-practice and current system constraints for patient flow in tobacco cessation.

of continuous quality improvement (Figure 26.6). We have built the collaborative network around a monthly (often bimonthly) teleconference that has been the foundation of two-way communication between the central office and the regions participating in the improvement process.

The focus was placed on an evaluation of the data quality and process measures as the program was implemented. While reviewing the data quality, we noted that only about 10 percent of tobacco users placed on tobacco cessation medication returned for the first and second resupply (that is, resupply rate), below our early estimates of 35 percent to 45 percent of patients starting tobacco cessation medication. We arrived at the estimated rate by looking at short-term (one to two months) quit rates for medications in the population we serve but projected a slightly higher rate to account for the large financial subsidy the program assumed with regard to the cost of visits and the cost of medication. For most of our very low income patients, the cost of the medications would be a co-pay of five dollars to seven dollars, about five percent of the wholesale price, with a negligible charge for the visit.

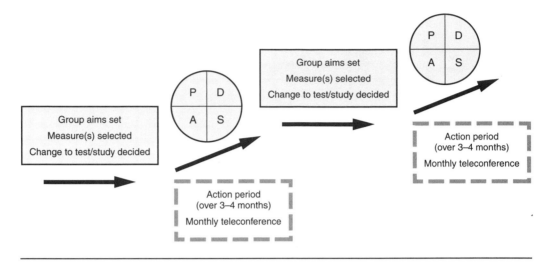

Figure 26.6 Continuous rapid cycle improvement.

Adapted from: "The Breakthrough Series: Institute for Healthcare Improvement Collaboration Model for Achieving Breakthrough Improvement," Innovation Series 2003, www.ihi.org.

Each region was instructed to implement a patient tracking system and appointment reminder system specifically for tobacco cessation patients receiving medication. Some regions with small local health departments developed a simple Excel spreadsheet with phone call reminders. Others utilized the tracking and appointment reminder system in the current PTBMIS administrative and billing system. One region centralized the patient tracking and appointment reminder system to one person overseeing multiple local health departments in the region.

STEP 3. STUDY

All regions tracked the percentage of patients receiving tobacco cessation medication that had a return visit for resupply and continued counseling. The group decided to allow a 15-day grace period for patients to return for a second visit. If a patient agreed to tobacco cessation treatment and received a 30-day supply of medication, then the patient had up to 45 days after receiving the first medication supply to receive the second. The results are highlighted in Figure 26.7.

Region 3 has shown the greatest improvement (return rate nearly doubled) with the simple excel spreadsheet and telephone reminder system. The improvement was not limited to one type of change. Region 1 showed modest improvement with implementing the PTBMIS patient reminder system, which generates a form letter two weeks prior to an appointment. The low-technology solution of an Excel spreadsheet and telephone contact was more consistently adopted (100 percent) by the local health departments in each of the counties in region 3 in comparison to the limited adoption of the PTBMIS system in region 1.

The other important short-term measure followed by the program is the tobacco screening rates (that is, percent of eligible patients who are screened for

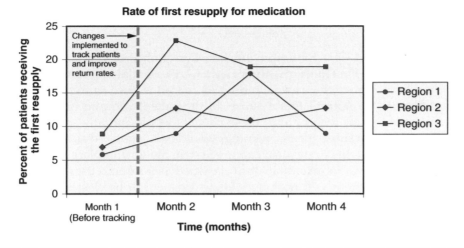

Figure 26.7 Percentage of patients returning within 45 days for a second 30-day supply of tobacco cessation medication.

tobacco use); the screening rates have been consistently high across the regions. Initial screening by the clerical staff is greater than 97 percent, and follow-up screening and tobacco use classification by a healthcare provider is greater than 93 percent. The screening process identifies the subset of the population currently using cigarette tobacco (approximately 33 percent of all screened patients, age 13 years and older, utilizing the Tennessee public health system for clinical services). Cigarette use among local health department patients (33 percent) is higher than in the general Tennessee population (25 percent).

STEP 4. ACT

Each of the 13 regions were given options as to the process by which they would track patients and encourage program compliance; however, each region was encouraged to modify their tracking methods for patients in the tobacco cessation program to target increasing resupply return rates. Region 3's approach (Excel spreadsheet plus telephone reminders) was the most successful of the approaches at increasing resupply rates, and the team has decided to spread this simple patient reminder system to other participating regions. Notwithstanding these efforts, resupply rates continue to be below the target goal of 35 percent to 45 percent; thus, additional rapid-cycle improvements are under review.

STEP 5. KNOWLEDGE CAPTURE, EDUCATION, AND QI ADVANCEMENT

Knowledge Capture. Documenting what does not work is just as important as documenting what does. Failures can provide invaluable learning opportunities for given populations that inform the next QI process. To document the improvement process, both successes and failures, we have started summarizing the efforts of each region into a one-page storyboard.

Lessons Learned. The Tennessee Tobacco Cessation Project was not without its lessons learned. First, data quality reviews were essential to troubleshoot the data capture system and the understanding of and adherence to the protocols. Most significantly, we noticed that a subset of the patients figured out how to avoid being screened for tobacco use; these patients would initially screen *positive for tobacco* use but in subsequent screenings would be categorized as *never having used tobacco*. Internal edits to the data capture system are now in place to prevent illogical classifications; for example, once classified as a tobacco user by a healthcare provider, the system will no longer allow a patient to be classified as one who never used tobacco.

Second, modifications to protocols were needed after the program launched. Large, more traditional public health departments did not have sufficient staffing levels of prescribing-level providers to supply prescription tobacco cessation medication to patients. While having physicians and advanced practice nurses on staff, the metropolitan health departments have most of the high-level providers in either administrative roles or in very limited patient caring roles such as in a tuberculosis (TB) clinic. To adjust, the program added more types of over-the-counter tobacco cessation medications, which could be supplied along with counseling by nursing staff via strict protocol to patients meeting the program criteria. In addition, smaller health departments referred patients who wanted prescription tobacco cessation medication to larger health departments with more physicians and advanced practice nurse staff. A useful tool we are generating from this second lesson learned is a Web-based survey to capture activity levels (administrative versus patient care) of staff. The Web-based survey also is being used to track a provider's knowledge, current practices, and attitudes prior to and after protocol implementation.

Education and QI Advancement. In Tennessee, initial improvement team members are forming a core group of quality improvement champions and experts that will provide the foundation for development of more public health QI initiatives. These local champions will introduce improvement model and PDSA methods and terminology. For many in Tennessee's public health system, as is likely across the country, the concepts of rapid-cycle improvement are not new. Many are doing QI in small ways without even knowing it. Tennessee's champions are QI teachers, trainers, and facilitators working to develop dynamic solutions to public health challenges at local, regional, and state levels.

Acknowledgement: Thank-you to Ellen Omohundro, PhD, for statistical support and for critical review of this chapter.

Chapter 27

Risk Management: Optimizing Scarce Resources

Grace L. Duffy and John W. Moran

WHAT IS RISK?

Risk is nothing more than the probability of the occurrence of an adverse consequence multiplied by the value (cost) of that adverse consequence. In public health situations, some programs or treatment strategies are simply too important to cease or scale back drastically within the community (number of deaths from diabetes or asthma if program funding is cut beyond a certain level, for example). The decision process for balancing scarce public health funding is not an easy one.

Figure 27.1 shows the progression of a commitment to action followed by the generation of risks consequent to the action. Continuing with the action causes risk closure, resulting in either a negative result being experienced, or the successful outcome of the action because of risk mitigation techniques.

Interest in risk management is growing and, according to some, approaching the level of interest in quality management. In this chapter, we will explore why the migration to risk management is occurring and what public health can do to position itself to take advantage of this shift.

Risk can be defined as the combination of the probability of an event and its consequences. Risk management is increasingly recognized as being concerned

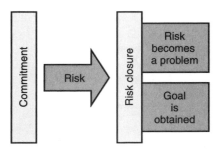

Figure 27.1 Risk is the possibility of a problem.

Source: L. Westfall, "Risk Management" (Presentation, ASQ World Conference on Quality and Improvement, Houston, TX, 2008).

with both positive and negative aspects of risk. Therefore this chapter considers risk from both perspectives.

In the safety field, it is generally recognized that consequences are only negative and therefore the management of safety risk is focused on prevention and mitigation of harm. In public health, risk can also be considered from the positive outcomes of communitywide assessments, expanding community partnerships, or inclusion of additional stakeholders focused on the success of targeted initiatives.

A complementary benefit analysis goes hand-in-hand with risk analysis in that there is a method for directly comparing the expected benefit to the potential risk in financial terms or in future relationships with the community. A risk matrix is offered later in this chapter as a tool for conducting a risk–benefit analysis.

The analysis of risk involves determining adverse event precursors and determining their probability. If the consequence (cost) is unacceptable after analysis, the analysis is usually transformed into a series of mitigations to reduce probability of the event precursors(s).[1]

Figure 27.2 illustrates the balance required during risk assessment. On the one side is the probability of a problem occurring and the anticipated loss due to that occurrence. On the other side of the scale is the reward of success and the benefit to be gained by the health department as a result of the intended action or decision. One of the responsibilities of leadership is the constant balancing of resources, people, and relationships to maximize positive health outcomes within the community.

Several generic definitions of risk are provided by major organizations accessible through the Internet:

- Risk of something happening that will have an effect on objectives; measured in terms of consequences and likelihood. (AS/NZS 4360: 1999. www.wales.nhs.uk/ihc/documents/A.4.1.4_Australia_and_New_Zealand_Methodology_AS_NZ 4360_1999.pdf)

- Risk of a situation or circumstance that creates uncertainties about achieving program objectives. (FAA System Engineering Manual, www.faa.gov)

- Risk of an event occurring that will adversely affect the achievement of objectives. (Enterprise Risk Management—Integrated Framework, COSO, 2004, www.coso.org)[2]

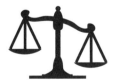

- Probability of a problem
- Loss associated with a problem
- Probability of a reward
- Benefit associated with the reward

Figure 27.2 Risk/reward balance.

- A general approach to risk assessment as defined on Wikipedia. (http://en.wikipedia.org/wiki/Risk_assessment)

This chapter is focused on business risk within public health rather than epidemiological risk as identified in the healthcare literature. The Wikipedia link has good information on the health risk issues.

WHAT IS RISK MANAGEMENT?

Risk management helps:

- Avoid disasters

- Avoid rework

- Avoid overkill

- Stimulates win/win solutions

Two of the above referenced Internet sources define risk management as:

- The culture, processes, and structures that are directed toward the effective management of potential opportunities and adverse effects. (AS/NZS 4360: 1999—"Risk Management")

- The identification, assessment, and response to risk to a specific objective. (Enterprise Risk Management—Integrated Framework, COSO, 2004, www.coso.org)

The value of risk management to public health is the ability to quantify risk and thereby make intelligent decisions based on analysis. One of the major characteristics of public health is that it exists within a community. Public health as a process does not stand alone. Variability and multifunctional controls are inherent within the concept of public health. This lack of centralized control increases the general incidence of risk within the public health environment. It is sometimes difficult to anticipate the risk of a local action on the outcomes in related, but more distant, communities and programs. Paul Epstein, et al. discuss approaches to risk management as it relates to measurement and controls in Chapters 17 and 18 of this text.

WHAT RISKS ARE THERE TO MANAGE IN PUBLIC HEALTH?

Risk management is not something just for the financial industry or large corporations. Public organizations are constantly assessing the risks of resource allocation, client relationships, and personnel policies. Some of the major areas of risk management revolve around the following areas:

- Client and community

- Technical

- Management

- Financial

- Contractual and legal

- Personnel

- Data and information

- Other resources

Risk management in a public health department (PHD) must extend beyond the department walls. The relationship with community partners is integral to the effectiveness of a PHD. Assessing priorities, opportunities, and threats related to use of resources, initiatives undertaken, and funding sources is a joint decision process for public health. This interrelated process makes risk management a more complex discussion among a multitude of stakeholders. Table 27.1 gives examples of risks the authors have experienced within each of the bulleted areas above.

Risk management is a central part of any organization's strategic management. It is the process whereby organizations methodically address the risks attached to their activities with the goal of achieving sustained benefit within each activity and across the portfolio of all activities. Its objective is to add maximum sustainable value to all the activities of the organization.

Risk management should be a continuous and developing process woven throughout the organization's strategy and implementation. It should address methodically all the risks surrounding the organization's activities—past, present, and future. Figure 27.3 illustrates a suggested flow from risk analysis through a final discussion of potential alternatives to unacceptable consequences.

Some operational definitions related to managing risks that will be useful for our discussion are:

risk identification—identifies the sources of risk, risk events, and their potential consequences.

risk analysis—analyzes the causes and source of the risks and the likelihood that they will occur.

risk evaluation—determines whether risks need to be addressed and treated.

risk treatment—determines strategies and tactics to mitigate or control risks.

In Figure 27.3, risk identification leads directly into risk analysis as part of an initial assessment process. Identification and analysis are a somewhat iterative function of acknowledging a potential risk, gathering further data, making a deeper analysis, and finally having enough information to make a judgment as to the perceived impact of the identified risk.

Once risk assessment has been completed, a decision must be made on whether the anticipated consequences can be tolerated. If the answer is yes, proceed with the proposed action while measuring and evaluating that successful progress is made to outcomes. If evaluation indicates the actions are not acceptable against expectations, then further analysis is necessary to explore potential alternative solutions, thus reentering the risk assessment phase. Note that the evaluation of the accepted consequences of the risk-assessed action is subject to the expectations and needs of a multifunctional group of internal and external stakeholders impacted by the outcome of the action.

Table 27.1   Types of risks to public health departments.

Potential problems or risks resulting from:

Client and community	Technical	Management	Financial	Contractual and legal	Personnel	Other resources
Inability of client to pay even minimal recovery charges for services provided	Incomplete requirements or design for equipment or laboratory procedures	Insufficient project planning, tracking, and control	Inadequate allocation or grant funding	Potential safety liability to staff or clients	Not enough staff to handle committed project workload	Weak inventory process for medications and vaccines
High number of non–English speaking persons requiring service	New technologies	Lack of experience or training	Limited grant-writing knowledge among staff	Rigid requirements for project outcomes by outside regulating body	High turnover of registered nursing staff	Clinic locations no longer within areas of highest need
Low response from local volunteers	New standards or processes	Conflict	Already stretched project budget	Existing legal complication with process	Insufficient quality training	Staff spread out too much across locations
Competition for scarce grant funds	General changes in requirements and environments	Organizational issues	Funding for project under outside control	Insufficient legal counsel available	Weak team leader skills	Laboratory equipment poorly maintained

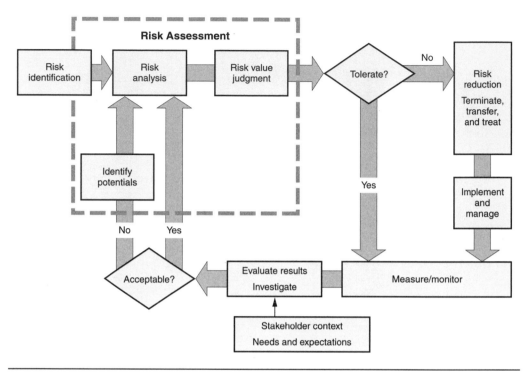

Figure 27.3 The risk management process.

If the risk value judgment is not tolerable, discussion immediately begins on mitigation activities such as reducing risk through terminating the project, transferring some risk to others, or treatment of the risk through validated improvement processes. Once the intolerable level of risk has been reduced, the ensuing actions are measured, monitored, and evaluated in the same fashion as the earlier tolerable risk alternative.

The consideration of risk must be integrated into the culture of the organization with an effective policy and program led by senior management. Effective risk management provides a basis for translating strategy into tactical and operational objectives, as well as assigning responsibility throughout the organization. Each manager and staff member is responsible for the management of risk as part of their job description. The management of organizational risk supports accountability, performance measurement, and reward, thus promoting operational efficiency at all levels.

Risk management protects and adds value to the organization and its stakeholders through supporting the organization's objectives by:

- Developing and supporting people and the organization's knowledge base

- Ensuring that action takes place in a consistent and controlled manner

- Improving decision making, planning, and prioritization by comprehensive and structured understanding of program activity, volatility, and project opportunity and threat

- Contributing to more efficient use of resources

- Reducing variation in nonessential areas of the department

- Protecting and enhancing assets and department image

Recently, many large financial institutions, despite having risk management departments, have suffered massive losses from a failure to understand the risks they took on. All organizations, not just financial ones, need to have better methods to assess and monitor their risks. Quantifying financial, operating, technological, and strategic risk is far from trivial, and much can be learned to make organizational risk management more effective. Risk management also requires effective systems for internal control, management control, and governance.

MITIGATING RISKS IN THE PUBLIC HEALTH COMMUNITY

Managing risk plays a significant role in an organization's success. The ability to synthesize information and make decisions may be a good leader's most important skill. Conversely, procrastination and indecisive leadership are hazardous for an organization. Identifying risk and the potential for adverse effects in a public health situation is a critical element of community support.

Why is it difficult to assess risk effectively? Uncertainty has quite a lot to do with it. Often, leaders don't have the data we need to make informed assessments. Frequently, we will have partial or incomplete data; this may give us some idea of what to do, but with considerable room for error. Often the risks and rewards of different programs are uncertain or completely unknown. It is not easy to manage the risk assessment process while fighting institutional inertia (which can easily lead to paralysis). A good strategy is to break the assessment down into steps.

The steps for an effective risk assessment are:

Step 1: *Analyze the risk involved.* How important are the outcomes of the program under consideration, and what are the potential consequences? (See Figure 27.3)

Step 2: *Perform a cost–benefit analysis.* A leader should avoid exposing the organization to unnecessary risk if the consequences are unacceptably large. Since risks are rarely known with certainty, a leader may perform several cost–benefit analyses, adjusting the probability of different outcomes. With this, the leader can calculate the expected benefits or cash flows under different risk scenarios.

Step 3: *Create the momentum for the decision.* Finally, it is often a good idea to build consensus for the decision to accept or reject the risk rather than imposing it unilaterally. This involves cooperation with all stakeholders in the decision. The simple act of consulting someone makes him or her feel valued and will frequently work wonders in getting the person on board with you.

The principal disadvantage of this type of consensus-building is that it can be time-consuming, especially if the leader's decision is unpopular. If it is critical to take action quickly, a leader may not have time to mount this sort of lobbying campaign. Thus, when confronting a choice a leader has a range of options. He or she may decide:

- To make the assessment and decision unilaterally

- To consult only the stakeholders

- To build a consensus by getting input from a variety of sources

- To delegate the assessment to someone else, either by taking a vote or by assigning responsibility to another individual

A good leader may use a variety of these options depending on the organizational culture, the decision at hand, and his or her personal leadership style. Each type of risk assessment brings its own benefits and shortcomings, but a strong and efficient leader is one who understands the true need of the organization and conducts the risk assessment and decision-making process accordingly.

The authors have learned a useful approach for involving others in the risk assessment and management process from Dr. Stephen R. Covey.[3] The most effective area in which to manage risk is that in which we have the strongest control. As seen in Figure 27.4, the area of control is in the center of the circle of influence. Process owners and those who control the resources that support public health programs have the best opportunity to assess and anticipate areas of risk to those programs. We call the shots, we own the environment.

The next most effective area in which to manage risk is where we have strong partnerships with clients, community, corporate sponsors, and related agencies. This area is one in which we have some level of influence over the use of resources and the eventual outcomes of the programs in which we are involved. We may not own the resources, but we can use our relationship with others to guide the positive outcomes of activities and decision making.

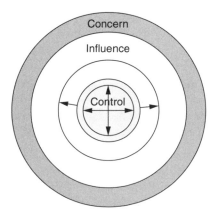

Figure 27.4   Control and influence.
Source: S. R. Covey, *The Seven Habits of Highly Effective People* (New York: Simon & Schuster, 1990).

The outer loop of concern is the area of highest level of risk for both positive and negative consequences of decisions or actions. Areas where we are interested in the outcomes but have little or no ability to guide and influence the actions of others require a complex set of relationships. As leaders we are often on the edges of the activity and outcomes for programs such as this. We must be very careful not to commit scarce resources, personnel, or reputation on the outcomes of programs where we see potential but are unable to influence or control what happens.

Table 27.2 provides a planning matrix to assist PH leadership in identifying levels of control and influence surrounding anticipated action. Examples within Table 27.2 illustrate situations where the authors have been faced with finding

Table 27.2   Risk assessment: level of control and influence.

Action	Outcome	Control	Influence	Outside our control and Influence
Translate application and instructions into Spanish	Septic system permit application in format that can be read and understood by Hispanic contractors	X		
Design and execute a MAPP communitywide assessment	Hard data and validated community preferences for effective local public health program planning		X	
Plan for changes to budgets and funding cuts anticipated by new state administration	Operational plan to balance local resources to maximize LPH community needs and requirements			X (State actions are outside our control, not plan)

For each action, identify the expected outcome and check which column(s) apply. From this, identify the area(s) of risk and develop a ranking of the actions to focus on to either mitigate the potential risk of negative consequences or improve your ability to control or influence positive outcomes for the quality improvement project to be started. Suggested legend for assessing levels of influence and control:

Symbol	Meaning
E	Extreme risk—Senior leadership involvement in continued monitoring of progress to jointly identified outcomes
H	High risk—Management responsibility should be specified for both resource commitment and monitoring of successful outcomes
M	Moderate risk—Manage by increasing level of influence through partnerships or committed resources
L	Low risk—Manage by routine process

ways to influence collaboration on complex projects through expanding public health department stakeholder involvement. Where there is little influence and no control over a situation, alternative methods for flexibility must be designed into the activity, or the activity must be restructured or abandoned.

TOOLS TO SUPPORT RISK MANAGEMENT IN PUBLIC HEALTH

A key risk management tool is the risk level matrix.[4] For each risk, the consequences and likelihood of occurrence are estimated. These data are then entered into a risk level matrix (See Table 27.3). Comparing the consequence of the occurrence with the likelihood indicates a level of extreme, high, medium, or low risk potential to the organization.

Once the level of concern is ascertained, preventive actions can be implemented for the extreme risks and high risks. Organizations can then use their internally defined preventive and corrective action processes.

Force Field Analysis

Force field analysis as described in Chapter 14 is a tool frequently used to address different perspectives of risk to a project or activity outcome. As seen in Figure 27.5, the opportunities and risks of reducing staff dedicated to syphilis testing in Orange County Florida Health Department (see Chapter 24) were listed by

Table 27.3   Risk level matrix.

	Consequences				
Likelihood	**Insignificant**	**Minor**	**Moderate**	**Major**	**Catastrophic**
A (Almost certain)	H	H	E	E	E
B (Likely)	M	H	H	E	E
C	L	M	H	E	E
D (Unlikely)	L	L	M	H	E
E (Rare)	L	L	M	H	H

Symbol	Meaning
E	Extreme risk—Immediate action; senior management involved
H	High risk—Management responsibility should be specified
M	Moderate risk—Manage by specific monitoring or responses
L	Low risk—Manage by routine process

Source: S. Liebesman, PhD, "Risk Management: A Tool for Improving Quality Management," *Quality Management Forum* (Milwaukee: American Society for Quality, 2008).

Move DIS resources from syphilis to gonorrhea testing	
+	–
• Address current epidemic of gonorrhea among pregnant females • Recognize DIS staff for exceeding department goals • Repair image of department within local community • Balance DIS resources among different STDs	• Remove needed resources from syphilis testing requirement • Reduce performance against national syphilis incidence • Risk reduction in grant funding for STD testing in general

Figure 27.5   Force field analysis.
Refer to Chapter 25 for full 2006 case study on OCHD STD unit.

senior management on a force field analysis form. Leadership then proceeded to maximize the benefits of staff reassignment while minimizing the risks of diluting the emphasis placed on the county's syphilis numbers.

EXAMPLES OF RISK MANAGEMENT IN PUBLIC HEALTH

All managers have a duty to reduce risk to their organizations. It is often an unspecified duty, but it comes with the manager title. There are many ways to reduce risk: one unfortunate human tendency is to "reduce" it by denying that risk exists. In our shrinking, flat earth, this is not a good approach. The best approach is to apply our skills to intelligently defining and mitigating risks. Quality professionals have the skills to define risk and control it. This is a clear need in our world today, and worthy of our time and talent.

—Douglas C. Wood, CQI, CMQ/OE,
finance for improvement expert

Traditional PHD objectives and metrics certainly have a home in a risk management perspective for increasing and sustaining stakeholder value, including the objective of funding growth and productivity improvements. Departments should have process objectives to manage and mitigate the risks associated with their strategies. Embedding risk management objectives in strategy maps and measurement scorecards should be a high priority where increases in knowledge and professional expertise could add substantial value to an organization. Reviews of a PHD's risk position should be part of the monthly leadership and strategy review meetings. Detailed examples of strategy maps and scorecards are offered in Chapters 17 and 18 of this text.

Recent news events have focused business leaders on the importance of looking after all their stakeholders. Although funding is fundamental to long-term department success, it is no longer acceptable to drive PHDs exclusively through financial controls. Other factors must be considered to ensure that the operation of the department remains successful during the medium term. Clients, employees, legislation, litigation, and local and worldwide opinions can and do all significantly affect the health and prosperity of any local, county, or state health department.

Governments in North America, Europe, and Asia are increasingly focusing on corporate governance and internal controls. As a result, organizations will have to demonstrate that they have structured management systems in place to review and prioritize all their stakeholders' needs as well as manage the business risks they face. Many view these issues as related initiatives that must be adopted as additional business functions.

Chapter 10 in this text discusses the NACCHO initiative for accreditation on a national scale. This self-assessment and accreditation project is designed to establish a threshold level of standardized services, infrastructure, community, and larger stakeholder relationships to minimize operational risk by sharing best practices and learning from peer public health organizations.

Encouraged by such standards as ISO 9001:2008, many departments are adopting a process-based approach and applying it to all their activities. It has become an essential tool in helping them understand their communities' needs and expectations. Quality management and improvement is no longer the exclusive domain of manufacturing operations; the process approach has proved invaluable to service organizations such as local governments, healthcare institutions, and financial organizations. As an additional benefit, management standards require that companies build a cycle of continuous improvement into everything they do.

Health departments that have implemented these standards and evolved with them have seen that they help manage conflicting priorities in a structured way. The challenge for these organizations is to recognize what is not being done and where development is required to build upon systems already in place.

In addition to ISO 9001:2008, two other risk-based approaches to management systems have been introduced in the environmental standard ISO 14000 and the occupational health and safety system OHSAS 18001. With these, organizations are encouraged to identify and evaluate all the environmental and occupational risks they face. Significant risks with severe consequences must be managed, either by eliminating them or reducing their frequency and/or severity.

By adopting these process- and risk-based approaches, organizations can improve their understanding of stakeholder requirements and expectations. Departments that do so will also be in a better position to manage the way in which they interact with their physical environments and look after the health and safety of people at work. Standards offer a method of measuring progress against objectives, which in turn helps drive continual improvement, competitiveness, and success in an increasingly demanding environment.

IDENTIFYING AND EVALUATING RISKS

Risks can be seen positively as program opportunities, such as investing in an innovative new service, moving into new geographical segments, or partnering with another service provider. Organizations that can effectively manage these risks are much more likely to protect and enhance their community reputation and expand their funding opportunities.

In a more traditional—that is, negative—sense, risk is usually seen as a potential for loss, whether it's lost funding, litigation, claims, or harm to people, property, or the environment.

In fiercely competitive manufacturing industries that use just-in-time techniques, late delivery from a supplier means production downtime and unhappy customers. Claims for lost revenue and damage to reputation ricochet down the supply chain, destroying the financial viability of otherwise successful businesses. Aside from the obvious negatives incurred when people or the environment are injured, the inevitable and damaging press coverage that follows can destroy shareholder confidence and business value. Public health examples of emotional media coverage of unmet individual needs, environmental crises, and epidemic outbreaks are just as damaging to our funding and partner and client well-being.

The risks associated with less tangible assets, such as an organization's reputation, must also be carefully evaluated. Reputations take years and significant financial investments to build but only seconds to destroy. For example, air traffic controllers have recently charged the pilots of some low-cost airlines in the United Kingdom with putting efficiency above other criteria. Would you fly with an airline with a poor safety record?

Organizations that have successfully applied the environmental management system standard ISO 14000 have reviewed their operations with respect to significant environmental issues (for example, air and water emissions, waste management, land contamination, raw materials and natural resources, and other local environmental and community concerns). Charleston, South Carolina Commissioners of Public Works (CPW) (now named the Charleston Water System) was the first water or wastewater system to receive certification to the ISO 14000 standard in 1999. As part of the process, the standard helps Charleston Water System respond to a common stakeholder expectation: managing risk and preventing loss with respect to the environment. Many of the functions of the Charleston Water System are paralleled within health department environmental health units.

Organizations that have successfully applied OHSAS 18001 have identified hazards and performed risk assessments relating to routine and unusual activities performed by anyone who has access to the workplace, even subcontractors and visitors. They have also extended this examination to workplace facilities, whether the organization or an outside supplier provides them. Organizations that adopt this standard not only establish a culture of risk management, but also address another key stakeholder concern: the people within the organization.

Essentially, the challenge to organizations is to master the risk assessment process and apply it departmentwide. Once the process is adopted for obvious concerns, such as those related to waste management or heavy equipment, it can be used to evaluate less tangible assets—like reputation management. Again, the environment in which an organization works—and this includes the stakeholders who influence how it operates—is a key prerequisite and shouldn't be forgotten.

MANAGING RISK THROUGH AN INTEGRATED SYSTEM

Once risks have been identified, the PHD must decide how it plans to tolerate, terminate, transfer, or treat them. Treating a risk is often the most complicated choice because it requires control and measurement. These form the foundation of an effective management system. Refer back to the discussion surrounding Figure 27.3 for an overview of the full risk management process.

Difficulties arise when an organization determines that a risk falls outside its management system's usual scope. For example, a risk might be identified in information security and how information is collected, stored, maintained, accessed, and communicated throughout the department and to other stakeholders. By adhering to the requirements agreed upon by industry and applying appropriate management system safeguards, such as those outlined in the NACCHO self-assessment described in Chapter 10, the organization can improve its current system and mitigate significant risks.

Another aspect of managing risks through treatment is maintaining the balance between competency and procedure. Organizations that have implemented quality improvement processes are aware that it is often more appropriate to manage a process through competent personnel rather than requiring them to follow meticulous, step-by-step instructions. This philosophy also applies to risk management: by its very nature, risk can not always be controlled through checklists.

Using the skills of a trained and highly competent staff is a very effective method of managing risk. Proper training and experience allow staff to identify inherent risks in given situations and quickly work out the most appropriate course of action. This implies a very different culture from one in which staff are expected to work methodically through detailed procedures before filling in the required documentation.

When managing risk, it may therefore be appropriate to build in checkpoints along a process to measure and identify potential risks. Staff competency can be matched to perceived risks at each stage in the process, ensuring that the risks are managed safely. Employee competency can be tested periodically, which will in turn help drive training programs and succession planning.

Most management system standards require that an organization measure its performance against objectives. For organizations that have successfully implemented management system standards, these measurements can be applied to risk management. Also, because processes are already in place to measure and analyze information, additional data required for risk management can be more readily obtained. For example, a department might decide that using a particular piece of equipment beyond its warranty period is an unacceptable risk. To monitor and continuously evaluate this risk, the department can determine from the associated operating processes the number of uses anticipated, and from those figures the corresponding amount of use expected until the warranty period expires. A process can then be developed to ensure that when the equipment exceeds the established warranty period it is safely disposed of or recycled.

Any department using an integrated approach that includes risk management will be able to provide objective evidence to senior leadership, who can use the information to ensure the organization's health and implement continuous improvement through management review. Applying a management system standard ensures a structured approach to fact-based decisions about the organization's future.

ONE SYSTEM FOR BEST PRACTICES

Is risk management an independent issue, something that must be managed separately from everyday operations? Evidence indicates that most health departments are already managing risk through their traditional management system standards.

Building upon what is already in place is often the most appropriate way forward. Perhaps the true challenge for departments today isn't identifying and managing risk but figuring out how to establish a culture based on a single integrated management system that can be used to apply best practices.

Internationally recognized standards can help organizations assess all their stakeholders' needs and expectations. The results of internal and external audits to these standards can be used to drive organizational risk management. The whole system must have a continual improvement focus in line with strategic objectives in order to safeguard the organization's future prosperity. Such a system could be described as a total business management system.

One such total business system is described by the Food and Drug Administration's strategic action plan, "Protecting and Advancing America's Health: Responding to New Challenges and Opportunities" (August 2003):

> The FDA has identified efficient risk management as the primary way to make the most effective use of agency resources and address these challenges. Efficient risk management requires using the best scientific data, developing quality standards, and using efficient systems and practices that provide clear and consistent decisions and communications for the American public and regulated industry. The FDA has long led the way in the science of risk management, and this ability is more important than ever, given the expanding complexity of the agency's challenges and the need to reduce the health risks facing the public at the lowest possible cost to society.
>
> The principal objective of this strategic action plan is to do as much as possible to improve the health outcomes of the American public. Only by becoming consistently more productive at what the agency does—always working to get the most public health bang for its regulatory buck—can the FDA have any chance of fulfilling its increasingly complex public health mission.
>
> Use science-based, efficient risk management in all agency regulatory activities, so that the agency's limited resources can provide the most health promotion and protection at the least cost for the public.

This statement from the FDA could just as easily have been penned by senior leadership of a local public health department. Chapter 16 on Lean Six Sigma in public health discusses a number of tools available to maximize the use of scarce agency resources while focusing on the highest priority activities to meet community needs.

Chapter 28

The Ethics of Quality Improvement

Kathleen F. (Kay) Edwards

INTRODUCTION

Ethics issues can arise in QI efforts due to the possible inadvertent causing of harm, resource allocation that may seem unexplainable, and possible unfair treatment of patients.[1] Engaging in QI activities in healthcare settings, including public health, means among other things establishing a clear ethics base so "disincentives" for QI activities can be ended and the perception of the above inequities can be reduced.

Most public health practitioners know that there are ethical reasons for having a public health system; when the roots of public health are recalled, for instance, the two key foci were protecting vulnerable populations and protecting citizens from environmental assault. There are ethics theories and principles that relate to public health research, practice, and education. Helping improve the quality of and length of people's lives is often stated as a major reason for public health agencies' existence. If doing the most good for the most people has an ethics root, then improving life quality and length should also probably be included under that goal.

It may come as no surprise that people who want to improve the quality and length of the lives of others also rely on an ethics base to support the philosophy and concepts of a quality improvement program. The connection is that if helping people help themselves and helping the community to improve its health status are worthy societal goals, then using quality improvement concepts and tools to help society reach its goals will also partially spring from an ethics base. There are *social arrangements* that hold healthcare workers and managers responsible for the quality of healthcare products and services, and the same social arrangements need to be in place to assure that QI activities meet requirements for the "ethical conduct of QI."[2]

A final introductory thought is that as people and organizations evolve in a given field, the accreditation of the work of that field generally assumes that the practitioners of it will improve their own practice in that field.

ETHICS PRINCIPLES AS FOUNDATIONS FOR QI

Quality improvement concepts and tools can be linked to several ethics principles. These four ethics principles also support health services in general.[3] Respect for persons is the first principle and it has four elements. The first element of respect for persons is known as *autonomy*. It is shown by providing information to health-care industry clients so that they can make informed decisions for themselves regarding their health and well-being. It also can be shown by allowing healthcare units and departments to select their own QI projects and approaches to problem solving.

The second element of respect for persons, *truth telling*, requires individuals to be honest in all that they do. In speaking the truth, respect is shown for the other person, even when sharing the information may cause harm to the other. In QI discussions, problems and issues can be uncovered that some may wish not to be revealed. The ethics principle of respect for persons would argue for disclosure of the information. The concept of *speaking truth to power*, discussed later in this chapter, would suggest that QI efforts also may lend themselves to courageous speaking out when areas in need of improvement are identified.

The third element of respect for persons is *confidentiality*. Protecting the confidentiality of information of patients and others also shows respect for persons. In QI efforts, confidentiality is supported by not revealing patients' names or other identifying information to those who do not have a valid reason to know them.

The fourth element of respect for persons is *fidelity*, and it's demonstrated in QI efforts by keeping one's word and doing one's duty. If a commitment to a particular unit of a public health agency is made based on QI project findings, the keeping of the commitment shows respect for the unit's employees. If a community is promised a certain outcome pending the results of the QI project's work, under the ethics principle of fidelity the community can expect that the agreement will be honored by the public health agency involved.

In addition to respect for persons, there are other ethics principles also linked to QI efforts in public health. *Beneficence*, which suggests conferring benefits, relates to acting with charity and kindness. When QI activities are being planned and implemented, the ways that target populations to be assessed or served are selected, how data are gathered, analyzed, and presented, and any follow-up from the QI activities should be based on acting toward the population and its public health workers with charity and kindness.

Beneficence also has another dimension—*utility*, or balancing the benefits and harms of an action. Utility is the ethics foundation for cost–benefit and risk–benefit analyses. In QI efforts, however, if one is focused on providing public health services for the greatest good, utility should not serve as the basis for overriding patients' or communities' interests.

The third ethics principle related to QI efforts in public health is *nonmaleficence*. This principle means doing no harm, to customers and employees. There often is needed a delicate balance of ethics principles in QI efforts, since moving forward with some data-driven decisions in public health may cause a loss of jobs and departmental strife, even when the goal of the public health decision is to better serve other people, the community. Researchers on the ethics of QI in other healthcare settings, for instance, have found no ethics requirement to allow a healthcare worker to not participate in a QI activity in case it might prove the worker incompetent or unnecessary.[4]

The fourth ethics principle that can be linked to QI efforts is *justice*. When considering the possible resource allocation and human resources aspects of QI efforts, justice is a part of the discussion. Since definitions of fairness can vary depending on the context of the discussion, the final analysis of the application of justice to QI efforts should probably focus on the consistent application of ethics principles in decision making, using the same criteria determined ahead of time.[5]

ETHICS CONSIDERATIONS IN PUBLIC HEALTH QI ACTIVITIES

Having identified various ethics principles that can provide an ethics foundation for public health quality improvement work, the next part of this discussion focuses on specific ways that public health settings can use ethical quality improvement approaches to advance public health goals and objectives.

As accreditation of public health settings becomes an implemented feature of the public health landscape, links with standards for agency and worker performance become even more important. Healthcare clinical services and research have generally been associated with quality improvement efforts, such as having informed consent by patients before administering medications, treatments, and experimental therapies. Research in the healthcare setting has usually had to seek approval based on some form of review board where the protection of patients, staff, communities, and facilities has been a key consideration in the approval process.

Society and academic/research bodies, for example, the Institute of Medicine, have asked if U.S. patients are safe and whether care is being provided as well as it can be. Recipients of healthcare products and services, including public health services, want to know if the care they receive is up to the standard that the community expects. Many stakeholders of public health also want to know, for instance, if funding for public health programs and services is being well spent. They also want to know if the public health agencies that are implementing decisions about the lives, safety, and overall health of the community are staffed by workers capable of providing appropriate public health services, meaning that these workers have the requisite knowledge, skills, and abilities to carry out public health's mission, goals, and objectives.

Though there can be varying views about the strategies and methods that can or should be used to reach public health agency accreditation standards, some of the bases for accreditation stem from society's and individual people's desire to be treated fairly, with respect, and in ways that do not harm them. Each of these bases flows from the ethics principles discussed above.

Other examples of the role of ethics in quality improvement focus on the choice of QI activities. When local, state, and regional health departments decide between competing priorities as to which of them will be chosen for continuous quality improvement efforts, this means, *de facto*, that other priorities will not be selected for QI. As QI projects are chosen, the ethics principles of fairness and doing no harm need to be considered, along with available data on community indicators of health and illness. For priorities not selected for QI efforts at one point in time, there may be a need to create a list of pending priorities that may be next up on the QI agenda—pending changes in the public health milieu, as always.

Sometimes public health workers say that they can not stop long enough in their daily tasks to think about or implement QI processes. The QI work may first appear to be an additional burden, as opposed to a useful tool that can, in the long run, help ease the public health workload and increase the efficiency and effectiveness of public health work.

It is generally been found to be true that as with other types of investments, in the beginning of any QI change effort there can be a dip in productivity while processes are put in place that improve the tasks already being done. When workers see that the QI efforts have a positive return, then the buy-in for QI can increase, as can productivity. Getting used to anything new requires change management skills that public health workers use regularly and well.

The fair allocation of time, funding, and other resources is a perennial concern of public health practitioners. In thinking about QI efforts and also about ethics, some public health agencies have decided that using QI can help them save money. For instance, by looking for the root causes of an issue or problem via the use of the *fishbone* (or Ishikawa) diagram QI tool, public health agencies can identify the causes of a certain event, including the deeper reasons for a particular problem, potentially leading to a more productive outcome, saving time, energy, and also funding.

One particular public health agency, for example, found that when it examined the reasons for a workplace morale issue, one of the deeper reasons that emerged via the use of a root cause analysis was a lack of understanding of the agency's true mission. Once that issue was on its way to being addressed satisfactorily in the minds of the agency's workers, the sense of poor worker morale was dissipated.

SUCCESSFUL APPROACHES TO QI AS LINKED TO ETHICS, AND SOME THINGS TO AVOID

Here are some relevant tips, techniques, and things to avoid in order to be effective with QI as it relates to ethics and public health.

As QI tools are used to increase public health's productivity and successful outcomes, the need for an ethics base for these tools continues to be apparent. As most public health QI activities are interpreted, they are not, strictly speaking, called research, and this is an important distinction to be made when one considers the ethics oversight needed for research in healthcare settings in the United States.

Deciding if a QI activity is research or not can be challenging, though researchers have mentioned that most QI efforts are *not* research. Here is some definitional guidance that may help: if the goal of the QI activity is to assess the success of an established program, and the results of the QI activity will be used to improve the program, it is not considered research.

Researchers in QI in healthcare, and of the ethics of human subjects research, have developed a set of ethical requirements to protect human participants—both healthcare patients and healthcare workers—in QI activities. These are:

    a. Social or scientific value should justify the resources expended.

    b. Participants are fairly selected.

    c. There is a favorable risk–benefit ratio.

    d. Respect for participants is shown.

    e. Participant and worker consent is informed.

    f. There is independent review of the ethical conduct of QI.[6]

When public health, and other healthcare, agencies are considering QI activities, they will want to determine whether the projects are also research, since if they are research projects, and humans are involved as participants, then human subjects research guidelines may be called for. There is a goal of having the U.S. federal level of government exempt, or not require, that human subjects research guidelines be applied when the model for the QI activity is for program review and evaluation for service or program improvement, as in QI activities.

If the QI activities are designed to produce both local improvements and also new and enduring knowledge about people and how they function, and those activities involve human subjects, these can be termed "overlap projects," and the activity may need review by both a QI approval process and an internal review board (IRB) process.

For organizations that carry out a large number of overlap projects, one suggestion in the literature is to establish specialized QI IRBs.[7]

What also may be useful for public health agencies engaging in QI activities to know is the following CDC guidance on distinguishing research from nonresearch efforts. If the criteria below are met, the public health program is *not* considered research:

    1. If the intent of the project is to identify and control a health problem or improve a public health program or service

    2. If the intended benefits of the project are primarily for the clients or the participants' community

    3. If the data collected are needed to assess and/or improve the program or service, the health of the participants, or the participants' community

    4. If the knowledge generated does not extend beyond the scope of the activity

    5. If the project activities are not experimental[8]

An example of a nonresearch public health QI effort would be gathering data on the attendance of public health workers at continuing education sessions in order to lay the foundation for a system of positive record keeping that showed the agency's support for and participation in professional trainings, as a possible part of accreditation requirements.

EVALUATION OF THE ETHICS OF PUBLIC
HEALTH QI ACTIVITIES

Healthcare QI ethics oversight procedures must allow QI activities to remain flexible and be integrated into ongoing public health service delivery. QI methods in public health should have supervisory procedures in place that focus on resource use, impact expected methods and any additional patient risk, compared with usual public health services risk.[9]

In evaluating the ethics of public health QI activities, the recommendations of the 2006 report on the use of QI methods in healthcare, sponsored by the U.S. Agency for Healthcare Research and Quality (AHRQ) and the Hastings Center, and summarized in the Lynn, Baily, et al. article cited in the endnotes for this chapter, may be useful.

The recommendations, adapted by the author of this book chapter, for the public health setting are:

1. Assure that the professional and organizational responsibility for QI in public health settings is clearly laid out and shared.

2. Design QI efforts so that recipients of public health services know that they may or may not be expected to participate in QI activities as part of service receipt.

3. Public health agencies should use resources and guidance on best practices of QI methods and for sharing of QI results.

4. If human subjects research is a part of a public health QI model, the management and supervision of the QI activities and QI human subjects research may need to develop new models of internal management and supervision of these processes.

5. As external accountability for QI in public health settings expands, accrediting bodies may seek even more effective methods for managing QI and assuring that accreditation requirements meet ethics standards.

In considering how to evaluate QI activities and their impact on healthcare settings, an example from other settings in the healthcare industry may also be instructive. One major healthcare industry accrediting body is the Joint Commission, formerly called the Joint Commission on the Accreditation of Healthcare Organizations (JCAHO). At its Web site (http://www.jointcommission.org/), the Joint Commission provides examples of standards that imply an ethics base for evaluating the quality of care.

Here's an example from the Joint Commission's Web site, for ethics standards categories for ambulatory surgery centers:

Ethics, Rights, and Responsibilities

Overview

An organization's adherence to ethical care and business practices significantly affects the patient's experience of and response to services. The standards in this chapter address the following processes and activities related to ethical care and business practices:

- *Managing the organization's relationships with patients and the public in an ethical manner*

- *Considering the values and preferences of patients, including the decision to discontinue services*

- *Helping patients understand and exercise their rights*

- *Informing patients of their responsibilities in services*

- *Recognizing the organization's responsibilities under law[10]*

In the Joint Commission's information on its Web site related to home health care and performance improvement, there is no apparent explicit statement re the ethics of QI in relation to Joint Commission accreditation of home health agencies, but there are many standards that imply an ethics base.[11]

A final thought when evaluating QI activities in public health is that the researchers who examined QI in other healthcare settings[12] mentioned that there has not been much published on QI ethics scandals.

SUMMARY

As the chapter on the ethics of quality improvement in public health settings concludes, you may want to consider some of the points the chapter covered.

In order for QI efforts to succeed, public health workers often need to work as a team in pursuit of common goals. The ethics of teamwork is strengthened by showing respect for persons by, for example, allowing stakeholders to have their say before decisions about QI efforts are made, and by truth telling in all QI dealings.

Another summary thought about the ethics of QI initiatives emphasizes how public health workers often speak and write about the need to reduce disparities in public health research, planning, education, and services. To the extent that QI efforts can help inform agency decisions that impact health disparities and risk factors, key roles for champions of QI in public health will include strong advocacy and targeting of the elimination of health disparities.

A final thought relates to truth telling, as included under the ethics principle of respect for persons. *Speaking truth to power* is a concept that can mean public servants giving unbiased advice about the policies they wish to pursue. And in the case of QI projects, the findings of a QI program can reveal to a community aspects of public health products and services that may need change, including additional resources or redirection of them. Some of these findings may not be palatable to citizens or elected officials. The choices that jurisdictions and their leaders make that impact the health of communities may need to be informed by truth being spoken to communities and their leaders, even when the cost of speaking that truth may be high. The ethics of QI require speaking truth to power and also encouraging the use of data-driven results, enhanced by the experience and insights of public health workers, to prove the worth and value of QI activities.

Enjoy your ethics journey as you engage in public health QI pursuits.

Bibliography

Edwards, K. "Ethics and Social Responsibility As Management Issues." Chapter V in
    C. Mann and K. Gotz, eds., *The Development of Management Theory and Practice in the
    United States*, 3rd ed. Boston: Pearson Custom Publishing, 2005.

Gostin, L. "What Does Social Justice Require for the Public's Health? Public Health Ethics
    and Policy Imperatives." *Health Affairs* 25, no. 4 (2006): 1053–61.

National Bioethics Advisory Commission. *Ethical and Policy Issues Involving Human
    Participants*. Bethesda, MD: U.S. Government Printing Office, 2000: 36–37.

Nelson, W., and P. Gardent. "Ethics and Quality Improvement." *Healthcare Executive* 23,
    no. 4 (2008): 40–42.

Scholtes, P., B. L. Joiner, and B. Streibel. *The Team Handbook*, 2nd ed. Madison, WI: Oriel,
    2000.

J. H. Zenger, E. Musselwhite, K. Hurson, and C. Perrin. *Leading Teams: Mastering the New
    Role*. Zenger-Miller, 1994.

Endnotes

Chapter 1

1. Wikipedia, http://en.wikipedia.org/wiki/culture (accessed May 26, 2008).
2. C. Collet, J. DeMott, and J. W. Moran, "Introduction to Critical Processes" (A GOAL/QPC Application Report No. 92-01A, 1992): 2.
3. "PDF: Two Steps to CTQ Identification," adapted from an ASQ training presentation by Treffs, Rabeneck, and Rabeneck (April 7, 2006), www.sixsigmaforum.com (accessed February 17, 2009).
4. R. S. Kaplan and D. Norton, *The Balanced Scorecard* (Boston: Harvard Business School Press, 1996).

Chapter 2

1. Public Health Foundation, *Turning Point Survey on Performance Management Practices in States: Results of a Baseline Assessment of State Health Agencies* (Seattle, WA: Turning Point National Program Office at the University of Washington, 2002).
2. Florida Public Health Indicators Data System, http://hpeapps.doh.state.fl.us/phids/phids.asp (accessed 11/14/02), "MMWR Weekly," 1992; 41(14) 240. www.cdc.gov/mmwr/preview/mmwrhtpm/00016515.htm and "Reported Tuberculosis in the United States," 1998. www.cdc.gov/nchstp/tb/pubs/slidesets/surv/surv1998/html/surv4.htm (accessed 11/14/02).
3. Ibid.
4. Centers for Disease Control and Prevention, *National Vital Statistics Report* 42, no. 2 (1991) and *National Vital Statistics Report* 48, no. 11 (2000).
5. P. Lichiello, *Guidebook for Performance Measurement* (Seattle, WA: Turning Point National Program Office, 1999): 48. www.turningpointprogram.org/Pages/lichello.pdf. Based on H. P. Hatry, M. Fall, T. O. Singer, and E. B. Liner, *Monitoring the Outcomes of Economic Development Programs* (Washington, DC: The Urban Institute Press, 1990).
6. Results of 1991–2000 Baldrige Award Recipients 10-Year Common Stock Comparison, National Institute of Standards and Technology, www.nist.gov/public_affairs/factsheet/stockstudy.htm (accessed 11/14/02). The seven criteria include leadership, strategic planning, customer and market focus, information and analysis, human resource focus, process management, and business results. More information is

available online at www.nist.gov/public_affairs/factsheet/baldfaqs.htm. For examples of ways public health agencies have used this proven performance management model, see Chapter 5 on Baldrige.

7. Frequently Asked Questions and Answers About the Malcolm Baldrige National Quality Award, National Institute of Standards and Technology, www.nist.gov/public_affairs/factsheet/baldfaqs.htm (accessed 11/14/02).

8. A. Donabedian, "The Quality of Care. How Can It Be Assessed?" *Journal of the American Medical Association* 260 (1988) 1743–48.

9. A. Handler, M. Issel, and B. Turnock, "A Conceptual Framework to Measure Performance of the Public Health System," *American Journal of Public Health* 91 (2001): 1235–39.

Chapter 3

1. Parts of this chapter are based on the following publications by John W. Moran: "Developing an Organization's Strategic Intent and Operational Plan," *The Quality Management Forum* 21, no. 1 and "The Pitfalls Associated with Strategic and Operational Planning," *The Quality Management Forum* 20, no. 4.

2. G. Hoffherr, J. Moran, and G. Nadler, *Breakthrough Thinking in Total Quality Management* (Englewood Cliffs, NJ: Prentice Hall, 1994): 50–52.

4. "Sony's Heartaches in Hollywood," *Business Week,* December 5, 1994, 44.

5. "Why Companies Fail," *Fortune,* November 14, 1994, 52.

6. Ibid, 52.

7. G. P. Bohan, "Focus the Strategy to Achieve Results," *Quality Progress* (July 1995): 89–92.

Chapter 4

1. Public Health Foundation. 2001. http://www.phf.org.

2. N. Kanarak and J. Stanley. "Local Public Health Agency Performance and Community Health Improvement." (Presentation at the Public Health Services Affiliate Academy of Health Second Annual Meeting, 2003).

3. G. P. Mayes et al. "Getting What You Pay For: Public Health Spending and the Performance of Essential Public Health Services," *J Public Health Manag Pract* 10, no. 5 (2004): 435–43.

4. North Carolina, *North Carolina Accreditation*, http://nciph.sph.unc.edu/accred/ (2008); Michigan, "Embracing Quality in Local Public Health: Michigan's Quality Improvement Guidebook," *Michigan Accreditation*, http://www.accreditation.localhealth.net (accessed October 28, 2008); Missouri. "Missouri Voluntary Local Health Agency Accreditation Program," (updated 2006), *Missouri Accreditation*, http://www.michweb.org/accred.htm (accessed October 28, 2008).

5. Institute of Medicine, *The Future of the Public's Health in the 21st Century* (Washington, DC: National Academies Press, 2003).

6. Centers for Disease Control and Prevention, *The Futures Initiative* (2008b). http://www.cdc.gov/futures/.

7. American Public Health Association, National Association of State and Territorial Health Officials, National Association of City and County Health Officials, National Association of Local Boards of Health, "Exploring Accreditation: Final Recommendations for a Voluntary National Accreditation Program for State

and Local Public Health Departments," 2007. http://www.rwjf.org/pr/product. jsp?id=18599.

8. PHF, "Improving Public Health Infrastructure and Performance through Innovative Solutions and Measurable Results," http://ww.phf.org (accessed 2008).

9. Institute of Medicine, *The Future.*

10. Centers for Disease Control and Prevention, National Public Health Performance Standards System (2008a). http://www.cdc.gov/od/ocphp/nphpsp/.

11. National Association of County and City Health Officials, "Operational Definition of a Local Public Health Department," 2008. http://www.cdc.gov/od/ocphp/nphpsp/.

12. PHAB, 2009. www.phaboard.org.

13. Insitute of Medicine, *The Future of Public Health* (Washington, DC: National Academies Press, 1998).

14. Ibid.

15. PHAB, 2009.

16. W. Riley and R. Brewer, "Review and Analysis of Quality Improvement (QI) Techniques in Police Departments: Application for Public Health," *Journal of Public Health Management and Practice* 15, no. 2 (2009): 141–51.

17. B. L. Joiner, *Fourth Generation Management: The New Business Consciousness* (New York: McGraw-Hill, 1994).

18. J. Kouzes and B. Posner, *The Leadership Challenge* (San Francisco: Jossey-Bass, 2002).

19. D. Lighter and D. Fair, *Quality Management in Health Care: Principles and Methods* (Sudbury, MA: Jones and Bartlett, 2004).

20. W. Riley, "The Multi-State Learning Collaborative and the Minnesota Public Health Collaborative for Quality Improvement," http://www.health.state.mn.us/divs/cfh/ophp/consultation/mlc2/showcase/presentations/2008d1session2.ppt (accessed November 20, 2008).

21. Joiner, *Fourth Generation Management.*

22. D. T. Boe et al., "Improving Service Delivery in a County Health Department WIC Clinic: An Application of Statistical Process Control Techniques, *American Journal of Public Health* (in press).

23. T. Pyzdek, *The Six Sigma Handbook* (New York: McGraw-Hill, 2003).

24. J. Liker, *The Toyota Way* (New York: McGraw-Hill, 2003).

25. *The Breakthrough Series: IHI's Collaborative Model for Achieving Breakthrough Improvement,* IHI Innovation Series white paper (Boston: Institute for Healthcare Improvement, 2003). Available on www.IHI.org.

26. PHAB, 2009.

27. M. M. Godfrey et al., "Planning Patient Centered Services," in E. C. Nelson, P. B. Batalden, and M. M. Godfrey, eds., *Quality By Design: A Clinical Microsystems Approach* (San Francisco: Jossey-Bass, 2007).

Chapter 6

1. A. Donabedian, "Evaluating the Quality of Medical Care," *The Milbank Quarterly* 44 (1966): 166–203.

Chapter 8

1. Quote from Tews et al., *Embracing Quality in Local Public Health*, Michigan Quality Improvement Guidebook, 2008.

Chapter 9

1. J. Lynn, M. Baily, and M. Bottrell, et al., "The Ethics of Using Quality Improvement Methods in Health Care," *Annals of Internal Medicine* 146, no. 9 (2007): 666–73.
2. P. Daly and M. Watkins with C. Reavis, *The First 90 Days in Government: Critical Success Strategies for New Public Managers at All Levels* (Boston: Harvard Business School Press, 2006).
3. B. Bumes, "Kurt Lewin and the Harwood Studies: The Foundations of OD," *The Journal of Applied Behavioral Science* 43, no. 2 (June 2007): 213–30.
4. E. Dent and E. Powley, "Employees Actually Embrace Change: The Chimera of Resistance," *Journal of Applied Management and Entrepreneurship* 8, no. 1 (January 2003): 40–57.
5. C. Musselwhite, *Change Style Inventory* (Greensboro, N.C.: Discovery Learning, 2003).
6. J. Gelatt, "Leadership. Chapter II" in C. Mann and K. Gotz, eds., *The Development of Management Theory and Practice in the United States*, 3rd ed. (Boston: Pearson Custom Publishing, 2005).
7. J. Byrnes, "Manage Paradigmatic Change," *Harvard Business School Working Knowledge* (July 4, 2005). Found at: http://hbswk.hbs.edu/archive/4887.html.
8. L. Lewis et al., "Communicating Change," *Harvard Management Communication Letter* (1999).

Chapter 10

1. Institute of Medicine, Committee for the Study of the Future of Public Health, *The Future of Public Health* (Washington, DC: National Academies Press, 1988). http://www.ncbi.nlm.nih.gov/pubmed/2715336.
2. Public Health Services Steering Committee, *Public Health in America* (1994). http://www.health.gov/phfunctions/public.htm.
3. Institute of Medicine, *The Future of the Public's Health in the 21st Century* (Washington, DC: National Academies Press, 2003).
4. Centers for Disease Control and Prevention. *Futures Initiative* (2004). www.cdc.gov/futures/.
5. Public Health Accreditation Board, Exploring Accreditation Steering Committee, *Exploring Accreditation Full Report: Final Recommendations for a Voluntary National Accreditation Program for State and Local Health Departments* (Washington, DC: PHAB, Winter 2006–2007). http://www.phaboard.org/Documents/FullReport.pdf.
6. American Society for Quality, *Quality 101*, self-study course, 2001.
7. T. Bornstein. *Quality Improvement and Performance Improvement—Different Means to the Same End?* QA Brief 9, no. 1 (Spring 2001): 6–12. http://www.reproline.jhu.edu/english/6read/6pi/pi_qi/pdf/qiandpi.pdf.
8. Institute of Medicine, *The Future.*
9. Institute of Medicine, *21st Century.*
10. National Association of County and City Health Officials, *Project Public Health Ready State Implementation Information* (Washington, DC: NACCHO, 2008).

Chapter 11

1. S. Kessler, *Total Quality Service: A Simplified Approach to Using the Baldrige Award Criteria* (Milwaukee: ASQ Quality Press, 1996).

Chapter 13

1. D. Besterfield, *Quality Control*, 8th ed. (Englewood Cliffs, NJ: Prentice Hall, 2008).
2. A. Rickmers and H. Todd, *Statistics: An Introduction* (New York: McGraw-Hill, 1967): v.

Chapter 14

1. ASQ Statistics Division, *Improving Performance through Statistical Thinking* (Milwaukee: ASQ Quality Press, 2000).
2. J. Evans and W. Lindsay, *Managing for Quality and Performance Excellence* (Mason, OH: Thompson Publishing, 2007).

Chapter 16

1. Public Health Foundation, "Turning Point: From Silos to Systems." http://www.phf.org/pmqi/silossystems.pdf
2. G. Byrne, D. Lubowe, and A. Blitz, *Driving Operational Innovation Using Lean Six Sigma* (Somers, NY: IBM Global Business Services, 2007).
3. R. T. Westcott, *The Certified Manager of Quality/Organizational Excellence Handbook*, 3rd ed. (Milwaukee: ASQ Quality Press, 2005).
4. Ibid.
5. Byrne, Lubowe, and Blitz, *Driving*.

Chapter 17

1. In the book and Web site, the authors use the term "engaging citizens" for this "core community skill." But they stress that they do not mean "citizens" in the legal sense. Instead, they consider all people who want to help improve their community to be "a community's citizens," regardless of their legal status. And they encourage professionals to substitute other terms for "citizens" if they are working in communities or situations where "citizen" is a charged word that may keep them from reaching people they want to engage. As this can be a common situation in public health, we have made such a substitution here, changing "engaging citizens" to "engaging the community." See P. D. Epstein, P. M. Coates, and L. D. Wray, *Results That Matter: Improving Communities by Engaging Citizens, Measuring Performance, and Getting Things Done* (San Francisco: Jossey-Bass, 2006): xiii–xiv. Also see the Web page http://www.resultsthatmatter.net/site/definitions/communitycitizens.php.
2. Epstein et al., 5–9 and http://www.resultsthatmatter.net/site/governance/index.php.

Chapter 18

1. E. Eng, "What Defines Community-Based Participatory Research: A Review and Synthesis." (Presented at the American Public Health Association 2004 Annual Meeting.) Available at http://apha.confex.com/apha/132am/techprogram/paper_87674.htm (accessed 8/30/08).

Chapter 21

1. H. J. Harrington, "Creating New Middle Managers," *Quality Digest* (August 2002): 14.
2. J. Bauer, G. Duffy, R. T. Westcott, *The Quality Improvement Handbook* (Milwaukee: ASQ Quality Press, 2002): 53.
3. Zenger, et al. *Leading Teams, Mastering the New Role* (New York: McGraw-Hill, 1994).
4. J. Dorman, "Creating and Leading Effective Team Building Sessions" (Presentation to Trident Area Community of Excellence, Charleston, SC, 1994).
5. P. Scholtes, B. L. Joiner, B. Streibel, *The Team Handbook*, 2nd ed. (Madison, WI: Oriel, 2000): 6-4–6-7.

Chapter 22

1. E. Salas, T. L. Dickenson, S. A. Converse, and S. I. Tannenbaum, "Toward an Understanding of Team Performance and Training," in R. W. Swezey and E. Salas, eds., *Teams: Their Training and Performance* (Norwood, NJ: Ablex, 1992).
2. S. A. Mohrman, S. G. Cohen, and A. M. J. Mohrman, *Designing Team Based Organisations* (San Francisco: Jossey-Bass, 1995).
3. E. Salas, D. E. Sims, and C. S. Burke, "Is There a 'Big Five' in Teamwork?" *Small Group Research* 36, no. 5: (2005): 555.
4. J. Hackman, *Leading Teams: Setting the Stage for Great Performances* (Boston: Harvard University Press, 1987).
5. C. P. Alderfer, "An Intergroup Perspective on Group Dynamics," in J. Lorsch, ed., *Handbook of Organizational Behavior* (New York: Marcel Dekker, 1987).
6. W. E. Deming, *Out of the Crisis* (Boston: MIT Press, 1986).
7. B. Tuchman, "Developmental Sequence in Small Groups," *Psychological Bulletin* 63 (1965): 384.
8. B. Fried and W. R. Carpenter, "Understanding and Improving Team Effectiveness in Quality Improvement," in C. P. McLaughlin and A. D. Kaluzny, eds., *Continuous Quality Improvement in Healthcare,* 3rd ed. (Sudbury, MA: Jones and Bartlett, 2006): 154–79.
9. M. Brassard and D. Ritter, *The Memory Jogger II: A Pocket Guide of Tools for Continuous Quality Improvement and Effective Planning* (Salem, NH: Goal/QPC, 1994).
10. Ibid.
11. W. Riley, H. Parsons, K. McCoy, and D. Anderson, *Evidence Based Practice and Public Health Systems Research: A Systematic Assessment of a Statewide Quality Improvement Training and Implementation Project* (in press).
12. P. R. Scholtes, B. L. Joiner, and B. J. Streibel, *The Team Handbook,* 2nd ed. (Madison, WI: Oriel, 2001).
13. Fried and Carpenter, *Understanding.*
14. T. Ohno and N. Bodek, *Toyota Production System: Beyond Large-Scale Production* (Portland, OR: Productivity Press, 1998); J. Womack and D. Jones, *Lean Thinking: Banish Waste and Create Wealth in Your Corporation,* 2nd ed., revised and updated (New York: Free Press, 2003).
15. J. Liker, *The Toyota Way* (New York: McGraw-Hill, 2003).
16. C. Argyris, "Teaching Smart People to Learn," *Harvard Business Review* 69 (1991): 99.
17. W. Riley, "The Multi-State Learning Collaborative and the Minnesota Public Health Collaborative for Quality Improvement," http://www.health.state.mn.us/divs/cfh/ophp/consultation/mlc2/showcase/presentations/2008d1session2.ppt (accessed November 20, 2008).
18. E. Nelson, P. B. Batalden, and M. M. Godfrey, eds., *Quality by Design: A Clinical Microsystems Approach* (San Francisco: Wiley, 2007).

19. P. B. Batalden, E. C. Nelson, J. J. Mohr, M. M. Godfrey, T. P. Huber, L. Kosnik, et al., "Microsystems in Health Care: Part 5. How Leaders are Leading," *Joint Commission Journal on Quality and Safety* 29, no. 6 (2003): 297.
20. E. Nelson et al., *Quality by Design.*
21. Salas, Sims, and Burke, "Is There."
22. B. L. Joiner, *Fourth Generation Management, the New Business Conciousness* (New York: McGraw-Hill, 1994).
23. Ibid.
24. P. B. Batalden and P. K. Stolz, "A Framework for the Continual Improvement of Health Care," *Journal on Quality Improvement* 19, no. 10 (1993): 424.
25. Deming, *Out of the Crisis.*

Chapter 25

1. G. J. Langley, K. M. Nolan, T. W. Nolan, C. L. Norman, and L. P. Provost, *The Improvement Guide* (San Francisco: Jossey-Bass, 1996).
2. Institute for Healthcare Improvement, *The Breakthrough Series: IHI's Collaborative Model for Achieving Breakthrough Improvement* (IHI Innovation Series white paper. Boston: IHI, 2003).

Chapter 26

1. D. M. Berwick, "Errors Today and Errors Tomorrow," *NEJM* 348 (2003): 2570–72.
2. M. C. Fiore, W. C. Bailey, S. J. Cohen, et al., *Treating Tobacco Use and Dependence,* clinical practice guideline (Rockville, MD: U.S. Department of Health and Human Services, Public Health Service, 2000).
3. J. O. Prochaska and W. F. Velicer, "The Transtheoretical Model of Health Behavior Change," *American Journal of Health Promotion* 12 (1997): 38–48.
4. G. Starr, T. Rogers, M. Schooley, S. Porter, E. Wiesen, and N. Jamison, *Key Outcome Indicators for Evaluating Comprehensive Tobacco Control Programs* (Atlanta, GA: Centers for Disease Control and Prevention, 2005).

Chapter 27

1. T. Davis, "Letters," *Quality Digest* (August 2008).
2. G. Hutchins, "Risk Management: The Future of Quality," *Quality Digest* (June 2008).
3. S. R. Covey, *The Seven Habits of Highly Effective People* (New York: Simon & Schuster, 1990).
4. H. Ozog, IOMOSAIC Corporation, "Designing an Effective Risk Matrix." www.IOMOSAIC.com. As identified by Dr. Sanford Liebesman, Quality Management Forum (Spring 2008).

Chapter 28

1. J. Lynn, M. Baily, and M. Bottrell, et al., "The Ethics of Using Quality Improvement Methods in Healthcare," *Annals of Internal Medicine* 146, no. 9 (2007): 666–73.
2. Ibid.
3. B. Longest and K. Darr, *Managing Health Services Organizations,* 5th ed. (Baltimore: Health Professions Press, 2008).
4. Lynn et al., 2007.

5. R. Bernheim, "Ethics in Public Health Practice and Management," Chapter 5 in L. Novick, C. Morrow, and G. Mays, eds., *Public Health Administration: Principles for Population-Based Management* (Boston: Jones and Bartlett, 2008).

6. Lynn et al., "Ethics."

7. Ibid.

8. Centers for Disease Control and Prevention, "Guidelines for Defining Public Health Research and Public Health Non-Research." Revised October 4, 1999. www.cdc.gov/od/science/regs/hrpp/rsearchDefinition.htm. (accessed 11/28/08).

9. Lynn et al., "Ethics."

10. Joint Commission, http://www.jointcommission.org/NR/rdonlyres/A88E7A36-0C20-4C37-B67D-CD8638538E09/0/ASC_stdsampler_07.pdf and at http://www.jointcommission.org/NR/rdonlyres/B729AA75-D9D7-46C1-ACC8-67B0DB95AE79/0/OME_PI.pdf (accessed 11/28/08).

11. Ibid (accessed 2/17/09).

12. Lynn et al., "Ethics."

About the Authors

Stephanie B.C. Bailey, MD, MSHSA, is chief of public health practice of the Centers for Disease Control and Prevention (CDC), U.S. Department of Health and Human Services.

As chief of public health practice, Dr. Bailey is responsible for assuring that the U.S. public health system is strong and that CDC provides leadership in building and supporting public health infrastructure and improving overall public health system performance. The Office of the Chief of Public Health Practice serves as an advocate, guardian, promoter, and conscience of public health practice throughout CDC and in the larger public health community.

Dr. Bailey holds a BA from Clark University, Worchester, Massachusetts, an MD from McHarry Medical College, Nashville, Tennessee, a master's of science in health services administration from the College of St. Francis, and performed her residency in internal medicine at Grady Memorial/Emory University, Atlanta, Georgia.

Prior to Dr. Bailey's career at CDC, she served for 11 years as the director of health of Nashville and Davidson County Public Health Department, Nashville, Tennessee. Dr. Bailey is a past president of the National Association of County and City Health Officials (NACCHO) and past chair of the National Public Health Leadership Society. She has been appointed to four national committees by the secretary of health and human services. She has received many awards, among them the APHA Roemer Award, AMA's Nathan Davis Award, the 2007 Balderson Lifetime Public Health Leadership Award, and the 2008 Southern Health Association's Howell Special Meritorious Service to Public Health Award. Since 2006, she has served on the editorial board for the *Journal of Public Health Management and Practice.*

Leslie M. Beitsch, MD, JD, joined the faculty at the Florida State University College of Medicine in November 2003 as professor of health policy and director of the Center for Medicine and Public Health.

From June 2001 until November 2003, Dr. Beitsch was the commissioner of the Oklahoma State Department of Health. In that role he provided oversight for 2500 employees and a budget of $260,000,000. Dr. Beitsch served as deputy secretary and assistant state health officer for the Florida Department of Health from 1997 through 2001. He provided guidance and direction for public health programs, the county health departments, and the state laboratory and pharmacy. Prior to this appointment, Dr. Beitsch served as assistant state health officer and division director for family health services from October 1991 through August 1997, focusing on maternal and child health. From October 1989 through October 1991, Dr. Beitsch was medical director of the Broward County Health Department in Ft. Lauderdale.

Dr. Beitsch has been an active member in several organizations. Recent interests have focused on accreditation and quality improvement for state and local health departments through the Multi-State Learning Collaborative and the Centers for Disease Control and Prevention. Dr. Beitsch served as a steering committee member for the Exploring Accreditation Project, and as its research and evaluation workgroup chair. He has participated as a member of committees representing the Association of State and Territorial Health Officials (ASTHO) and committees advising the Centers for Disease Control and Prevention. He is past chair of the board of directors for the Public Health Foundation (PHF) and the Public Health Leadership Society. He has recently been recognized for his contributions by ASTHO (2007 Alumni Award) and PHF (2008 Theodore Erwin Award).

Carlton Berger, MPA. Like the Baldrige National Quality Award Program, Carlton Berger recently began a third decade of public service. He has worked in nonprofit and public disciplines including organizational development, performance management, business assistance, emergency preparedness, and public health evaluation.

He is the author of *Quality Improvement Through Leadership and Empowerment,* which achieved a global distribution of 65,000 copies. The book is recognized on SkyMark Corporation's "All-Time Great Books on Management" list and is available at www.leadandempower.com.

Ron Bialek, MPP, is president and CEO of the Public Health Foundation (PHF). Under his leadership over the past 11 years, PHF has focused its efforts on developing and implementing innovative strategies for improving performance of public health agencies and systems. Initiatives include creating AARO—the Alliance for Achieving Results and Outcomes—to provide quality improvement technical support, tools, and training to public health professionals, developing the consensus set of Core Competencies for Public Health Professionals through the Council on Linkages between Academia and Public Health Practice, creating the nation's most comprehensive public health learning management system—TRAIN—linking together 23 states and the U.S. Medical Reserve Corps, and developing consumer-oriented county health profiles—the Community Health Status Indicators initiative—for all counties in the United States.

Before joining PHF, Mr. Bialek was on the faculty of the Johns Hopkins University School of Public Health for nine years and served as director of the Johns Hopkins Health Program Alliance. He also spent three years in the Maryland Department of Health and Mental Hygiene as executive assistant to the assistant secretary for health regulation. Mr. Bialek received his BA in political science and MA in public policy from Johns Hopkins University.

Dorothy Bliss, MA, is a principal planner at the Minnesota Department of Health. She supports Minnesota's local health departments through the clarification of concepts, critical thinking, and the translation of data into meaningful information. She is an experienced researcher, writer, and editor and has authored or contributed to dozens of state reports and publications, including Minnesota's public health goals, and articles published in the Robert Wood Johnson Foundation Turning Point newsletter. She has an MA in sociology from the University of Minnesota. She may be reached at dorothy.bliss@state.mn.us

Paul Borawski. Known as a creative and innovative "early adopter" in the field of quality, Paul Borawski has been called "the man behind the curtain" at the American Society for Quality (ASQ). As executive director and chief strategic officer, Paul's influence and progressive managerial concepts are what drive the 62-year-old organization based in Milwaukee, Wisconsin. Paul has served as a facilitator, theme weaver, and author, and has served on a dozen corporate boards. He has led startups, wind-downs, turnarounds, and every phase of an organization's lifecycle.

Paul's 20 years of CEO experience and a track record of accomplishments have made ASQ the world's largest and most respected organization of its kind. ASQ has been named "a best place to work" and "a model organization." A frequent speaker, Paul has delivered his inspirational message of quality on five continents and is the recipient of numerous honors and recognitions. He was named "one of the most influential people in the field of quality" by *Quality Digest* magazine in 2005. The European Organization for Quality awarded him the Georges Borel medal in 2006 for his contributions to the European Community.

Debra Burns, MA, is director of the Office of Public Health Practice at the Minnesota Department of Health, where she and her staff work to strengthen and maintain Minnesota's public health infrastructure. She has more than 20 years of management, planning, and policy analysis experience in public health and has overseen many systemwide initiatives. She has an MA in public affairs from the University of Minnesota, Humphrey Institute of Public Affairs.

Susan R. Cooper, MSN, RN, made Tennessee history on January 20, 2007, when she became the first nurse to serve as the commissioner of the Tennessee Department of Health. She is a master's prepared registered nurse, who received both her bachelor's and master's degrees from the Vanderbilt University School of Nursing. Her priorities are to protect, promote, and improve the health of all Tennesseans. Cooper first came to the state in 2005 as a special policy and health advisor to Governor Phil Bredesen. She was charged with development of the Health Care Safety Net and later assumed leadership of Project Diabetes and Get Fit Tennessee, a program developed to address the threats of type II diabetes facing the youth of Tennessee.

Liza Corso has worked for the Centers for Disease Control and Prevention since June 2002. She serves as team lead in the Office of Chief of Public Health Practice, where she oversees activities related to the National Public Health Performance Standards Program, CDC's support for the advancement of state and local agency accreditation, and activities related to quality improvement and accreditation readiness in the field. During 2004–05, Liza also served as a member of the CDC Futures Initiative Governmental Public Health Infrastructure Work Group, which explored opportunities for building the public health infrastructure in the areas of workforce, accreditation, and preparedness.

Before joining CDC, Liza worked for the National Association of County and City Health Officials (NACCHO), where she served as program manager for the development and initial implementation of the mobilizing for action through planning and partnerships (MAPP) process, NACCHO's role in the development of the NPHPSP, APEXPH, and other projects related to strengthening public health infrastructure. Prior to joining NACCHO in 1994, Liza worked for the National Public Health and Hospitals Institute conducting research on a variety of topics related to public hospitals.

In addition to serving on numerous national advisory committees and work groups as part of her professional duties, Liza has served as a volunteer community member of the Healthy Dekalb Steering Committee, which oversaw Dekalb County's MAPP process, as well as a member of the Community Basics Advisory Board for the United Way of Metropolitan Atlanta. Liza has a master of public administration from the Maxwell School at Syracuse University and a bachelor of arts from the University of Richmond.

Natasha Coulouris, MPH, is the health officer and director of Saginaw County, Michigan, Department of Public Health. She holds a master's of public health degree from the University of Michigan, School of Public Health, Health Behavior/ Health Education Program. Her most current accomplishments in public health are: participation in the MLC-1, 2, and 3 quality improvement committees and helping define the framework for this initiative, experience with strategic planning/ CQI facilitation, national social marketing, and health education campaigns, and participation in NACCHO National CQI Workshop and Peer Assistance Network Agency Lead, NACCHO Pilot Accreditation Grant.

Penney Davis, MPH, joined the National Association of County and City Health Officials (NACCHO) in 2006 as part of the Infrastructure and Systems Team. Penney serves as the senior analyst for the Accreditation Preparation and Quality Improvement and Regionalizing Public Health Services projects. Penney facilitates the use of quality improvement techniques and provides technical assistance to local health departments preparing to participate in the voluntary national accreditation program. As part of NACCHO's support of national accreditation, Penney also contributes to the Public Health Accreditation Board's work groups and committees.

In addition to working at NACCHO, Penney serves on George Washington University's School of Public Health alumni board of directors and volunteers with the Washington Area Clinic Defense Task Force. Penney earned her bachelor of arts in sociology from the University of Arkansas at Fayetteville, and her master of public health in global health promotion from George Washington University in Washington, D.C. Penney may be reached at pdavis@naccho.org.

Grace L. Duffy, MBA, CLSSMBB, provides services in organizational and process improvement, leadership, quality, customer service, and teamwork. She designs and implements effective systems for business and management success.

Her clients include government, healthcare, public health, education, manufacturing, services, and not-for-profit organizations. She is coauthor of *The Quality Improvement Handbook, The Executive Guide to Improvement and Change,* and *Executive Focus: Your Life and Career.* Grace holds a master's in business administration from Georgia State University and a bachelor's in archaeology and anthropology from Brigham Young University. She is an ASQ certified manager of quality/organizational excellence, certified quality improvement associate, and certified quality auditor. Grace is a certified Lean Six Sigma Master Black Belt and manager of process improvement. She is an ASQ fellow and past vice president of ASQ.

During her 20 years with IBM, Grace held a series of positions in technical design, services, management, and process improvement. She helped design and deliver IBM's executive quality training in the late 1980s. Grace retired from IBM in 1993 as head of corporate technical education. Grace served with Trident Technical College in Charleston, South Carolina, for 10 years as department head for business, curriculum owner, and instructor for Trident's Quality and Corporate Management programs and as a dean for management and performance consulting to private industry. Grace is a member of ASTD, ISPI, and ASQ. Grace can be reached at grace683@embarqmail.com.

Kathleen F. (Kay) Edwards, PhD, is professor and program director, healthcare administration, Graduate School, University of Maryland University College (UMUC), Adelphi, Maryland. Kay also guides research of doctoral students in the healthcare industry and taught strategic planning in the UMUC online MBA program.

She has over 35 years of experience in public health practice and teaching, as well as strong leadership and management skills, honed through managing a major statewide public health program, serving as a county health officer in a medium-sized county, serving as an assistant commissioner in a large city health department, and successfully carrying out management and consulting roles in another large health department.

Kay provides consultation and training for public health and other executive leadership groups on quality improvement in public health, effective communication, ethics, conflict management and negotiation, organizational management and change, strategic thinking and planning, including situational analysis, and succession planning, including pay for performance.

Her special organizational interests include public health leadership, public health strategic thinking and planning (for example, SWOT), public health partnerships, public health change management, including quality improvement processes (for example, PDCA), the changing nature of the U.S. healthcare system, health care management and leadership, teamwork, negotiation/conflict resolution, succession planning, and ethics/corporate social responsibility. To get in touch with the author, contact the Public Health Foundation at www.phf.org.

Julia Joh Elligers, MPH, joined NACCHO in 2003 and is a senior analyst on the Public Health Infrastructure and Systems team. She provides trainings and technical assistance to local jurisdictions using mobilizing for action through planning and partnerships (MAPP). MAPP is a community-based strategic planning process for improving public health. Julia also provides training and technical assistance to communities using the National Public Health Performance Standards

Program (NPHPSP) local assessment. NPHPSP measures local public system capacity to deliver essential public health services. As a senior analyst, Julia is also responsible for evaluating the effectiveness of the MAPP and NPHPSP projects and researching the extent to which MAPP and NPHPSP improve public health practice and outcomes.

In addition to working at NACCHO, Julia is pursuing her doctoral degree in government and politics at the University of Maryland, College Park. Her academic work focuses on how national, state, and local politics affect governmental public health capacity. Julia received her bachelor of arts degree in biology and public policy from Cornell University and her master of public health degree in health policy and management from Columbia University Mailman School of Public Health. Julia can be reached at jjoh@naccho.org.

Paul D. Epstein, Principal, Epstein & Fass Associates, has over 25 years' experience in public service performance measurement and improvement, strategy management including balanced scorecards, and sharing innovation. In 2003, he received the American Society for Public Administration's (ASPA's) Harry Hatry lifetime achievement award for distinguished performance measurement practice. Mr. Epstein has assisted local, state, federal, United Nations, and nonprofit agencies, and helped entire local governments develop performance measures. Recently, he has assisted a partner firm, Insightformation, in automating local health department accreditation standards. For the Public Health Foundation, he is devising ways to use those standards in health agency strategy management and performance improvement.

His best-practice research since the 1970s led to his many publications, including three books, *Using Performance Measurement in Local Government* (1984 and 1988), *Auditor Roles in Government Performance Measurement* (lead author, 2004), and *Results That Matter* (lead author, 2006). The "effective community governance model" and practices in *Results That Matter,* which combine citizen engagement and results measurement, have provided valuable templates for evaluating organizations' practices in communities in the United States and abroad. Mr. Epstein is a consulting member of the Governmental Accounting Standards Board's performance measurement research team. In 1993 he was tapped by Vice President Gore's National Performance Review to assist in federal reinvention.

Before he started Epstein & Fass, he was manager of citywide productivity improvement for the New York City mayor's office, where he played a critical role in integrating efficiency improvement with the budget process, leading to over a billion dollars in annual productivity savings and revenue. He has an engineering degree from MIT, has trained thousands of public officials, and has taught graduate public management courses at NYU, Baruch College, and the University of Hartford. Paul may be reached at Epstein & Fass Associates at epstein@epstein-andfass.com.

Erica Farmer, MA, CLSSMBB, is originally from Maryland, but has lived in Florida most of her life. She has a BA in music performance from Florida Southern College, a BS in business administration from the University of South Florida, and an MA in organizational management from the University of Phoenix. She is currently a member leader of the American Society for Quality section 1509 chapter in Orlando, Florida, and has achieved ASQ certifications for the quality improvement associate, Six Sigma Black Belt, and manager of quality/organizational excellence. She has also received the certified Lean Six Sigma Master Black Belt through the Harrington Group. Erica currently works as a process manager for State Farm Insurance Companies in Winter Haven, Florida. In her role she provides support and training in Lean Six Sigma and facilitates Lean Six Sigma project teams.

Erica serves as a Lean Six Sigma Master Black Belt coach to the Florida Department of Children and Families in a series of quality improvement assessments, analysis, and design projects. She is a mentor for the industrial engineering graduate students at University of Central Florida.

Jennifer R. J. Frost is director of program planning and development for the California Regional Health Information Organization (CalRHIO), a collaborative statewide initiative to improve the safety, quality, and efficiency of healthcare through health information technology and the secure exchange of health data. Previously, Ms. Frost was a community health planner with the San Mateo County Health Department, where she helped develop and lead countywide health policy planning and education. Ms. Frost also developed business plans and international applications for Bio-Source Therapeutics, a life sciences company. As a project associate with Epstein & Fass Associates, Ms. Frost helped manage design and implementation of performance measurement, strategic management plans and reports, and balanced scorecards for organizations across the country, including Los Angeles County Public Health. She also mapped how Epstein & Fass's effective community governance model applies to public health. Ms. Frost was a program developer for Health People: Community Preventive Health Institute in the South Bronx where she was responsible for monitoring and evaluation, grant management support, and policy research. Her international experience includes program implementation, process development, strategic management planning, and policy analysis for the New York-based Medical Relief Alliance, in addition to on-site research in Kilgoris, Kenya. Ms. Frost has a bachelor of science in health systems from Georgetown University, and a master of public administration in health policy and management from New York University's Robert F. Wagner Graduate School of Public Service. Ms. Frost can be reached at epstein@epstein-andfass.com.

Sarah Gillen, MPH, is the associate director for the National Network of Public Health Institutes (NNPHI). She directs the implementation of NNPHI's programs and membership services to 28 public health institutes. Sarah joined NNPHI in June 2005 to lead the development of the Multi-State Learning Collaborative for Accreditation and Performance Assessment programs, which is now in its third phase. Prior to joining NNPHI, Sarah served as HIV/AIDS program manager for Nos Petits Freres et Soeurs in Port-au-Prince, Haiti. Sarah is a graduate of Saint Mary's College in Notre Dame, Indiana, and she received a master of public health degree from Tulane University in New Orleans, Louisiana.

Christina Harrington is emergency preparedness director for the Saginaw County, Michigan, Department of Public Health. She holds a bachelor of science in physiology from Michigan State University. Her most current accomplishments in public health are as a member, Continuous Quality Improvement Core Team for Saginaw County PHD and as team leader, NACCHO Pilot Accreditation Grant.

Jim Hinson is the area 7 STD program manager for the State of Florida Department of Health. He oversees the Orange, Osceola, and Brevard County STD operations. Mr. Hinson graduated from the University of Alabama with a BS degree in business education. After three years of teaching/coaching, he worked in wholesale and then retail business for 10 years.

He began his career in the public health STD field with the State of Florida Department of Health in Orange County in 1989 as an STD DIS (disease intervention specialist). He was promoted to supervisor in 1993, and then to surveillance supervisor in 1997. In 2000, he was promoted to a management position at the Seminole County Health Department, in charge of the STD and HIV programs (patient care and prevention). In 2005, he was promoted to area 7 manager for district 7.

His functions include STD surveillance, screening, clinical operations, field activities, and education/public awareness with the following goals: identifying diseases in the community, assuring notification and treatment of those infected, interviewing infected persons to identify where the disease came from and others that may have been exposed to the disease, activities to notify, examine, and treat those exposed persons and other at-risk individuals, and educating persons about STDs and how to prevent their spread. He communicates with the Bureau of STD in Tallahassee and federal CDC staff on a continual basis.

Dennis D. Lenaway, PhD, MPH. As director of the Office of Public Health Systems Performance within the Office of the Chief of Public Health Practice, Centers for Disease Control and Prevention, Dr. Lenaway individually provides the leadership and overall management of CDC's efforts toward building the nation's public health system and improving operational capacity of state and local public health departments. Previously, Dr. Lenaway served as the director for the Division of Public Health Systems Development and Research, Public Health Practice Program Office at CDC, and spent 16 years as the epidemiologist for the Boulder County Health Department, Boulder, Colorado. Dr. Lenaway received his MPH and PhD in epidemiology from the University of Washington School of Public Health and Community Medicine.

Marlene "Marni" Mason is a managing consultant with MCPP Healthcare Consulting, based in Seattle, Washington. She has extensive experience in the assessment and improvement of public health practice, the development of performance standards for public health, in health plan preparation for NCQA accreditation, and in operational and clinical improvement in general healthcare, public health, and behavioral health organizations. She also has expertise in assessment and compliance with performance standards such as the National Committee for Quality Assurance (NCQA), the National Performance Standards for Public Health, and the Baldrige Criteria for Performance Excellence. As an excellent communicator who quickly builds trust and instills a spirit of cooperation in achieving desired results, she has a proven track record in managing and facilitating the integration of management and decision-making processes.

Recently, Marni has been traveling across the United States teaching quality improvement methods and tools to public health leaders in many states. Marni has consulted with 25 local and state public health QI teams in Washington and with four local QI teams in Michigan as part of the Multi-State Learning

Collaborative. She contributed to the QI guidebook developed by the Michigan Accreditation Continuous Quality Improvement Collaborative (MACQIC) titled *Embracing Quality in Local Public Health.* She has also coauthored several articles regarding performance management in public health, including "Quality Measurement and Performance Standards in Washington State" for the *Journal of Public Health Management and Practice.* Marni lives in the Seattle area and spends her free time sailing with her husband, gardening, traveling, and enjoying time with her extended family.

Bridget K. McCabe, MD, MPH, is a licensed pediatrician with fellowship training in health services research. Dr. McCabe currently serves as the director of the Division of Quality Improvement and Public Health Accreditation for the Tennessee Department of Health. In this role, she oversees quality improvement and public health accreditation efforts in the state of Tennessee, which includes 89 rural and six metropolitan county health departments and 13 regional health offices. Dr. McCabe previously served as a clinical fellow at Children's Hospital Boston and the Harvard Center for Child and Adolescent Health Policy at Massachusetts General Hospital. She holds a bachelor of arts degree in biology, a medical doctorate with distinction in a special field of neuroscience, and a master of public health in clinical effectiveness, all from Harvard University. She completed her internship and residency training at Children's Hospital Boston; in addition, she completed a Harvard Pediatric Health Services Research Fellowship in general pediatrics where she worked with members of the Institute for Health Care Improvement. Her areas of research have focused on improving care for chronic diseases affecting children and have led to publications and presentations at national meetings.

Kim McCoy, MS, MPH, is a principal planning specialist at the Minnesota Department of Health. She is the Minnesota coordinator for the Multi-State Learning Collaborative program. She has worked in federal, state, and local public health, and began her public health career as a presidential management fellow at the Centers for Disease Control and Prevention. Degrees: MPH in public health administration, MS in health services research, University of Minnesota. Kim may be reached at Kim.Mccoy@state.mn.us.

Jennifer McKeever, MSW, MPH, is a program manager with the National Network of Public Health Institutes (NNPHI). Prior to joining the NNPHI team in 2006, Jennifer oversaw HIV testing and community-based programs across the state of Louisiana for the Office of Public Health and was the program director of a residential facility for persons living with HIV. Jennifer received a master of social work and a master of public health from Tulane University.

John W. Moran, MBA, PhD, CMC, CQM, CQIA is a senior quality advisor to the Public Health Foundation. He brings to PHF over 30 years of quality improvement expertise in developing quality improvement tools and training programs, implementing and evaluating quality improvement programs, and writing articles and books on quality improvement methods. Dr. Moran is a retired senior vice president of information systems, administrative and diagnostic services at New England Baptist Hospital. He was previously chief operating officer of Changing Healthcare, Inc., specializing in management consulting and educational support to healthcare organizations. For 21 years, Dr. Moran was employed at Polaroid Corporation where he worked in various senior management capacities in manufacturing, engineering, and quality. His last position was as the director of Worldwide Quality and Systems.

Dr. Moran has authored numerous articles, case studies, and textbooks in healthcare, quality function deployment, and process redesign. His most recent books include *The Public Health Quality Improvement Handbook, Executive Focus: Focusing Your Life and Career, The Executive Guide to Improvement and Change, Action Strategies for Healthcare Leaders, The Quality Function Deployment Handbook, Management Development and Training, The Future Focused Organization, Breakthrough Thinking,* and *Growing Teams.*

Dr. Moran has been active in the American Society for Quality (ASQ) as a fellow of the society and serving as division chair, vice chair of technology, and chair of the ASQ Certification Committee, and a member of the Standing Review Board of Quality Press. Dr. Moran is an ASQ certified manager of quality/organizational excellence (CMQ/OE). He is a certified management consultant (CMC) by the Institute of Management Consultants. Dr. Moran is a 1993–2001 RIT/USA Today Quality Cup judge in healthcare and a member of the Malcolm Baldrige board of examiners. He was a founder and past member of the board of directors of the Massachusetts Quality Award. Dr. Moran has a BS, MBA, MS, and PhD in Education from Walden University in 1977. For 20 years Dr. Moran was an adjunct professor in the Graduate and Undergraduate School of Engineering at the University of Massachusetts at Lowell.

He may be reached at the Public Health Foundation at (202) 218-4423 and by e-mail at jmoran@phf.org.

Helen M. Parsons, MPH, is a research assistant at the University of Minnesota, School of Public Health. She specializes in health outcomes and quality improvement, which she has applied to research on a variety of chronic diseases, including depression and cancer. She was involved in implementing a statewide quality improvement program for local public health agencies in Minnesota, a collaboration between the University of Minnesota, the Minnesota Department of Health, and local public health agencies. Her previous research includes studying the effectiveness of implementing mass depression screening programs for adolescents as well as factors that influence health outcomes in colorectal cancer patients. She is a doctoral student in health services research at the University of Minnesota where she earned her MPH in public health administration and policy.

Cheryl Plettenberg, EdD, is substance abuse director for the Saginaw County, Michigan, Department of Public Health. Her most recent accomplishments in Public Health are as a member, Continuous Quality Improvement Core Team, NACCHO Pilot Accreditation Grant, and co-chair, Saginaw County Community Health Assessment, 1998–2004.

William Riley, PhD is associate dean, School of Public Heath, University of Minnesota. He specializes in the area of quality improvement and quality control and safety. He teaches healthcare quality improvement, finance, and process control. Dr. Riley has over 20 years' experience as a senior healthcare executive and has held the position of president and CEO of several healthcare organizations, including an integrated delivery system, a large multispecialty medical group, and a health plan joint venture. In these capacities, he has had extensive experience developing and implementing effective quality control systems, as well as leading numerous process improvement initiatives. He is the author of numerous studies and articles related to quality control, patient safety, and healthcare management. He has consulted nationally on numerous quality improvement projects. Dr. Riley is currently the principal investigator on a multiyear study leading an interdisciplinary team of physicians, nurses, and administrators to improve patient safety and develop innovative safety training programs.

Patricia Ritter is office manager, environmental health services for the Saginaw County, Michigan, Department of Public Health. Her most current accomplishments in public health are as co-facilitator, "MOD squad" 2 thru 4, member, Continuous Quality Improvement Core Team, NACCHO Pilot Accreditation Grant, and as a participant in a National Environmental Public Health Performance Standards (NEnvPHPS) workshop.

Pamela Russo, MD, MPH, is a senior program officer on the Robert Wood Johnson Foundation Public Health Team, which is committed to strengthening the public health system to enable it to protect and promote health. She is the lead on the foundation's programs in accreditation and quality improvement in public health agencies, and also focuses on the translation of evidence to policy change in public health.

Russo came to the Foundation in November 2000 from the Cornell University Medical Center in New York City, where she was an associate professor of medicine, director of the clinical outcomes section, and program codirector for the master's program and fellowship in clinical epidemiology and health services research. Over her 10 years at Cornell, she was the primary investigator on multiple NIH- and AHRQ-funded research projects, and her research and teaching often focused on the methodology for developing scales to measure outcomes.

She earned an MD from the University of California, San Francisco, and completed her residency in primary care general internal medicine at the Hospital of the University of Pennsylvania in Philadelphia, followed by a fellowship in clinical epidemiology and rheumatology at Cornell University Medical Center and the Hospital for Special Surgery. She earned an MPH in epidemiology from the University of California, Berkeley, School of Public Health and a BS from Harvard College.

Alina Simone, MPA, is an associate consultant with Epstein & Fass Associates. She focuses on government and community applications of best practices in community outcome and service performance measurement, community engagement, strategy management, and results-based organizational and community learning. She conducted research for the book *Results That Matter* based on the effective community governance (ECG) model, which brings together community engagement and performance measurement for continuous community improvement. She has over 10 years' experience working with nonprofit and public organizations in the United States and abroad as an executive director, evaluator, best-practice researcher, policy advocate, and consultant. She was on the Epstein & Fass design team that developed ECG best-practice assessment tools, including tools for assessing citizen roles, for use in training, consulting, and evaluation projects, including an evaluation of community services and engagement in Los Angeles County. She also adapted ECG and community balanced scorecard tools for use in Russia, and has provided evaluation, consulting, and training to local government and nonprofit teams developing outcome indicators and governance improvement initiatives in Siberian communities that range from small villages to a city of 250,000. She has assisted a partner firm, Insightformation, in automating local health department accreditation standards. She has also worked on public performance measurement projects for the Governmental Accounting Standards Board and the Institute of Internal Auditors (IIA). For U.S., Russian, and international organizations she has created, or helped create, Web sites that disseminate best practices, including a site promoting auditor practices to improve government performance management for the IIA. Ms. Simone holds a master's in public administration from the Wagner Graduate School of Public Service at New York University. She received a David L. Boren graduate fellowship from the federal government, a Sara's Wish Foundation scholarship, and an NYU public service scholarship. She may be reached through Epstein & Fass Associates at epstein@epsteinandfass.com.

Jessica A. Solomon, MCP, joined the National Association of County and City Health Officials (NACCHO) staff in January 2003 and serves as program manager for the Accreditation Preparation and Quality Improvement and Regionalizing Public Health Services projects. Her work includes managing several projects through grants from the Robert Wood Johnson Foundation and a cooperative agreement with the Centers for Disease Control and Prevention. As part of NACCHO's support of national accreditation, Ms. Solomon also works closely with the Public Health Accreditation Board on program development and communications.

Previous project work at NACCHO includes the Operational Definition of a Functional Local Health Department, Community Design Partnership project, and several projects related to environmental health.

Ms. Solomon received a master of community planning with a specialization in planning policy from the University of Maryland School of Architecture, Planning, and Preservation. She also holds a bachelor of science in geography from Ohio University, with a major in urban/regional planning. Prior to joining NACCHO, Ms. Solomon worked with the water treatment plant in the city of Athens, Ohio, as they partnered with the Ohio EPA to draft a wellhead protection plan. Ms. Solomon may be reached at jsolomon@naccho.org.

Cathy R. Taylor, DrPH, MSN, RN, is assistant commissioner, Tennessee Department of Health's Bureau of Health Services Administration, where she oversees administration of primary care and disease prevention services and programs in Tennessee's 89 rural and six metropolitan county health departments and 13 regional offices. Dr. Taylor previously served as assistant professor of nursing at Vanderbilt University School of Nursing, director of the McHarry-Vanderbilt Alliance Disease Management Program, and in various other administrative and clinical venues. She was appointed by Governor Phil Bredesen to chair the Tennessee Center for Diabetes Prevention and Health Improvement Board in 2006, and has served as a consultant on projects for organizations including the U.S. Department of Health and Human Services and the Maternal and Child

Health Bureau's Leadership Institute. Dr. Taylor is a member of the American Diabetes Association, the American Nurses Association, and the American Public Health Association. She has earned numerous grants and awards, and her work has been included in professional publications such as *Diabetes Care, Maternal and Child Health Journal* and *Concepts and Models for Service Learning in Nursing*. Dr. Taylor earned a doctor of public health degree from the University of Alabama at Birmingham and completed a postdoctoral fellowship at Vanderbilt University. She holds a master of science in nursing from the University of Tennessee at Memphis, a bachelor of science in nursing from the University of Alabama at Huntsville, and a bachelor of science from Middle Tennessee State University.

Tamara Theisen, ASCP, is laboratory director for the Saginaw County, Michigan, Department of Public Health. She holds a bachelor of science in medical technology with minors in biomedical science and chemistry from Western Michigan University.

Tamara is ASCP (American Society of Clinical Pathology) certified. Her most current accomplishments in public health are as co-facilitator, "MOD squad" 2 thru 4, and member, Continuous Quality Improvement Core Team, NACCHO Pilot Accreditation Grant.

Barbara J. Volz, MEd, MPH, CCPS, has worked in public health for the last 19 years. Her original degrees in chemistry and education have been supplemented with her most recent degree, a master's in public health. Barbara is currently supporting the Wagoner County, Oklahoma, Health Department. She has used her knowledge to organize the first countywide exercise of public health preparedness in Wagoner County and is currently directing a countywide initiative in tobacco control as well as an initiative in the county schools to impact fitness and nutrition in young children. Her responsibilities also include helping her health department become ready for accreditation.

Fredia Stovall Wadley, MD, MSHPA, is medical director for Delmarva Foundation, a quality improvement organization in Easton, Maryland. Prior to her position with Delmarva, Dr. Wadley spent 28 years in public health service in Tennessee at the local, regional, and state level including eight years as director of Nashville/Davidson County Health Department, and eight years from 1995 through 2003 as Tennessee's state health commissioner. Dr. Wadley has served as a delegate to APHA and AMA, been president of the Tennessee Public Health Association and the Southern Health Association, and won multiple public health awards for her service. She was a member of the National Academy of Sciences and Institute of Medicine's committee that produced the 2004 report *Our Children's Health, the Nation's Wealth: Assessing and Improving Children's Health,* has been on the faculty of four medical schools, and served on multiple ASTHO committees. Dr. Wadley's interest now is in bringing quality improvement and health data integration skills to the public health workforce. She assisted PHF in developing a quality improvement e-training module on childhood obesity for TRAIN. Dr. Wadley may be contacted at wadleyf@dfmc.org or at her office at 410-763-6200.

Lyle D. Wray, PhD, is senior resource consultant for Epstein & Fass Associates. He serves as executive director of the Capitol Region Council of Governments based in Hartford, Connecticut. He has a BA, MA, and PhD from the University of

Manitoba, Winnipeg, Canada. As county administrator of Dakota County, Minnesota, for five years, he led the county to performance management with monthly graphic performance reports of key results against budget and performance targets. As county administrator and, before that, human services director, he was involved in a pre-paid Medicaid demonstration initiative, expert systems development for public health case management, and restructuring of public health administration and finance. Dr. Wray headed developmental disabilities services in Newfoundland and Labrador, and outcomes measurement in the Minnesota Department of Human Services. For 11 years, Dr. Wray was executive director of the Citizens League, a civic organization that identifies important state and regional policy issues and advocates for solutions developed through citizen research. During that period, he teamed with Paul Epstein and others to co-lead the Sloan Foundation–funded research on citizen engagement and public performance measurement and coauthor the related book, *Results That Matter* (2006), which features the effective community governance (ECG) model. *Results That Matter* includes many examples of governments and nonprofits making community engagement more effective by helping citizens play multiple roles, a concept Dr. Wray pioneered and first published in ICMA's *Public Management*. Dr. Wray teaches graduate courses in public service outcomes measurement, e-government, and public service reform. He can be reached at Epstein & Fass Associates at epstein@epsteinandfass.com.

Index

Model for Improvement, 59
Montgomery Measures Up!, 67
moving organization, versus stuck
  organization, 295
Multi-State Learning Collaborative, 347
musical chairs, planning pitfall, 50

N

Nashville Jail Syphilis Demonstration
  Project, 141
Nashville/Davidson County, Tennessee,
  syphilis reduction case study, 139–44
  implementation, 142–44
  sustainability, 144
National Association of City and County
  Health Officials (NACCHO), 245–46,
  253
  Operational Definition of a Functional
    Local Health Department, 84–86,
    116–118, 121
National Public Health Performance
  Standards Program (NPHPSP), 20, 119,
  121, 123–25, 244–45
Nightmare on Elm Street, planning pitfall, 45
no linkage, planning pitfall, 30–31
no way to achieve it, planning pitfall, 40–41
nominal group technique, 175–76
non-health agency, assigned community
  health issue with public health
  implications, 258
nonmaleficence, ethics principle, 414–15
North Central District Health Department,
  Idaho, accreditation preparation
  process, 122–23
Northern Kentucky Independent District
  Health Department, accreditation
  preparation process, 123–25

O

OHSAS 18001 occupational health and safety
  system, 408
O.K. Corral, planning pitfall, 47–48
online collaboration software, 267
Operational Definition of a Functional
  Local Health Department, 84–86,
  116–118, 121
operational planning, 25–51
  pitfalls, 29–51
operational plans, 27
operationalizing improvement, 326–30
Orange County Health Department (OCHD),
  Florida
  process improvement efforts, 276

STD quality improvement case study,
  331–46
teams in, 294
organizational improvement frameworks,
  276
organizational structure for quality
  improvement
  building formal, 284–85
  formal and informal, 323–24
Osborn, Alex Faickney, 162
outcome measure, 74–75
outcomes
  critical-to-business, 7
  quality improvement, communicating,
    278–79

P

Pareto, Vilfredo, 176
Pareto chart, 176–78
parks and recreation departments, role in
  community results compact, 269
Patient Tracking and Billing Management
  Information System (PTBMIS), 392, 394
performance, managing, to improve health,
  15–24
performance data, in performance
  improvement, 18–19
performance feedback
  tailoring multiple cycles to government
    systems, 246–47
  use of in decision making, 242–48
performance improvement, 71
  using data, 18–19
performance indicators, 21
performance management
  adding community engagement to, for
    "governing for results" system,
    247–48
  alignment of with agency priorities,
    289–90
  community-focused, 235–49
  components of, 18–19, 20–22
  and ECG model, 237–38
  results in other fields, 17
  results in public health, 15–16
  role of leadership in, 283–92
  role of leadership in structuring, 287
  system, 19–20
performance management cycle, 22–24
Performance Management National
  Excellence Collaborative (PMC) survey,
  15–16
*Performance Management Practices in States:
  Results of a Baseline Assessment of State
  Health Agencies*, 15–16